W9-CNF-634

AVOIDING COMMON SURGICAL ERRORS

AVOIDING COMMON SURGICAL ERRORS

EDITORS

LISA MARCUCCI, MD
Clinical Assistant Professor of Surgery
East Tennessee State University
Johnson City, Tennessee

MICHAEL J. MORITZ, MD
Chief, Section of Transplantation Services
Lehigh Valley Hospital
Allentown, PA

HERBERT CHEN, MD
Chief, Endocrine Surgery
Assistant Professor, Division of General Surgery
University of Wisconsin
Madison, Wisconsin

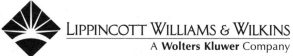

LIPPINCOTT WILLIAMS & WILKINS
A **Wolters Kluwer** Company
Philadelphia • Baltimore • New York • London
Buenos Aires • Hong Kong • Sydney • Tokyo

Acquisitions Editor:	Brian Brown
Developmental Editor:	Nancy Winter
Managing Editor:	Joanne Bersin
Project Manager:	Bridgett Dougherty
Senior Manufacturing Manager:	Benjamin Rivera
Design Coordinator:	Rica Clow
Associate Director of Marketing:	Adam Glazer
Production Services:	Schawk, Inc.
Printer:	R. R. Donnelly—Crawfordsville

© 2006 by Lippincott Williams & Wilkins
530 Walnut Street
Philadelphia, Pennsylvania 19106-3621 USA
351 West Camden Street
Baltimore, Maryland 21201-2436 USA
LWW.com

Library of Congress Cataloging-in-Publication Data
Avoiding common surgical errors/editors. Lisa Marcucci, Michael J. Moritz. Herbert Chen.
   p.; cm
  Includes bibliographical references and index.
  ISBN 0-7817-4742-2 (alk. paper)
  1. Surgical errors—Prevention. I. Marcucci, Lisa. II. Moritz, Michael J. III. Chen, Herbert.
  [DNLM: 1. Medical Errors—prevention & control. 2. Surgical Procedures. Minor—methods. 3. Peer Review, Health Care. WO 500 A961 2005]
RD27.85.A86 2005
617—dc22
                                              2005022798

10 9 8 7 6 5 4 3 2 1

This book is dedicated to these truly exemplary physicians and surgeons

Colonel Philip Lisagor, MC
Major Stephen A Lawson, MC
Major Carolyn V Smith, MC
Major David T Ward, MC

and

With sincere appreciation to Cary Moritz and Ariel, Marshall, and Ethan Moritz for their patience with the time-consuming research, writing, and editing of this volume.

All men make mistakes, but only wise men learn from their mistakes.

Winston Churchill

An expert is someone who knows some of the worst mistakes that can be made in his subject and how to avoid them.

Werner Karl Heisenberg

An expert is a man who has made all the mistakes which can be made in a very narrow field.

Niels Bohr

All men make mistakes, but married men find out about them sooner.

Red Skelton

Morbidity & Mortality Conference (M&M) is a fixture in Surgery departments at teaching hospitals. This exercise in peer review, self-examination, and self-criticism, preceded by decades the increasingly formalized processes of quality assessment and improvement. As such, the editors have been attending M&M's collectively for over 50 years. The errors included in this book have been gleaned from this environment and selected for a variety of reasons, including: very preventable errors that should never occur again (no one should lose a guide wire); a change in practice (DVT prophylaxis begins before anesthetic induction); and recurring yet preventable errors (abdominal complaints in compromised patients).

The editors would like this book to be viewed as a conversation between practitioners striving to give patients the best care. We are not experts in every area covered in this book, but are colleagues trying to aid others in decreasing errors and improving outcomes. We are not naïve enough to believe that these complications will not occur again, but we do earnestly believe that physicians want to improve so that these complications can be minimized. It is our hope that by providing a portable, compact compendium of avoidable errors, the motivation to achieve excellence amongst students and physicians will make this volume of interest to surgical practitioners and thus, will improve overall patient care. When available, we have attempted to include the evidenced-based arguments for the care we suggest. However, regretfully, since very little of what is done by physicians in the practice of medicine is evidenced-based (because the data just do not exist) we have used practice-based recommendations in many instances. It is our hope that following editions will be able to increasingly incorporate evidenced-based conclusions as the data are compiled.

Although many people have contributed to helping us put together this list of errors, we would like to specifically thank Nadine Semer, MD and Mark Lockett, MD for their review of the manuscript and editorial help. The editors would like to invite our readers to send us their comments and suggestions at marcucci50@hotmail.com.

Were we to coin our own quotation about our motivation in writing this book, it would be:

Learn from others' mistakes—it is safer for the patient and better for the surgeon than learning from your own.

LISA MARCUCCI, MD
MICHAEL J. MORITZ, MD
HERBERT CHEN, MD

HEATHER ABERNATHY, MD
Staff Anesthesiologist
Department of Anesthesiologist
Madison Anesthesiology Consultants, LLP
Department of Anesthesiology
Meriter Hospital
Madison, WI

RACHAEL A. CALLCUT, MD
Post-Graduate Trainee in General Surgery
Department of Surgery
University of Wisconsin-Madison
University of Wisconsin Hospital & Clinics
Madison, WI

SUE-MI CHA, MD
Resident, Department of Surgery
Hahnemann Hospital
Drexel University College of Medicine
Philadelphia, PA

HERBERT CHEN, MD
Chief, Endocrine Surgery
Assistant Professor
Division of General Surgery
University of Wisconsin
Madison, WI

X. D. DONG, MD
Surgical Oncology Fellow
Department of Surgery
University of Pittsburgh
Fellow, Department of Surgery
University of Pittsburgh Medical Center
Pittsburgh, PA

DIANE L. FERRARA, MSN, CRNP, RNFA, APRN,BC
Registered Nurse First Assistant
Department of Nursing
Thomas Jefferson University Hospital
Philadelphia, PA

JAMES HERRINGTON, MD
Clinical Instructor of Surgery
Department of Surgery
Temple University College of Medicine
Fellow, Department of Surgery
Division of Vascular Surgery
Temple University Hospital
Philadelphia, PA

JACK RYAN HUDKINS, MD
Department of General Surgery
East Tennessee State University
Resident, Department of Surgery
Johnson City Medical Center
Johnson City, TN

HARSH JAIN, MD
Department of Surgery
Drexel University College of Medicine
Resident, Department of Surgery
Hahnemann University Hospital
Philadelphia, PA

GREGORY KENNEDY, MD, PHD
Department of Surgery
University of Wisconsin
Surgical Resident, Department of Surgery
University of Wisconsin Hospitals and Clinics
Madison, WI

JAMES F. KIRKPATRICK III, MD
Surgical Resident
Department of Surgery
East Tennessee State University
Johnson City, TN

ADRIAN L. LATA, MD
Resident, Department of Surgery
Hahnemann University Hospital
Philadelphia, PA

AHMED G. MAMI, MD, FRCS (GLASG.)
Research Fellow in Pediatric Surgery
Department of Pediatric Surgery
St. Christopher's Hospital for Children
Philadelphia, PA

LISA MARCUCCI, MD
Clinical Assistant Professor of Surgery
East Tennessee State University
Johnson City, Tennessee

CATHERINE MARCUCCI, MD
Assistant Professor of Anesthesiology
Department of Anesthesiology
University of Maryland Medical System
Baltimore, MD

KENNETH MEREDITH, MD
Department of Surgery
University of Wisconsin-Madison
Resident, Department of Surgery
University of Wisconsin Hospital and
Clinics
Madison, WI

MICHAEL J. MORITZ, MD
Chief, Section of Transplantation Services
Lehigh Valley Hospital
Allentown, PA

DMITRIY A. NIKITIN, MD
Department of Surgery
Drexel University College of Medicine
Hahnemann University Hospital
Philadelphia, PA

ASHRAF I. OSMAN, MD
Chief Resident, Department of Surgery
Drexel University College of Medicine
Hahnemann University Hospital
Philadelphia, PA

RICHARD PUCCI, DO
Attending Surgeon,
Section Minimally
Invasive Surgery
Department of General Surgery
Good Samaritan Hospital
Suffern, NY

RAMON RIVERA, MD
Laparoscopic Fellow
Institute for Minimally Invasive Surgery

Department of Surgery
Washington University School of Medicine
St. Louis, MO

NEIL SANDSON, MD
Clinical Assistant Professor
Department of Psychiatry
University of Maryland Medical System
Director, Division of Education &
Residency Training
Sheppard Pratt Health System
Baltimore, MD

NADINE B. SEMER, MD, FACS
Plastic Surgeon
Southern California Permanente Medical
Group
Venice, CA
Assistant Adjunct Professor
Department of Preventative and
Restorative Dental Sciences
University of California at San Francisco
San Francisco, CA

MICHAEL SILBER, DO
Department of Surgery
Drexel University College of Medicine
Resident in General Surgery
Department of Surgery
Hahnemann University Hospital
Philadelphia, PA

MARK S. SNEIDER, MD
Surgery Resident
Department of Surgery
East Tennessee State University
Johnson City, TN

PATRICK SCHANER, MD
Jefferson Medical College
General Surgery Resident
Department of Surgery
Thomas Jefferson University Hospital
Philadelphia, PA

JUSTIN M. YOUNG, DDS, MD
Resident, Jefferson Hospital
Jefferson Medical College
Department of Oral and
Maxillofacial Surgery
Thomas Jefferson University Hospital
Philadelphia, PA

TABLE OF CONTENTS

PREFACE vii
CONTRIBUTORS ix

EMERGENCY DEPARTMENT

1   Remember the classic triad for a ruptured abdominal aortic aneurysm—hypotension, pulsatile abdominal mass, and severe abdominal/back pain *Lisa Marcucci, MD* 1

2   Look for a ruptured aneurysm or aortic dissection in any patient who complaints of flank pain *Harsh Jain, MD* 5

3   Consider aortic injury or thoracic great vessel injury if a patient has fractures of the first or second ribs *Ahmed G. Mami, MD* 8

4   Evaluate the patient for mediastinal or heart injuries if a sternal fracture is present *Adrian Lata, MD* 10

5   Have a high index of suspicion for nerve injures in humeral fractures and dislocations *Ahmed G. Mami, MD* 14

6   Give prophylactic antibiotics on initial evaluation of an open fracture *Lisa Marcucci, MD* 17

7   Have a high index of suspicion for compartment syndrome after tibial fractures *Lisa Marcucci, MD* 19

8   Line up the vermilion border when repairing a lip laceration *Nadine Semer, MD* 21

9   Do not shave the eyebrow when repairing a laceration to this area *Nadine Semer, MD* 23

10 Use absorbable sutures when repairing a laceration on a young child *Nadine Semer, MD* 25

11 Do not use staples when repairing a facial laceration *Nadine Semer, MD* 26

12 Admit a knee dislocation for observation if an arteriogram is not performed to rule out popliteal artery injury *Michael J. Moritz, MD* 27

13   Do not incise and drain an abscess in the antecubital fossa, groin, or neck in the emergency room *Mark S. Sneider, MD* 29

14   Treat a perirectal abscess in a diabetic as a surgical emergency *Michael J. Moritz, MD* 31

15   Make a wide incision when draining an abscess *Nadine Semer, MD* 34

16   Do not close a human bite on the hand *Michael J. Moritz, MD* .. 36

17   Do not discard a traumatically amputated body part (finger, ear, lip) until a plastic surgeon has evaluated it for possible replantation *Nadine Semer, MD* 38

18   Do not allow a traumatically amputated tissue segment to become immersed unprotected in ice/cold saline *Nadine Semer, MD* 40

19   Counsel the patient to stop smoking when treating a hand injury, soft tissue injury, or fracture *Nadine Semer, MD* 41

20   Elevate an injured or infected hand *Nadine Semer, MD* 42

21   Admit a patient with second degree burns to the dorsum of the foot *Nadine Semer, MD* 43

22   Strongly consider electively intubating a patient who has suffered inhalation burn injuries or significant burn injuries to the face or mouth *Michael J. Moritz, MD* 45

23   Make sure tetanus prophylaxis is up-to-date with stab and gunshot wounds, burns, frostbite, corneal injury with metallic implants, and bite wounds *James Kirkpatrick, MD* 47

24   Do not debride tissue on initial evaluation in a patient with a frostbite injury unless there are signs of surrounding infection *Nadine Semer, MD* 49

25   Cover eyelid lacerations promptly with a damp dressing while waiting for ophthalmology or plastics to evaluate the patient *Michael J. Moritz, MD* 51

26   Be alert for duct and facial nerve injury in facial and cheek lacerations *Justin Young, MD* 54

27   Remember to account for all missing teeth after maxillofacial trauma *Justin Young, MD* 57

28 Completely undress a patient when examining them for traumatic injury *Michael J. Moritz, MD* 59

29 Do not nasotracheally intubate or place a nasogastric tube in a patient who has or may have facial or skull fractures *Michael J. Moritz, MD* 61

30 Do not blame hypotension on an intracranial injury in a trauma setting unless all other causes have been ruled out *X. D. Dong, MD* 63

31 Obtain a chest radiograph, pelvic radiograph, and lateral, anterior-posterior, and open mouth cerivical-spine films (or the computed tomography equivalents) in blunt trauma or a fall *Michael J. Moritz, MD* 65

32 Do not clear a neck based on lack of tenderness if patient has distracting pain or is intoxicated *Richard Pucci, MD* 68

33 Obtain lumbar spine radiographs in patients with a positive seat belt sign *Lisa Marcucci, MD* 71

34 Do a rectal exam before inserting a urinary catheter in male trauma *Michael J. Moritz, MD* 73

35 Do not rule out intra-abdominal trauma by clinical exam if the patient is intoxicated or has altered sensorium *Michael Silber, DO* 76

36 Be aware that it is possible to bleed to death from a scalp wound *X. D. Dong, MD* 77

37 Close the galea as a separate layer when repairing a full-thickness laceration to the scalp *Nadine Semer, MD* 79

38 Do not remove a knife that is penetrating tissue unless you have a direct intraoperative vision and control *James Herrington, MD* 81

39 Explore an expanding retroperitoneal hematoma caused by trauma should be explored *X. D. Dong, MD* 82

40 Do not give disulfiram (antabuse) or metronidazole (Flagyl) to a patient who has alcohol in his or her system *Michael J. Moritz, MD* 85

41 Have an extremely low threshold for mechanical control of the airway in Ludwig's angina *Lisa Marcucci, MD* 87

42   Treat myoglobinuria with copious intravenous saline fluid
Rachael A. Callcut, MD 89

43   Consider and exclude the highly lethal diagnosis of midgut volvulus
in an infant with bilious vomiting *Michael J. Moritz, MD* 91

44   Consider the possibility of an underlying malignancy when
treating a woman with breast inflammation or abscess
Michael J. Moritz, MD 93

45   Wear gloves when examining a patient in the emergency
room *Michael J. Moritz, MD* 97

46   Promptly dispose of your own sharps after doing a bedside
or emergency room procedure *Michael J. Moritz, MD* 100

OPERATING ROOM

47   Institute deep vein thrombosis prophylaxis before the
induction of anesthesia *Diane L. Ferrara, RN, PA and
Michael J. Moritz, MD* 102

48   Do not use chlorhexidine to prep the face (to avoid corneal
and middle ear injury) *Sue-Mi Cha, MD* 107

49   Prep and drape both legs to the midfoot when doing
vascular procedure on an extremity *Michael J. Moritz, MD* 109

50   Use meticulous attention to correct positioning when
placing a patient in the lateral decubitus position
Ashraf Osman, MD 111

51   Do not inject any substance into a patient in the operating
room without first informing the anesthesiologist
Catherine Marcucci, MD 114

52   Do not move an intubated patient (especially the patient's
head and neck) without first obtaining permission from the
anesthesia staff *Catherine Marcucci, MD* 116

53   Repair a common bile duct injury as close to the hilar plate
as possible *Adrian Lata, MD* 117

54   Remember the Pringle Maneuver (the use of which in
hepatic trauma is less successful than generally thought)
will not control a replaced or accessory left hepatic artery
or control hepatic venous bleeding *Michael J. Moritz, MD* 119

55   Do not allow a patient to bleed to death from a liver injury
Michael J. Moritz, MD 122

56   Have a low threshold for converting a laparoscopic
cholecystectomy to an open cholecystectomy
Michael B. Silber, DO 125

57   Know the three places where small bowel antimesenteric fat
is found when "lost" among loops of bowel
Michael J. Moritz, MD 128

58   Free up the bowel proximally and distally when repairing
an enterotomy to avoid fistula formation *X. D. Dong, MD* 130

59   Make sure that the red rubber catheter in a Witzel
jejunostomy is going distally in the small bowel lumen
Michael J. Moritz, MD 132

60   Avoid undue traction on the left renal vein when exposing the
neck of an aortic aneurysm *Michael J. Moritz, MD* 135

61   Remember that inferior polar arteries to the right kidney
cross the infrarenal inferior vena cava *James Herrington, MD* ... 138

62   Use clips for hemostasis sparingly and with care in
proximity to where vascular clamps might be used
Michael J. Moritz, MD 140

63   Check the jaws of a vascular clamp before applying
James Herrington, MD 142

64   Obtain proximal and distal control before exploring a
vascular wound *Michael J. Moritz, MD* 145

65   Do not use a permanently non-absorbable suture on the
bladder or ureter *Michael J. Moritz, MD* 147

66   Never think you know where the bladder is—it can look
a lot like the colon *Michael J. Moritz, MD* 149

67   Avoid initially grabbing the appendix or tip of appendix
when doing a laparoscopic appendectomy
Michael J. Moritz, MD 151

68   Do not initially close the skin completely after doing
fasciotomy for compartment syndrome *James Herrington, MD* . 153

69   Use blunt dissection when doing an emergency venous
cutdown *Michael J. Moritz, MD* 156

70   Make sure that breast biopsy sites are bone dry before closing *Michael J. Moritz, MD* 159

71   Place the marking stitches to orient specimen *before* excising a lesion that might be malignant *Michael J. Moritz, MD* 161

72   Do not do a shave biopsy on a lesion suspicious for melanoma *X. D. Dong, MD* 163

73   Handle sutures with proper technique to decrease fascial dehiscence *Ramon Rivera, MD* 168

74   Do not reach onto the scrub nurse's table without permission *Michael J. Moritz, MD* 170

75   Do not call the anesthesiologists or nurse anesthetists "anesthesia" or "Dr. Anesthesia" *Catherine Marcucci, MD* 171

MEDICATIONS

76   Make sure that intravascular medications are not inadvertently placed in the extravascular space and extravascular medications are not placed intravascularly *Michael J. Moritz, MD* 172

77   Do not give a verbal order for a medication without inquiring about the patient's allergies *Rachael A. Callcut, MD*................. 177

78   Do not prescribe a Kayexalate-sorbitol enema to a kidney transplant patient *Dmitriy Nikitin, MD* 179

79   Remember to change the dosage when converting from the intravenous (IV) to the oral (PO) form of immunosuppressive and other drugs in transplant patients *Dmitriy Nikitin, MD* 181

80   Do not allow St. John's wort to be co-administered with cyclosporine, tacrolimus, or sirolimus *Neil Sandson, MD* 184

81   Do not prescribe a non steroidal anti-inflammatory drug (NSAID) or an aminoglycoside to a patient with cirrhosis *Michael J. Moritz, MD* 186

82   Be cautious when using Demerol in patients with renal insufficiency *Michael J. Moritz, MD* 188

83   Remember that antibiotics can have severe and irreversible side effects with even short courses *Michael J. Moritz, MD* 189

84 Consider prescribing Lactobacillus (or other probiotic
therapy) when a patient receives any dose of antibiotics
Lisa Marcucci, MD 192

85 Check peak and trough levels when dosing aminoglycosides
and trough levels in select situations when dosing
vancomycin *Harsh Jain, MD* 195

86 Avoid long courses of antibiotics with significant
anti anaerobic activity to lessen the risk of vancomycin
resistant enterococcus *Michael J. Moritz, MD* 199

87 Do not prescribe intravenous vancomycin to treat
Clostridium difficile *Michael J. Moritz, MD* 202

88 Consider double-covering Pseudomonas infections
Michael J. Moritz, MD 204

89 Remember to give vaccines for *Haemophilus influenzae*,
Meningiococcus and Pneumococcus in patients who undergo
a splenectomy, and always have a high index of suspicion for
overwhelming postsplenectomy sepsis (OPSS) in patients
with splenectomy *Harsh Jain, MD* 207

90 Consider the use of fluconazole prophylaxis in intensive
care patients with severe pancreatitis, abdominal sepsis, or
need for multiple abdominal surgeries *Lisa Marcucci, MD* 210

91 Do not prescribe Viagra to a patient taking nitrates and
vice versa *Ashraf Osman, MD* 212

92 Do not prescribe hydrocodone (Vicodin, Lortab) or
tramadol (Ultram) to a patient who is taking fluoxetine
(Prozac), paroxetine (Paxil), or high-dose sertraline
(Zoloft) *Neil Sandson, MD* 214

93 Do not prescribe monoamine oxidase inhibitors (MAOIs)
to a patient who is taking a selective serotonin reuptake
inhibitor (SSRI) *Neil Sandson, MD* 215

94 Give prophylactic perioperative beta-blockers for patients
at risk for cardiac ischemia *Michael J. Moritz, MD* 216

95 Consider *N*-Acetylcysteine or sodium bicarbonate
prophylaxis along with adequate hydration to combat
contrast-induced nephropathy *Michael J. Moritz, MD* 219

96 Do not use "renal dose" dopamine *Lisa Marcucci, MD* 221

97 Stop metformin (Glucophage) before any elective surgery (however minor) or intravascular contrast study to avoid lactic acidosis *Michael J. Moritz, MD* 223

98 Make sure the heparin is removed from the intravenous flushes and heparin-coated lines are removed if a patient is diagnosed with heparin-induced thrombocytopenia *Heather Abernethy, MD* 225

99 Have a high threshold for administering Vitamin K intravenously *Michael J. Moritz, MD* 227

100 Do not push intravenous verapamil without the patient being monitored for cardiac rhythm and blood pressure *Richard Pucci, DO* 229

101 Be cautious when loading a patient with intravenous Dilantin *Ahmed G. Mami, MD* 231

102 Monitor the patient when using protamine to reverse heparin *Heather Abernethy, MD* 233

103 Check for history of migraine before giving Zofran *Michael J. Moritz, MD* 235

104 Become familiar with the antidotes to commonly prescribed drugs *Michael J. Moritz, MD* 237

105 Consider drugs as a possible cause of leukocystosis *Lisa Marcucci, MD* 243

LINES, DRAINS, AND TUBES

106 Do not draw blood proximal to an intravenous line that is infusing *Gregory Kennedy, MD, PhD* 246

107 Go above the rib when placing a chest tube or needle into the chest cavity *Heather Abernethy, MD* 249

108 Do not push a malpositioned chest tube into the thoracic cavity *Michael J. Moritz, MD* 251

109 Do not allow a patient to vomit around a nasogastric tube *Lisa Marcucci, MD* 253

110 Confirm correct placement of a Foley catheter by return of urine *Lisa Marcucci, MD* 255

111 Be reluctant to allow more then 500 mL to drain out of a newly placed catheter or drain at one time *Lisa Marcucci, MD and Kenneth Meredith, MD* 257

112 Obtain a drain study when the output from a drain in an abscess cavity decreases abruptly *Kenneth Meredith, MD and Lisa Marcucci, MD* 259

113 Release the suction on the bulb before removing a Jackson-Pratt drain *Lisa Marcucci, MD and Kenneth Meredith, MD* 260

114 Use a dedicated, upper body, single lumen central venous catheter for administration of parenteral nutrition *Lisa Marcucci, MD* 262

115 Be meticulous in technique when inserting and caring for central venous access catheters in the intensive care unit to lower the incidence of infection *Lisa Marcucci, MD* 264

116 Avoid the subclavian vein for central access of any type in a dialysis patient or possible dialysis patient *Michael J. Moritz, MD* 266

117 Do not enter the femoral artery or vein superior to the inguinal ligament when attempting a needle cannulation *Lisa Marcucci, MD and Kenneth Meredith, MD* 269

118 In a patient with a previously placed vena cava filter, do not use the J-tip on the guidewire when using the Seldinger technique to place a central venous catheter *Lisa Marcucci, MD* 271

119 Aim for the ipsilateral nipple when placing a central venous catheter in the internal jugular vein *Heather Abernethy, MD* 273

120 Advance the needle into the vein with the plunger pulled back gently when doing central venous access *Lisa Marcucci, MD* 275

121 Maintain control of the wire when putting in a central line using the Seldinger technique *Lisa Marcucci, MD* 277

122 Check for venous blood before dilating the tract when inserting a central venous catheter *Michael J. Moritz, MD* 279

123 Do not push the dilator in the entire length when using the Seldinger technique to insert a central venous catheter *Lisa Marcucci, MD and Kenneth Meredith, MD* 282

124   Secure a central line with anchoring sutures at four sites
Lisa Marcucci, MD 284

125   Do not insert, remove, or change a central line in the upper torso unless the patient is lying flat or is in the Trendelenberg position. *Michael J. Moritz, MD* 286

126   Obtain a chest radiograph before switching sides when attempting elective subclavian or jugular central line placement *Lisa Marcucci, MD* 288

127   Check for left bundle-branch block on an electrocardiogram before placing a pulmonary artery catheter *Michael J. Moritz, MD* 290

128   Be extremely cautious when manipulating the balloon used in pulmonary artery catheters *Lisa Marcucci, MD* 293

Wounds

129   Remember that the first symptom of a wound infection is pain, and the first sign is tenderness (*not* erythema) *Heather Abernethy, MD* 298

130   Consider the VAC dressing for difficult wounds *Michael J. Moritz, MD* 302

131   Examine the wound when a patient has a high fever, especially within 12 to 24 hours of surgery *Rachael A. Callcut, MD* 304

132   Do not debride a dry/black eschar overlying a decubitus ulcer in a bedridden patient who has no evidence of underlying cellulitis *Nadine Semer, MD* 305

133   Strongly consider the diagnosis of fascial dehiscence when a wound drains pinkish or salmon-colored fluid *Michael J. Moritz, MD* 306

Bleeding

134   Look for the source of a lower gastrointestinal bleed in the upper gastrointestinal tract *Rachael A. Callcut, MD* 310

135   Remember that bleeding in the right upper quadrant diagnosed by a bleeding scan can be from the hepatic flexure of the colon or the duodenum *Michael J. Moritz, MD* 313

136   Recognize herald bleeding and institute the appropriate diagnostic and therapeutic maneuvers *Michael J. Moritz, MD* .. 315

137 Discuss when and how to reanticoagulate a patient postoperatively with a senior member of the surgical team *Michael J. Moritz, MD* 318

138 Consider a retroperitoneal bleed if a patient has new onset flank pain, ecchymosis, or back pain *Michael J. Moritz, MD* 320

139 Do not presume that a gastrointestinal bleed in a patient with known cirrhosis is from varices *Michael J. Moritz, MD* 322

140 Have a high index of suspicion for liver injury in children who receive chest compressions *Mark S. Sneider, MD* 325

GASTROINTESTINAL TRACT

141 Mediastinitis from an esophageal perforation is a treatment emergency *Michael J. Moritz, MD* 328

142 During rectal examination, initially insert the fingertip just slightly and hold for several seconds *Rachael A. Callcut, MD* 332

143 Perform routine rectal exams *Rachael A. Callcut, MD* 333

144 Do not believe the old surgical dictum that it is not possible to reduce a hernia if it contains dead bowel *Michael J. Moritz, MD* 335

145 Do not use high-density barium for an initial contrast study when a gastrointestinal (GI) perforation or leak is suspected *Michael J. Moritz, MD* 338

146 Be cautious when evaluating the abdomen of a patient taking corticosteroids *Ramon Rivera, MD* 339

147 Do not allow a "negative CT" (computed tomography) to prevent you from taking a case of suspected appendicitis to the operating room if the diagnosis is supported clinically *Lisa Marcucci, MD* 341

148 Have a high index of suspicion for ischemic colitis if a patient has a bowel movement in the first 24 hours post operatively after an abdominal aortic repair *Michael J. Moritz, MD* 343

149 Do not do perform elective hernia repairs or hemorrhoidectomies in patients who have cirrhosis *Michael J. Moritz, MD* 345

150 Consider gastric dilatation when a patient is having respiratory difficulty *Rachael A. Callcut, MD* 347

151 Have a high index of suspicion for incarcerated or strangulated hernia if a patient has a bowel obstruction and no previous abdominal surgery *James Herrington, MD* 349

152 Consider an anastomotic leak, inadvertent enterotomy, or devitalized loop of bowel if tachycardia and/or tachypnea that is resistant to fluids occurs after abdominal surgery *Michael J. Moritz, MD* 354

WARDS

153 Consider consulting psychiatry on admission of the patient to evaluate for competency *Neil Sandson, MD* 358

154 Do not discharge a patient if he or she wishes to leave the hospital against medical advice *Michael J. Moritz, MD* 362

155 Investigate cardiac devices (pacemakers) before taking the patient to the operating room *Catherine Marcucci, MD* 364

156 Include the order "No procedures on _____ arm (the side operated on)" when writing postoperative orders for modified radical mastectomy and lumpectomy and axillary lymph node dissection *Harsh Jain, MD* 366

157 Order an ampule of naloxone (Narcan) to the bedside when writing orders for patient-controlled analgesia or if the patient is receiving continuous epidural narcotic infusion *Catherine Marcucci, MD* 368

158 Use 20 seconds of acupressure with your fingertip to decrease patient discomfort at the insertion site of a needle *Rachael A. Callcut, MD* 370

159 Do not attempt a radial and ulnar artery cannulation on the same side at the same sitting *Heather Abernethy, MD* 371

160 Make the decision to intubate based on the overall clinical picture *Jack Hudkins, MD* 374

161 Do not attempt to elucidate ischemic changes on an electrocardiogram that has a left bundle-branch block *Lisa Marcucci, MD* 376

162 Treat crepitus associated with a soft tissue infection with a high level of concern that may require definitive treatment in the operating room *James Herrington, MD* 378

163 Do not administer sterile water intravenously to correct hypernatremia *Lisa Marcucci, MD* 381

164 Consider physical restraints on combative hepatic encephalopathy patients *Michael J. Moritz, MD* 383

165 Diabetics often do not have chest pain in myocardial infarction and absence of angina can not be used to rule out signficant coronary artery disease *Rachael A. Callcut, MD* 386

166 Remember when reviewing Doppler ultrasound results that the superficial femoral vein is a component of the deep enous system *Patrick Schaner, MD* 388

167 Aggressively treat phlebitis from intravenous sites in immunosuppressed or heart valve patients *Gregory Kennedy, MD* 390

168 Assume that if a patient is not doing well post-operatively, there is an undiagnosed complication of your procedure until proven otherwise *Rachael A. Callcut, MD* 392

169 Examine the patient before switching pain medication when a patient complains of a lack of relief *Rachael A. Callcut, MD* ... 394

170 Do not discount a patient's complaint of neck or back pain *Michael J. Moritz, MD* 395

171 Be alert for abdominal sepsis in the morbidly obese patient *Adrian Lata, MD* 398

172 Consider an Addisonian state if it "looks like sepsis and smells like sepsis" but you cannot identify any offending microbes *Rachael A. Callcut, MD* 401

173 Do not put adhesive tape on a patient with fragile skin *Michael J. Moritz, MD* 403

174 Do a thorough head and neck examination when an anterior neck mass is discovered, and do a fine–needle aspiration of the mass as the first tissue diagnosis procedure *Michael J. Moritz, MD* 405

175 Stay up-to-date on the latest advanced cardiac life support (ACLS) protocols. *Lisa Marcucci, MD* 407

176 Always ask for help if you are uncertain of the best course of action *Michael J. Moritz, MD* 408

INTENSIVE CARE UNIT

177 Do not attempt to wean a patient on a ventilator with an abdominal binder in place *Lisa Marcucci, MD* 410

178 Strongly consider the use of smaller tidal volumes when ventilating patients with acute lung injury or acute respiratory distress syndrome *Lisa Marcucci, MD* 414

179 Allow a sedated patient to awaken every 24 hours *Michael J. Moritz, MD* 415

180 Maintain tight glucose control in the intensive care unit *Michael J. Moritz, MD* 417

LABORATORY

181 Obtain a pregnancy test on every female between the ages of ten and fifty years *Gregory Kennedy, MD* 420

182 Do not use a Hemoccult test kit to test for the presence of blood in gastric contents *Rachael A. Callcut, MD* 424

183 Do not disregard an even slightly elevated partial thromboplastin time (PTT) when the prothrombin time (PT) is normal *Lisa Marcucci, MD* 425

184 Remember that urine electrolytes, commonly used as an indicator of intravascular volume, are significantly altered after diuretics are given *Michael J. Moritz, MD* 428

185 Make sure that the labs drawn for tacrolimus and cyclosporin levels are timed appropriately *Michael J. Moritz, MD* 431

186 Know the risks of disease transmission and the universal donor and recipient types for transfusion (the universal donor for red cells is "O" negative and for fresh frozen plasma (FFP) is "AB" positive) *Michael J. Moritz, MD* 433

INDEX 437

EMERGENCY DEPARTMENT

OPERATING ROOM

MEDICATIONS

LINES, DRAINS, AND TUBES

WOUNDS

BLEEDING

GASTROINTESTINAL TRACT

WARDS

INTENSIVE CARE UNIT

LABORATORY

REMEMBER THE CLASSIC TRIAD FOR A RUPTURED ABDOMINAL AORTIC ANEURYSM— HYPOTENSION, PULSATILE ABDOMINAL MASS, AND SEVERE ABDOMINAL/BACK PAIN

LISA MARCUCCI, MD

Making the diagnosis of a ruptured abdominal aortic aneurysm (AAA) is one of surgery's true emergencies. The condition is so grave that an estimated 50% to 70% of patients with a ruptured AAA do not survive to the emergency room. Ruptured AAAs account for approximately 15,000 deaths in the United States each year. The condition is common enough that every surgical intern can expect to manage at least one of these patients. Although there has been a significant overall reduction in deaths from heart attacks and strokes in the last three decades, the incidence of AAA (and thus of ruptured AAAs) is increasing. It is estimated that 10% of men over 70 years of age have an AAA; this condition is likely to become even more common in the aging population in the United States.

SIGNS AND SYMPTOMS

A prompt diagnosis is key to maximizing patient survival. The classic triad for a ruptured AAA is hypotension, a pulsatile abdominal mass, and acute onset of severe back or flank pain. However, only 50% of patients with ruptured AAAs present with this triad. One recent review documented the presence of a pulsatile mass in 83% of patients, abdominal and/or back pain in 72%, and hypotension in 48%. In addition, fewer than half the patients with a ruptured AAA have a known AAA. Other signs and symptoms of ruptured AAAs occur with variable frequency. These are: flank or periumbilical ecchymosis (Turner's and Cullen's sign, respectively); flank, groin, perineal, or testicular pain; paraplegia; and acute unilateral femoral or obturator nerve neuropathy. Further complicating the clinical presentation is that perforated viscus, mesenteric ischemia, and other causes of intraperitoneal hemorrhage can mimic the presentation of AAA.

How should a patient with this diagnosis be managed by the surgeon? There are two protocols for patient management. First, if the patient has the classic triad including hypotension, he or she should be taken to the operating room for emergency laparotomy without delay or further workup. The following steps should be taken with the utmost haste on the way to operating room:

1) Placing two large bore IVs peripherally or a large bore central venous introducer
2) Fluid resuscitation with crystalloid or colloid to a systolic pressure of 100 mm Hg
3) Ordering of 6 units of O negative non–cross-matched blood while typing and cross-matching is pending
4) Contacting a senior member of the surgical team
5) Inserting a Foley catheter

As other members of the team become available or as the operative procedure begins, the other steps that should be taken include:

6) Prepping the *awake* patient from neck to toes using the "pour" technique

7) Cross-matching of 6 to 10 units of packed red blood cells
8) Arranging for 6 units of platelets and fresh-frozen plasma
9) Administering intravenous antibiotics
10) Arranging an autotransfusion device
11) Increasing the ambient room temperature
12) Applying warming devices

The second scenario of ruptured AAA involves the patient who has a pulsatile mass and acute onset of abdominal or back pain but is clinically stable, which presents a greater diagnostic and management dilemma. Abdominal ultrasonography or computed tomography (CT) with intravenous contrast (first choice, if available) has become more widespread in this scenario. Computed tomography has a greater than 90% accuracy in diagnosing ruptured AAAs. Typical CT findings include extravasation of intravascular contrast material, retroperitoneal fluid collections, hematomas or mass lesions in the psoas muscle, ventral dislodgement of the kidney, and indistinct aortic wall margins. Ultrasound has the advantage over CT of being available at the bedside in some emergency rooms but requires an experienced user and is best at detecting large ruptures with significant extravasation. Of critical importance when obtaining these tests is close observation by a surgeon to monitor for clinical deterioration. If this event occurs, the imaging tests should be terminated at once, and the patient should be taken emergently to the operating room.

One final note is that, if the patient is being seen and evaluated by residents, senior attending staff should be notified immediately if the diagnosis of a ruptured AAA is even remotely considered.

SUGGESTED READINGS

Cameron JL, ed. Current Surgical Therapy. 7th Ed. Philadelphia: Mosby, 2002:813–817.

Ernst CB, Stanley JC, eds. Current Therapy in Vascular Surgery. 3rd Ed. St. Louis: Mosby, 1995:224–226.

LOOK FOR A RUPTURED ANEURYSM OR AORTIC DISSECTION IN ANY PATIENT WHO COMPLAINS OF FLANK PAIN

HARSH JAIN, MD

The patient who presents to the hospital with flank and/or back pain can be a diagnostic challenge. Although the differential diagnosis is lengthy, the most emergent diagnosis to be considered is a ruptured aortic aneurysm. The classical triad for a ruptured abdominal aortic aneurysm (AAA) is pain, hypotension, and a pulsatile abdominal mass. However, because most patients do not present in this manner, a high index of suspicion is essential. If a ruptured aneurysm is suspected, speed is of the essence. A lengthy workup in the emergency department may cost the patient's life.

Ruptured AAAs typically present with sudden onset of severe, constant, abdominal, back or flank pain that may radiate to the scrotum, chest, groin, or thigh. Abdominal aortic aneurysms can rupture into the peritoneal cavity or into the retroperitoneum. Frank intraperitoneal rupture causes hemodynamic collapse and has a higher mortality. Retroperitoneal ruptures are usually temporarily contained by adjacent structures. Other symptoms that may be seen are those associated with shock: pallor, diaphoresis, tachycardia, hypotension, and syncope.

SIGNS AND SYMPTOMS

The clinical presentation of ruptured AAA may be confused with renal colic. In renal colic, the pain is also sudden in onset, usually beginning in the flank region, with radiation to the lateral abdomen, inguinal region, and groin. There may be associated nausea and vomiting. In one study, 18% of patients with symptomatic AAA were initially diagnosed with renal colic in the emergency department.

A distinction must be made between aneurysm rupture and aortic dissection. **Aneurysms** occur throughout the aorta, most commonly in the infrarenal segment, and risk of rupture rises with larger size. **Dissection** is a different pathologic process whereby blood enters the aortic wall from the lumen through a disruption of the aortic intima (the "lead point") and spreads (i.e., dissects) radially and longitudinally along the aortic wall. Dissections most commonly occur in the thoracic aorta. A dissection causes ischemia when the intramural hematoma narrows or occludes aortic branches. Dissection can also present by perforating through the aorta (rupture) with hemorrhage or by disruption of the aortic valve with acute valvular insufficiency. Unlike ruptured AAAs, most acute aortic dissections are managed with control of hypertension and beta blockade to decrease aortic shear forces, with surgery reserved for ischemic complications or hemorrhage. A chronic dissection weakens the aortic wall and can lead to the development of an aneurysm, which is also at risk of rupture.

Aortic dissection most commonly presents with pain. The pain is abrupt in onset and sharp, ripping, or tearing in nature. The pain is typically midline, either in the anterior or posterior thorax (front pain usually from the ascending aorta, back pain usually from the descending aorta), and does not commonly radiate to the neck, shoulder, or arm. Abdominal pain is also present in 30% of patients. Extension of pain down the back, abdomen, hips, or legs indicates extension of the dissection distally.

WHAT TO DO

The workup of suspected aortic problems in the emergency department should be approached with care and speed and is dependent on the hemodynamic stability of the patient. An unstable patient with a known abdominal aneurysm or a pulsatile abdominal mass should be taken to the operating room *immediately*. A hemodynamically unstable patient in whom the diagnosis is unclear is a difficult problem. Expeditious surgical abdominal exploration may be lifesaving, thus any delay in surgery must be well justified. If immediately available, a bedside ultrasound may confirm the presence of an aneurysm but may not discern the presence or absence of rupture. A rapid computed tomography (CT) scan will be diagnostic, but first be sure the patient is stable enough to tolerate the scan. A hemodynamically stable patient with an unknown diagnosis can undergo a CT scan, which will show an aneurysm, its extent, and the involvement of the iliac arteries—all of which can be useful in planning repair. Of critical importance is timeliness of the workup. If the CT scan cannot be obtained on an urgent basis, this test should be abandoned. In one recent review, all patients with ruptured AAA who underwent a diagnostic workup lasting more than 5 hours died.

Similar to patients with abdominal lesions, those patients with a suspected thoracic aortic dissection or aneurysm should be evaluated with the imaging modality that is most readily available at that facility. Computed tomography scan, transesophageal echocardiography (TEE), and angiography each have advantages and disadvantages.

Magnetic resonance imaging (MRI) is rarely used due to time constraints. The workup must be expeditious. Untreated proximal aortic dissection has a mortality of 1% to 3% per *hour*, with an inhospital mortality of 25% during the first 24 hours.

SUGGESTED READINGS

Borrero E, Queral LA. Symptomatic abdominal aortic aneurysm misdiagnosed as nephroureterolithiasis. Ann Vasc Surg 1988;2:145–149.

Khan IA, Nair CK. Clinical, diagnostic, and management perspectives of aortic dissection. Chest 2002;122:311–328.

Townsend CM, Beauchamp RD, Evers BM, eds. Sabiston Textbook of Surgery 16th Ed. Philadelphia: WB Saunders, 2001: 1357–1372.

3

CONSIDER AORTIC INJURY OR THORACIC GREAT VESSEL INJURY IF A PATIENT HAS FRACTURES OF THE FIRST OR SECOND RIBS

AHMED MAMI, MD

When attempting to diagnose traumatic aortic or great vessel injury, one must consider that the first two ribs are shorter, thicker, and stronger than the lower ribs and are also protected by the clavicle and shoulder girdle. Fractures of these ribs indicate an injury delivering a substantial amount of kinetic injury (from a rapid decelerating force such as a high speed motor vehicle accident or from a fall from a significant height). Because of the magnitude of energy transfer, first and second rib fractures have been associated with severe chest and aortic injuries; 5% to 15% of these fractures have concomitant aortic or thoracic great vessel injuries. Because specific signs and symptoms of great vessel injury may be absent, a high index of suspicion is needed to make the diagnosis promptly while the patient's life can still be saved. All chest radiographs in the trauma setting should be inspected for these fractures and for the other radiographic signs associated with aortic injury (see page 9).

WHAT TO DO

If ribs 1 or 2 are fractured, the surgeon is obligated to definitively rule out great vessel injury. Aortography, with a sensitivity and specificity approaching 100%, has traditionally been the gold standard for diagnosis of thoracic aorta injury. Other diagnostic modalities include transesophageal echocardiography (TEE) and helical chest computer tomography (CT) scan. Transesophageal echocardiography has sensitivity, specificity, and diagnostic accuracy that are almost equal to aortography. Drawbacks to TEE include the need for specialized personnel and equipment, the necessity for esophageal instrumentation, and the limited view of certain portions of the aorta. Helical CT scan also has accuracy similar to aortography and is very sensitive, but is not as specific as aortography. However, this test is being used with increasing frequency in major trauma centers because it is easily and quickly obtained, provides good visualization of the thoracic great vessels, and is noninvasive. Whatever modality is used, care should be taken to inspect the area just proximal to the takeoff of the left subclavian artery, as the 10% to 20% of patients with aortic tears who survive to reach the trauma bay usually have an incomplete laceration at this site.

To briefly review, other chest radiographic findings that are associated with aortic injury include:

- Widened mediastinum
- Obliteration of the outline of the aortic knob
- Deviation of the trachea, nasogastric, or endotracheal tube to the right
- Obliteration of the space between the pulmonary artery and the aorta
- Inferior displacement of the left main bronchus
- Widened right paratracheal stripe
- Widened paraspinal interfaces
- Presence of a pleural or apical cap (usually on the left)
- Left hemothorax
- Fractures of scapula

The most common finding on chest radiographs in cases of traumatic aortic disruption is a widened mediastinum, which is present in approximately 90% of cases of traumatic aortic disruption. However, widened mediastinum is common in the trauma setting in the absence of aortic injury and can be related to radiologic technique and body habitus. Standard workup of a widened mediastinum to further delineate the presence of aortic injury is a computed tomography arteriogram; if this is equivocal, then it should be followed by a conventional arteriogram.

SUGGESTED READINGS

American College of Surgeons Committee on Trauma. Advanced Trauma Life Support Program for Doctors: Student Course Manual Chicago: American College of Surgeons, 1997.

Demetriades D, Asensio JA. Subclavian and axillary vascular injuries. Surg Clin North Am 2001;81:1357–1373.

Feliciano DV, Rozycki GS. Advances in the diagnosis and treatment of thoracic trauma. Surg Clin North Am 1999;79:1417–1429.

Hunt JP, Baker CC, Lentz CW, et al. Thoracic aorta injuries: management and outcome of 144 patients. J Trauma 1996;40:547–556.

4

EVALUATE THE PATIENT FOR MEDIASTINAL OR HEART INJURIES IF A STERNAL FRACTURE IS PRESENT

ADRIAN LATA, MD

Blunt trauma can fracture the sternum. An isolated sternal fracture is usually stable and of little concern, and most heal without intervention. The primary concern in evaluating the patient with sternal fracture is the risk of myocardial or great vessel injury from the force involved in the injury. The particular risk to individual vessels is partly a function of the anatomy of the sternum and where the fracture occurs.

The manubrium sterni, the heaviest and the densest portion of the sternum, overlies the internal mammary vessels, segments of the superior vena cava and left and right innominate veins, and the ascending and arch portions of the aorta. Fracture through the manubrium sterni or in the region of the sternomanubrial symphysis can tear the internal mammary vessels or injure the great vessels, with the resulting mediastinal hemorrhage manifesting as widening of the mediastinum on a chest radiograph (see *Figure 4.1*). Pericardial laceration, hemopericardium, pericarditis, or pericardial effusion may also occur.

The body of the sternum is thinner and less rigidly supported by the costosternal cartilages than is the manubrium. The area of the outflow tract of the right ventricle and the aortic valve occupy the space immediately deep to the uppermost portion of the body of the sternum; the right atrium and right ventricle are immediately posterior to the remainder. Fractures of the body of the sternum may result in pericardial or cardiac injuries that include myocardial contusion, laceration, or rupture and cardiac tamponade. Associated injuries to the lung (contusion, laceration) or ribs (fractures) with sternal fractures may cause hemothorax or pneumothorax. Major bronchus injury, fatal systemic fat embolism, and cervical, thoracic, or lumbar spinal fractures (secondary to flexion injuries) have been described in patients with fractures in the sternal body.

The xiphoid process varies greatly in size and shape. It is rarely fractured because of its protected position between the flare of the costal margins and the relatively flexible sterno–xiphoid joint. Because of the flexibility of the xiphoid and costal margins, blunt trauma

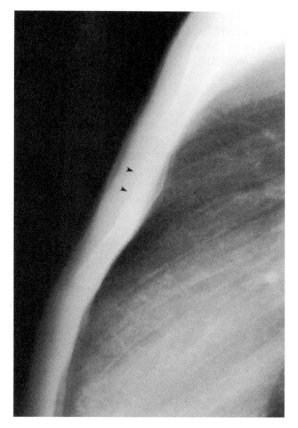

FIGURE 4.1. Sternal fracture (*arrows*) with surrounding soft tissue swelling.

to this area (with or without fracture of the sternum) may result in liver laceration, contusion or rupture of hollow organs (e.g., duodenal laceration), or pancreatic injury.

In sternal fractures, patients almost always complain of sternal pain. Physical examination may reveal deformity, tenderness, or ecchymoses overlying the sternum. Sternal fracture can be confirmed by either sternal view or lateral chest radiographs (see Figure 4.1). As computed tomography of the chest becomes more commonly used for evaluation of the thorax in trauma, more sternal fractures may be identified. As specific radiographic examination of the sternum is not a routine part of trauma assessment, the surgeon must have a high index of suspicion and a low threshold in initiating the search for these fractures. More critically injured patients, such as those requiring mechanical ventilation and sedation or those with associated head injuries who cannot complain of chest pain, may escape evaluation of the sternum. In these situations, occult sternal fractures often remain undiagnosed (along with the associated injuries) when other injuries become the focus of attention.

WHAT TO DO

Operative reduction and stabilization of sternal fractures is performed in patients with severe, unrelenting pain related to sternal fragment displacement. Steel wires or plates with anchoring screws are used to stabilize the sternal fragments. Dissection of the displaced sternal fragments can be hazardous because adhesions between the posterior table of the sternum and the right ventricle can form quickly.

The incidence of myocardial contusion in patients with sternal fractures has been reported to range from 1.3% to 62%. The reason for the wide variation in these findings lies in the lack of uniformity in defining myocardial contusion. Blunt cardiac injury or myocardial contusion has been defined by various investigators as follows: (1) CPK (creatine phosphokinase)-MB isoenzyme concentration of greater than 5% of total CPK enzyme level; (2) electrocardiogram (ECG) showing evidence of acute injury pattern; (3) ECG or telemetry revealing newonset arrhythmia requiring therapy; or (4) echocardiography showing wall-motion abnormalities. Treatment protocols are evolving, but it seems reasonable in patients with sternal fractures to provide further observation and testing if the patient has any of the findings listed above. In addition, anterior chest wall ecchymosis or contusion, complaints of sternal or substernal chest pain, sternal tenderness, or deformity to palpation should likewise prompt a period of observation and testing. If the patient remains stable and has an isolated sternal fracture and a normal ECG after 6 to 24 hours, he or she can usually be discharged home with analgesics and follow-up. If the patient is hemodynamically unstable, then an ECG, CPK-MB levels, echocardiography, intensive care unit admission, and continuous cardiac monitoring should be obtained.

One final note is that several recent small series have not reported a strong association between sternal fracture and thoracic visceral injury. This may be because the impact from the three-point seatbelt has become the most common cause of fracture, rather than contact with a vehicle steering wheel. This evolving mechanism of injury has been associated with a lower incidence of concomitant head, facial, and abdominal trauma and with a lower incidence of death after sternal fracture. Despite such encouraging information, the surgeon must remain vigilant for this injury.

SUGGESTED READINGS

Brookes JG, Dunn RJ, Rogers IR. Sternal fractures: a retrospective analysis of 272 cases. J Trauma 1993;35:46–54.

Chiu WC, D'Amelio LF, Hammond JS. Sternal fractures in blunt chest trauma: a practical algorithm for management. Am J Emer Med 1997;15:252–255.

Gibson LD, Carter R, Hinshaw DB. Surgical significance of sternal fracture. Surg Gynecol Obstet 1962;114:443–448.

Greenberg MD, Rosen CL. Evaluation of the patient with blunt chest trauma: An evidence-based approach. Emer Med Clin North Am 1999;17:41–62.

Harley DP, Mena I. Cardiac and vascular sequelae of sternal fractures. J Trauma 1986;26:553–555.

Roy-Shapira A, Levi I, Khoda J. Sternal fractures: a red flag or a red herring? J Trauma 1994;37: 59–61.

Sadaba JR, Oswal D, Munsch CM. Management of isolated sternal fractures: determining the risk of blunt cardiac injury. Ann R Coll Surg Engl 2000;82: 162–166.

HAVE A HIGH INDEX OF SUSPICION FOR NERVE INJURES IN HUMERAL FRACTURES AND DISLOCATIONS

AHMED MAMI, MD

Injuries of the humerus, including glenohumeral dislocations, humeral fractures (head, shaft, and supracondylar), and elbow dislocations may result in injury to any of the major nerves that traverse the arm.

AXILLARY NERVE

The axillary nerve is at risk for injury in shoulder dislocations (glenohumeral joint dislocations) and in proximal humeral fractures (see *Figure 5.1*). Proximal humeral fractures are more common in females than males (2:1) and most commonly occur in women with osteoporosis. The typical mechanism is a fall on an outstretched arm or directly onto the shoulder. In younger males, high-energy trauma is a typical mechanism for shoulder dislocation. Iatrogenic injury to the axillary nerve may occur during shoulder arthroscopy, arthroplasty, and open reduction/internal fixation of proximal humeral fractures.

The axillary nerve derives from the C5 and C6 nerve roots, via the upper trunk and the posterior cord of the brachial plexus. It emerges inferior to the subscapular and thoracodorsal nerves at the level of the humeral head, passes posteriorly through the quadrangular space (accompanied by the posterior circumflex humeral artery), and then winds around the neck of the humerus (medially, posteriorly, laterally, then anteriorly). Upon emerging from the quadrangular space posteriorly, the nerve innervates the teres minor muscle, divides into a medial branch that supplies part of the deltoid muscle and a patch of skin over the muscle, and an anterior branch that supplies the anterior two-thirds of the deltoid.

Patients with an injury to the axillary nerve may have an area of skin numbness overlying the deltoid. Such patients are usually unable to abduct the affected shoulder due to loss of function of the deltoid. However, arm abduction is sometimes possible despite deltoid paralysis if the patient uses the supraspinatus muscle with rotation of the scapula to effect shoulder abduction. Therefore, in a thorough examination for axillary nerve injury, the deltoid must be observed and palpated for contraction when arm abduction is attempted.

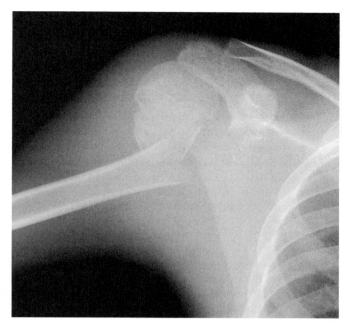

FIGURE 5.1. Fracture of the proximal humerus.

If axillary nerve damage has occurred, the shoulder should be rested until the orthopedic injury has healed. When clinically appropriate, the patient should then undergo an extensive rehabilitation program. Signs of nerve recovery may not appear for 3 to 6 months after the injury. If no recovery is observed by 6 months, surgical exploration may be indicated.

RADIAL NERVE

The radial nerve is vulnerable to injury from (or treatment of) midshaft humeral fractures or elbow dislocations and occurs in 10% to 15% of such injuries. Most nerve damage secondary to a fracture is due to contusion or a mild stretch (neuropraxic) injury and slow recovery can be expected.

The radial nerve is a continuation of the posterior cord of the brachial plexus and consists of fibers from C6–C8 and sometimes T1. It is primarily a motor nerve that innervates the triceps brachii, supinators of the forearm, and the extensors of the wrist, fingers, and thumb. Consequently, radial nerve injuries produce mainly motor deficits leading to "wrist-drop."

ULNAR NERVE

The ulnar nerve is susceptible to injury from dislocations of the elbow and in supracondylar and condylar fractures. The ulnar nerve arises from fibers of C8 and T1 via the medial cord of the brachial plexus. Interruption of the ulnar nerve proximal to the elbow results in paralysis of the flexor carpi ulnaris, the flexor profundus and lumbricals to the little and ring fingers, the interossei, the thumb adductor, and the short muscles of the little finger. The patient will be unable to make a fist.

OTHER NERVES

The other nerves that may be injured in humeral fractures are the median nerve and the musculocutaneous nerve. The median nerve may be injured by the protruding lower end of the proximal fragment of a humeral supracondylar fracture. This is usually a neuropraxic injury and can be managed expectantly. The musculocutaneous nerve is a branch of the lateral cord of the brachial plexus and is composed of fibers from C5 and C6. It may occasionally be injured by anterior dislocation of the shoulder or fractures of the humeral neck. Weakness of the biceps brachii is the only reliable finding on examination.

SUGGESTED READINGS

Beeson, MS. Complications of shoulder dislocation. Am J Emerg Med 1999;17: 288–295.

Bono CM, Grossman MG, Hochwald N, et al. Radial and axillary nerves: anatomic considerations for humeral fixations. Clin Orthop 2000;373:259–264.

Canale ST, ed. Campbell's Operative Orthopaedics 10th Ed. St Louis: Mosby, 2003: 3221–3286.

6

GIVE PROPHYLACTIC ANTIBIOTICS ON INITIAL EVALUATION OF AN OPEN FRACTURE

LISA MARCUCCI, MD

WHAT NOT TO DO

Most general surgeons have ceded the definitive care of open fractures to orthopedic surgeons. The best outcome for these injuries is dependent on prevention of infection, obtaining quick union of the fracture, and rapid restoration of function. However, it is still common for patients with this injury to be initially evaluated by general surgeons. Intravenous antibiotics should be given as soon as possible after the diagnosis of open fracture and then continued for 24 hours, with an additional 24 hours of coverage after operative treatment. Although clearly efficacious early in the treatment course, prolonged use of antibiotics (>3 days) has not been shown to prevent infection. Treatment regimens vary and it is common sense for general surgeons to administer the antibiotics recommended by their orthopedic colleagues. For general surgeons who do not see these injuries commonly, the typical recommendation is a parenteral first-generation cephalosporin for all open fractures unless an allergy is present. Alternately, some surgeons advocate a slightly more nuanced protocol as listed below:

Grade 1 injury—bone spike has pierced the skin or laceration is less than 1 cm; minimal crush injury; minimal communition; nonfarm environment.
second-generation cephalosporin (e.g., cefuroxime) 1–2 g q8hours for 48 hours
Grade 2 injury—skin laceration is greater than 1 cm but no extensive soft tissue damage, flaps, or avulsions; no vascular compromise; nonfarm environment.
cephalosporin 1–2g q8 hours for 48 hours
Grade 3 injury—significant crush injury and avulsion or vascular compromise; nonfarm environment.
cephalosporin 1–2 g q8hours for 48 hours *and*
gentamicin 1–2 mg/kg q8hours for 48 hours
Special situations—farm environment or other risk of fecal clostridial contamination.
cephalosporin 1–2 g q8hrs for 48 hours *and*
gentamicin 1–2 m q8hours for 48 hours *and*
penicillin G 4 million units q4hours for 48 hours

In penicillin allergy, vancomycin 1 g q12hours or clindamycin 900 mg q8hours for 48 hours can be used. In addition, some orthopedic surgeons use ciprofloxacin for grades 1 and 2 injuries instead of cephalosporin-based treatment plans.

SUGGESTED READINGS

Cochrane Database Syst Review 2004;(1)CD003764. J Am AcadOrthop Surg 2003;11(11):212–219.

Patzakis MJ, Bains RS, Lee J, et al. Prospective, randomized, double-blind study comparing single-agent antibiotic therapy, ciprofloxacin, to combination antibiotic therapy in open fracture wounds. J Orthop Trauma 2000;14:529–533. Available at: surgery.med.umich.edu. Accessed July 26, 2005.

7

HAVE A HIGH INDEX OF SUSPICION FOR COMPARTMENT SYNDROME AFTER TIBIAL FRACTURES

LISA MARCUCCI, MD

SIGNS AND SYMPTOMS

Compartment syndrome is a serious complication occurring after both acute and chronic injury. It occurs when the interstitial pressure in a closed fascial compartment rises sufficiently high so as to compromise tissue perfusion and cause nerve ischemia and myofascial necrosis. The clinical signs and symptoms are only variably present and include pain out of proportion to the injury, pain on passive range of motion of fingers or toes, extremity pallor, paralysis, paresthesias (especially the early loss of vibratory sensation), and loss of distal pulses.

WATCH OUT FOR

The injury that is most closely associated with compartment syndrome is a tibial fracture, especially tibial plateau fractures. Of interest is that the incidence of compartment syndrome is higher in closed fractures than in open ones. Compartment syndromes can result in any of the four leg compartments with tibial fracture but are most common in the deep posterior compartment followed by the anterior compartment. Specific clinical signs of a compartment syndrome in the deep posterior compartment are weakness of toe flexion and ankle inversion, decreased sensation on the plantar foot surface, and pain that may be referred to the posterior leg on passive toe extension (dorsiflexion). Specific clinical signs of anterior compartment involvement include decreased sensation in the skin web between the great and second toes, pain on passive toe flexion (plantar flexion), variable weakness in toe extension, and severe pain and tenderness over the anterior compartment muscles rather than the fracture site. In addition, any complaint of increased pain after reduction and casting should heighten suspicion of compartment syndrome. Importantly, clinical signs may not present for up to 24 hours.

WHAT TO DO

In addition to the clinical exam, the evaluation for compartment syndrome should include measurement of compartment pressures, especially if the patient is severely injured or has multiple injuries and is not able to reliably cooperate in a clinical exam. This is most easily accomplished using an 18-gauge side-ported needle or slit catheter attached to a handheld device such as that manufactured by Stryker Instruments (a simple needle causes consistently high readings). The measurement of compartment pressures should be performed or supervised by an experienced clinician, preferably the surgeon who would be performing the fasciotomies if indicated. It is important that all four leg compartments be evaluated, with care taken to obtain readings as close to the fracture site as possible, because readings taken at a distance tend to underestimate the pressure. Needle placement must be done sterilely to avoid the risk of infection in a fracture hematoma.

There is some controversy over how often and how long pressure readings should be obtained and what parameters should be used to diagnose compartment syndrome. The traditional teaching has been that a tissue pressure greater than 30 to 35 mm Hg is an indication for fasciotomy even with a normal clinical exam. This resulted in a fasciotomy rate of approximately 50% for tibial fractures. Recent reports have shown the safety of using a pressure differential between the tissue pressure and the diastolic pressure to determine need for fasciotomy. The consensus is when this differential falls below 20 to 30 mm Hg, fasciotomy is indicated. This results in a fasciotomy rate of 3% to 5%, with a high specificity for compartment syndrome. Although firm guidelines are evolving, it seems reasonable to take serial measurements every 6 to 12 hours for the first 24 to 36 hours to avoid missing a late developing compartment syndrome.

One final note is that there are multiple case reports of compartment syndromes developing after the initial period of evaluation or after repair where the diagnosis was missed (with disastrous results) due to patient-controlled analgesia obscuring a worsening clinical situation. If patient-controlled analgesia is prescribed or if patients are otherwise narcotized to the point of comfort, the clinician must pay meticulous attention to serial exams and with consideration of stopping or decreasing the narcotics.

SUGGESTED READINGS

McQueen M. Acute compartment syndrome. Acta Chir Belg 1998;98:166–170.
McQueen MM, Court-Brown CM. Compartment monitoring in tibial fractures: the pressure threshold for decompression. Br J Bone Joint Surg 1996;78:99–104.
O'Sullivan MJ, Rice J, McGuinness AJ. Compartment syndrome without pain! Ir Med J 2002;95:22.
White TO, Howell GE, Will EM, et al. Elevated intramuscular compartment pressures do not influence outcome after tibial fracture. J Trauma 2003;55:1133–1138.

LINE UP THE VERMILION BORDER WHEN REPAIRING A LIP LACERATION

NADINE SEMER, MD

In facial trauma, lacerations of the lip are common. To obtain the best cosmetic result, meticulous reapproximation of the anatomic sections must be fashioned. Even a 1 mm discrepancy will be noticeable and loupe magnification should be used during surgical repair of the lip.

External anatomy and landmarks of the lip are described as follows (see *Figure 8.1*):

- The white skin just before the red mucosal surface is the white roll.
- The line of red just next to the white roll is the vermilion border.
- The red part of the lip is divided into the outer dry mucosa and the inner wet mucosa (shiny and moist to the touch).

The first suture to place when suturing a laceration that crosses the vermilion border is the stitch to realign the vermilion border. There should be no hesitation in removing the stitch and placing it again if the border is not properly aligned. Absorbable suture (chromic is most commonly used) should be placed on the mucosal surface, and with care taken to not invert the edges. Unless repairing a laceration on a child, use fine nonabsorbable suture material (5-0 or 6-0 nylon or polypropylene) should be used on the skin. Nonab-

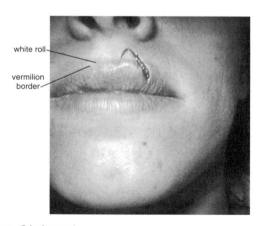

white roll

vermilion
border

FIGURE 8.1. Lip laceration.

sorbable skin sutures should be removed within 5 to 7 days to lessen subsequent scarring; absorbable sutures will come out on their own.

Of particular importance, when repairing lip lacerations, the underlying orbicularis oris muscle must be closely inspected. If this muscle is cut, it must be surgically repaired. Failure to reapproximate the muscle will lead to an unsightly depression in the lip. Absorbable suture material (chromic or Vicryl) in a figure-of-eight fashion works best.

One final note is that consideration should be given to obtaining a plastic surgery consult if the examining physician is not experienced in repairing these injuries and especially if the patient is a child or teenager.

SUGGESTED READINGS

Smith JW, Aston SJ, eds. Grabb and Smith's Plastic Surgery 4th Ed. Boston: Little, Brown & Company, 1991:338.

9

DO NOT SHAVE THE EYEBROW WHEN REPAIRING A LACERATION TO THIS AREA

NADINE SEMER, MD

The eyebrow is an important facial landmark and irregularities here can be quite noticeable. Most surgeons are eager to carefully and meticulously close wounds to this area to improve cosmesis. However, when preparing a wound for closure here, do not shave the eyebrow to provide an unobstructed view of the wound and ensuing closure. The hairs may not grow back, or they may grow back in an abnormal pattern that does not match the contralateral side.

If the wound affecting the eyebrow is large and gaping, the underlying muscle should be reapproximated if it is involved. A few deep dermal sutures should be used to help minimize an unsightly depression in the eyebrow scar. Absorbable sutures should be used for these layers. When closing the more superficial layers, care should be taken to place the minimum number of sutures needed for reapproximation. Sutures in the dermis and epidermis can destroy hair follicles with patchy loss of the eyebrow hair. If using a nonabsorbable suture for skin closure, use a different color than the patient's eyebrow color

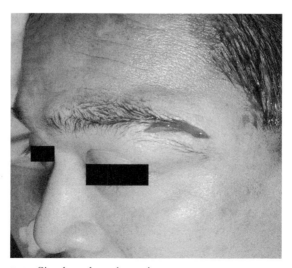

FIGURE 9.1. Simple eyebrow laceration.

to facilitate easier suture removal. Polypropylene is a good choice because most people do not have blue eyebrows. Absorbable suture such as chromic gut is also an acceptable choice.

SUGGESTED READINGS

Smith JW, Aston SJ, eds. Grabb and Smith's Plastic Surgery 4th Ed. Boston: Little, Brown & Company, 1991:330.

USE ABSORBABLE SUTURES WHEN REPAIRING A LACERATION ON A YOUNG CHILD

NADINE SEMER, MD

Suturing a laceration on a child is often difficult. Despite best efforts to soothe the child, there is usually much crying and squirming, and sedation may be necessary to allow for the best chance for optimal skin approximation to minimize the scar. The smallest suture size possible should be used to repair a laceration on a child. A laceration on the trunk or extremity should be repaired with a 4-0. For a laceration on the face, 5-0 or smaller is recommended.

Although there is less scarring with the use of nonabsorbable monofilament suture material (e.g., nylon and Prolene), these sutures still must be removed. Suture removal in a young child can be just as difficult for the surgeon and child as placing the sutures in the first place. Therefore, even on the face—where scarring concerns are the greatest—absorbable sutures should be placed on young children. Chromic gut or fast-absorbing gut sutures are best because they usually separate and fall off during bathing within 10 to 14 days. Consideration should also be given to placing a few deep dermal sutures as a first layer; these dermal sutures will support the closure if the absorbable sutures fall out sooner than planned.

To briefly review, four absorbable suture types are (fastest to slowest absorbable):

- Plain gut (7 to 14 days)
- Chromic gut (10 to 14 days)
- Vicryl or Dexon (multifilaments, 4 weeks)
- Monocryl (4 to 6 weeks)

DO NOT USE STAPLES WHEN REPAIRING A FACIAL LACERATION

NADINE SEMER, MD

To optimize aesthetic outcome when definitively repairing or closing a facial laceration, staples should never be used below the hairline. Some trauma surgeons suggest the use of staples on the face when large lacerations are present and attention must be rapidly diverted to other concerns. However, if at all possible, wounds on the face should be closed (even temporarily) with the smallest possible suture size. In general, nothing larger than 4-0 should be used for skin closure, with 5-0 or even 6-0 being optimal. Magnifying loupes make the use of smaller size sutures easier.

In adults and older children, nonabsorbable monofilament suture material is best (e.g., nylon or Prolene). In young children, absorbable suture is best to eliminate the trauma of suture removal. Surgical staples should not be used on the face because skin edges are difficult to align properly, and the staples will leave unsightly track marks on the skin.

WHAT TO DO

When repairing the facial wound, meticulous suture placement is needed. Each suture should be placed 1 to 2 mm from the wound edge and 1 to 2 mm apart. Skin edges should be everted to make certain there is adequate dermis-to-dermis approximation. Sutures should be removed 5 to 7 days after placement to obtain the best scar. After removal of sutures, Steristrips can be applied to help reinforce the skin closure.

ADMIT A KNEE DISLOCATION FOR OBSERVATION IF AN ARTERIOGRAM IS NOT PERFORMED TO RULE OUT POPLITEAL ARTERY INJURY

MICHAEL J. MORITZ, MD

SIGNS AND SYMPTOMS

Knee dislocation is an uncommon injury requiring significant blunt force. Because of the proximity of the popliteal artery, knee dislocation is associated with a significant incidence of injury to the artery. By the time the patient arrives in the hospital, knee dislocations have typically been reduced. If the dislocation has not been reduced, this must be done expeditiously so that distal perfusion can be accurately assessed. Hard signs of an arterial injury (distal ischemia and the "Ps" of pain, pallor, pulselessness) mandate rapid surgical intervention.

Knee dislocations are classified by the movement of the tibia relative to the femur. Anterior dislocations (see *Figure 12.1*) stretch the popliteal artery over the femoral condyles with the risk of intimal disruption. Posterior dislocations push the posterior edge of the tibial plateau backward to impinge on the artery and mechanically compress and damage it. Less common lateral or rotatory knee dislocations also may result in popliteal artery injury. Fractures adjacent to the knee (tibial plateau, distal femur) have a lower (but still significant) risk of vascular injury than do dislocations.

WATCH OUT FOR

Previously, all patients with knee dislocation or adjacent fractures underwent angiography, which showed that 25% of knee dislocations have popliteal artery injury severe enough to require immediate surgical intervention. Another 10 to 15% of patients with knee dislocations will have minor popliteal artery injuries that do not require surgery (spasm, small intimal flap), although some may require interventional radiologic procedures. Importantly, all patients requiring surgery will eventually manifest ischemia or pulse deficit on physical examination, although the examination can evolve over hours; thus, some patients can present with normal pulses that subsequently deteriorate.

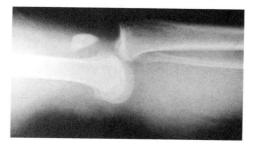

FIGURE 12.1. Anterior knee dislocation.

Currently, some surgeons maintain that major popliteal artery injury can be reliably excluded without arteriography on the basis of physical examination if the patient is observed for an adequate length of time (24–36 hours) by a qualified surgeon. Alternatively, a high quality ultrasound with duplex Doppler that is read by an experienced ultrasonographer and that shows no evidence of major vascular injury in the setting of a normal vascular examination is also reliable. As an adjunct, serial measurements of the ankle-brachial index (which should be normal; i.e., greater than or equal to 1.0) can be obtained to help detect evolving injury. In contrast to this strategy of close observation, many surgeons would not observe a knee dislocation without an ultrasound or arteriogram as the incidence of injury is high enough "to go looking for it."

SUGGESTED READINGS

Bynoe RP, Miles WS, Bell RM, et al. Noninvasive diagnosis of vascular trauma by duplex ultrasonography. J Vasc Surg 1991;14:346–352.

Miranda FE, Dennis JW, Veldenz HC, et al. Confirmation of the safety and accuracy of physical examination in the evaluation of knee dislocation for injury of the popliteal artery: a prospective study. J Trauma 2002;52:247–252.

Treiman GS, Yellin AE, Weaver FA, et al. Examination of the patient with a knee dislocation: the case for selective arteriography. Arch Surg 1992;127:1056–1063.

Do not incise and drain an abscess in the antecubital fossa, groin, or neck in the emergency room

Mark Sneider, MD

A surgeon commonly is called to the emergency room to evaluate a red, tender, and fluctuant mass in the antecubital fossa, groin, or neck. The typical history from the patient is that of a pulsatile, painful, and enlarging mass that may or may not be associated with signs of a systemic illness such as fever. In this situation, prompt incision and drainage (I and D) under local anesthetic in the emergency room is contraindicated as mycotic aneurysms must be included in the differential diagnosis, and inadvertent I and D of these lesions without proper planning can result in life-threatening hemorrhage to the patient.

WATCH OUT FOR

A mycotic aneurysm is a localized dilation of an artery at least 1½ times its normal diameter and is due to destruction of the vessel wall by infection. Direct bacterial inoculation secondary to penetrating injury is the usual source of this infection. These lesions are seen most commonly in intravenous (IV) drug users, in whom the femoral and brachial arteries are typically affected. All masses in these areas in possible IV drug users should be carefully evaluated for pulsation and bruit. Signs of mycotic aneurysm may be masked by overlying inflammation and cellulitis, and strong consideration should be given to assessment with ultrasound Doppler, computed tomography angiography, or arteriography before definitive treatment. In one reported series, 17% of mycotic aneurysms in IV drug users were misdiagnosed as cellulitis, abscess, or thrombophlebitis.

Effective treatment of mycotic aneurysm involves both surgical therapy and intensive antibiotic treatment. Surgical options include:

1) Ligation of the artery with exclusion and drainage of the diseased segment. This can usually be done safely in the radial, external iliac, and deep femoral vessels if there is good collateral blood supply to the involved extremity as documented by Doppler. With this approach, the wound is allowed to heal before a revascularization procedure is attempted.
2) In situ repair, bypass, or revascularization with autogenous tissue (typically a saphenous vein graft).

Broad spectrum antibiotic coverage (especially for *Staphylococcus* and *Streptococcus*) should be instituted empirically until blood and culture results are available with coverage narrowed as appropriate. Patients should receive a minimum of 4 to 6 weeks of antibiotic treatment.

One final note is that, if definitive radiologic study shows the vessels to be uninvolved, incision and drainage in the emergency room of a small to moderate size abscess in the antecubital, groin, or neck areas can be contemplated.

SUGGESTED READINGS

Cameron JL, ed. Current Surgical Therapy 7th Ed. Philadelphia: Mosby, 2001.

Tintinalli J, ed. Emergency Medicine 4th Ed. New York: McGraw Hill, 1996.

Spelman, D. Mycotic aneurysms Available at: www.uptodate.com. Accessed July 15, 2005.

TREAT A PERIRECTAL ABSCESS IN A DIABETIC AS A SURGICAL EMERGENCY

MICHAEL J. MORITZ, MD

WATCH OUT FOR

Perirectal abscesses present a wide spectrum of disease severity, from minor infections to major life-threatening infections. Particularly in neurologically or immunologically compromised patients, the severity of the infection can be greatly underestimated—these infections must be diagnosed and treated with great urgency. Although diabetics do not have the obvious defects that paraplegic or neutropenic patients do, perirectal abscesses in diabetics have a significant tendency to rapidly progress to deeper, more serious infections. When treatment (incision and drainage) is delayed, such patients are predisposed to develop Fournier's gangrene, a life-threatening disorder with a reported 9% to 43% mortality.

Anatomically, there are roughly five types of perirectal abscess listed in *Table 14.1* from right to left, in increasing order of the depth of the abscess and the magnitude of the surgery needed for drainage. With the exception of a superficial perianal abscess in a cooperative patient without significant comorbid conditions, all other perirectal abscesses should be admitted to the hospital for intravenous fluids, antibiotics, and emergency surgery under general or regional (not local) anesthesia. Factors contributing to excess morbidity and mortality of perirectal abscess include delay in treatment (even as little as several hours), inadequate initial drainage, and comorbid conditions.

WHAT TO DO

Appropriate management of perirectal abscess requires making the diagnosis, obtaining surgical consultation, admitting the patient for intravenous fluids (varying with the depth of the infection, the degree of toxicity, and comorbidities), antibiotics, and prompt surgical drainage of the abscess. Microbiology of perirectal abscesses typically includes anaerobes, most commonly *Bacteroides fragilis*, and Gram-negative enteric bacteria.

WHAT TO DO NEXT

After obtaining appropriate anesthesia and visualization of the area, the abscess is drained at its most superficial point via a generous incision (see *Figure 14.1*). The incision must be large enough to provide

	PERI-ANAL	**POST-ANAL**	**ISCHIO-RECTAL**	**INTER-SPHINC-TERIC**	**SUPRA-LEVATOR**
TABLE 14.1	**TYPES OF PERIRECTAL ABSCESS**				
Incidence	40%	5%	25%	25%	<5%
Symptoms	Painful perianal mass	Pain near coccyx	Buttock pain	Rectal fullness	Perianal and buttock pain
Fever & Leuko-cytosis?	No	Yes	Sometimes	Sometimes	Yes
Associated fistula?	Usually	No	Sometimes	Always	Always
Treat in ER?	Yes	No	Infrequently	No	No

adequate access to fully drain the abscess, to explore the space and insure that all loculations and extensions have been drained, and to allow the skin to remain open until deep spaces have healed. An incision that is too small will rapidly close, inviting a recurrence.

As mentioned above, the surgeon must be assiduous in preventing the occurrence of Fournier's gangrene. This is an aggressive syn-

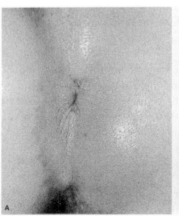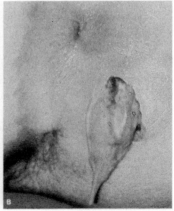

FIGURE 14.1. Anorectal abscess. A: A ripe ischiorectal abscess in the left posterior quadrant. B: The same abscess expressing pus immediately after incision.

ergistic infection of the perineum, involving the fascial planes, sub-cutaneous tissue, and skin. Underlying muscular structures are rela-tively less involved, but extensive infection can result in their de-struction as well. Most cases arise from colorectal disease (most commonly perirectal abscess), the urinary tract (usually urethral stricture), or from dermatologic conditions. The most common co-morbid condition is diabetes (20% of cases), followed by alcoholism, HIV/AIDS, leukemia, and other systemic conditions that impair host defenses. Rarely, Fournier's gangrene occurs as postoperative complication of hernia, genitourinary, or anorectal surgical proce-dures. As with other synergistic fasciitis infections, Fournier's gan-grene is a mixed synergistic infection ultimately dominated by anaer-obes. Full thickness loss of skin and subcutaneous tissue is commonplace. Aggressive surgery to excise nonviable infected tissues is essential, usually with multiple, staged procedures. Diversion of the fecal stream (diverting colostomy) may be needed to allow control of sepsis. Concomitant antibiotic therapy is important, but surgical treatment is primary and mandatory. Hyperbaric oxygen therapy may have adjunctive value, although its effectiveness is unproven.

SUGGESTED READINGS

Eke N. Fournier's gangrene: a review of 1726 cases. Br J Surg 2000;87:718–728.

Onaca N, Hirshberg A, Adar R, et al. Early reoperation for perirectal abscess: a preventable complication. Dis Colon Rectum 2001;44:1469–1473.

Roberts JR, Hedges JR, eds. Clinical Procedures in Emergency Medicine 3rd Ed. Philadelphia: WB Saunders, 1998:634–658.

Yaghan RJ, Al-Jaberi TM, Bani-Hani I. Fournier's gangrene: changing face of the disease. Dis Colon Rectum 2000;43:1300–1308.

MAKE A WIDE INCISION WHEN DRAINING AN ABSCESS

NADINE SEMER, MD

The distinction between cellulitis and an abscess is important as the treatments are different. **Cellulitis** is a diffuse soft tissue infection without a defined fluid collection and is treated with antibiotics alone. An **abscess** is a localized collection of pus that is treated by incision and drainage (I and D) and antibiotics. Usually, it is easy to differentiate the two clinically because an abscess is often fluctuant on exam. For deep abscesses that are not obviously fluctuant, ultrasound can be used to detect the underlying fluid collection.

WHAT TO DO

When an abscess is drained, the surgeon should not be timid: the abscess cavity must be fully opened for timely resolution of the infection. If only a small stab wound is used, the abscess cavity may not be fully drained, and the cavity may reform. Before opening the abscess, local anesthetic should be used, although its efficacy is usually reduced in the infected tissue due to hyperemia and an acidic pH. Thirty seconds of acupressure at the site of local injection should also be applied to provide additional analgesia before the incision is made. Alternatively, a nerve block (e.g., a digital block when the I and D is done on the fingertip) or general anesthesia/sedation (when the abscess is large) may be required. The area to be incised should be prepped with antibacterial solution. An incision with a knife (or cautery) is made at the area of the abscess wall that is thinnest (where it seems to "point"). The incision should be generous enough to allow complete drainage of the cavity and easy dressing changes. Some surgeons make a cruciate (cross-shaped) incision to allow the skin edges to gap open and prevent premature reapproximation. Immediately after opening the abscess, culture specimens should be obtained from the liquid removed from the abscess cavity with care taken not to contact the skin.

WHAT TO DO NEXT

After the abscess is opened and cultured, the wound should be gently probed with the tip of a finger or instrument to insure that any loculated collections are drained. The cavity is then irrigated with sterile saline or water and packed with gauze, using several layers of dry gauze on top. There are many acceptable types of packing, but iodine-impregnated gauze should be avoided as its use is more painful than noniodine gauze. The initial packing is allowed to remain in place for 24 hours with dressing changes every 12 to 24 hours thereafter. The gauze may be slightly dampened before removing to reduce patient discomfort. After the packing has been removed the abscess cavity should be rinsed with saline or water before repacking. One commonly used technique is to have the patient shower with the packing in place to allow it to become wet. This will facilitate removal. The patient then allows warm water to rinse the empty cavity for several minutes before re-packing the wound with a moist "wet to dry" gauze. With an ample incision and regular packing changes, even a large abscess cavity will gradually heal from the inside outward.

SUGGESTED READINGS

Beers MH, Berkow R, eds. The Merck Manual. 17th Ed. New Jersey: Merck Research Labs, 1999:1135–1136.

Root RK, ed. Clinical Infectious Diseases. New York: Oxford University Press, 1999:501–503.

16

DO NOT CLOSE A HUMAN BITE ON THE HAND

MICHAEL J. MORITZ, MD

Human and animal bite wounds are common, responsible for more than 1 million emergency room visits in the United States annually. Each bite wound potentially contaminates deep tissue spaces with flora present in saliva and traumatizes tissue via the significant forces generated by the mechanisms of these injuries. Physical trauma beyond the crush injury can include scratches, punctures, lacerations, and evulsions. The spectrum of known causative organisms from bite wounds has changed due to better techniques of anaerobic culture, with a greater importance now given to the polymicrobial nature of many of these infections.

WATCH OUT FOR

Human bite wounds are usually polymicrobial (>80%), with an average of more than 5 bacterial isolates per wound. Anaerobic isolates slightly outnumber aerobic ones. Anaerobes include Gram-negative microbes such as *Eikenella corrodens*, non-*fragilis Bacteroides* species, Gram-positive cocci, fusiform bacilli, and spirochetes. Most aerobic isolates are staphylococci, streptococci, and Gram-negative rods. *E. corrodens* is susceptible to penicillin, ampicillin, and the quinolones but resistant to oxacillin, methacillin, and sometimes cephalosporins.

Human bites, especially to the hand, occur in many settings. Sexual assault, fights, and rough sexual activity, in addition to the contribution of alcohol or illicit drug ingestion, often lead to two problems in diagnosis: (1) delayed presentation and (2) denial that the hand injury is from a bite. The astute physician should be suspicious of seemingly minor puncture wounds on the dorsal aspect of the 3rd, 4th, or 5th metacarpophalangeal (MCP) joints. The surgeon should not insist that the patient confess to a bite injury before giving appropriate treatment for such an injury and resulting infection.

Human bites to the hand have a very high risk of infection (at least 50% if no antibiotics are given). In addition to cellulitis, lymphangitis, and abscess formation, major underlying tissues at significant risk include the joint space (septic arthritis), bone (osteomyelitis), and tendons (tenosynovitis). Systemic spread of aggressive polymicrobial infections is a real risk. The risk of serious infection can be reduced to less than 10% with appropriate preventative antibiotics. These wounds should almost never be closed if the patient is not under the care of an experienced hand surgeon.

Animal bites to the hand are usually from dogs or cats. Anaerobic bacteria are also important in these bites. Dog bites that have been cultured average 3 organisms per wound with fewer anaerobic species per wound compared to human bites. The most common organisms are the *Pasteurella* species (which are Gram-negative facultative anaerobes), especially *P. multocida*. Most *Pasteurella* species are sensitive to penicillin, ampicillin, and azithromycin, and resistant to clindamycin and penicillinase-resistant penicillins.

WHAT TO DO

Parenterally, ampicillin in combination with sulbactam (Unasyn) or ticarcillin with clavulanate (Timentin) or ampicillin with clavulanate (Augmentin) provide reasonable coverage while culture and sensitivity results are pending. For penicillin-allergic patients, other possibilities include cefoxitin, tetracyclines, or the newer quinolones with anti-anaerobic activity (e.g., moxifloxacin and gatifloxacin).

Other important considerations for bites include tetanus prophylaxis; a booster is given if the patient has been adequately immunized previously and it has been less than 10 years from the patient's last booster. Otherwise, tetanus immunoglobulin and immunization is needed. For animal bites, consideration of rabies prevention is important for dogs, bats, and rodents (particularly raccoons and skunks).

Essential local care of the human bite wound involves thorough cleansing with water and an antiseptic soap, irrigation with saline, and debridement of devitalized tissue. Any concern of fracture, joint space involvement, or the presence of a foreign body mandates a radiograph. Facial wounds may be closable under some circumstances; however, the much higher infection rate of hand wounds, the proximity to tendon, joint, and bone, and the greater frequency of puncture wounds on the hand preclude closure of hand wounds. In fact, more widely opening the wound to establish better drainage is often the better choice. In general, any hand wound suspicious for a bite should be seen by a senior physician, consultation of a hand surgeon should be considered, and hospital admission for intravenous antibiotics or operative irrigation and debridement must be strongly considered.

SUGGESTED READINGS

Brook I. Microbiology and management of human and animal bite wound infections: an overview. Primary Care 2003;30:25–39.

Mollit DL. Infection control: avoiding the inevitable. Surg Clin North Am 2002;82: 365–378.

Perron AD, Miller MD, Brady WJ. Orthopedic pitfalls in the ER: fight bite. Am J Emer Med 2002;20:114–117.

17

DO NOT DISCARD A TRAUMATICALLY AMPUTATED BODY PART (FINGER, EAR, LIP) UNTIL A PLASTIC SURGEON HAS EVALUATED IT FOR POSSIBLE REPLANTATION

NADINE SEMER, MD

While working in the emergency room, you may encounter a patient who has suffered a traumatic amputation or avulsion of the scalp, finger, hand, ear, or digit. Even though it may appear on first inspection that there is little chance of saving the severed tissue, do not comprise the ultimate outcome by discarding it until it is seen by a plastic surgeon. Until this occurs, the amputated segment should be wrapped in a saline-moistened gauze and placed in a plastic bag, which is then placed in an iced saline solution.

Although the procedure to reattach an amputated part is highly technical and tedious, replantation should be attempted in most instances. Only a specially trained plastic surgeon can make the determination about whether an amputated segment can be replanted. Even if the entire tissue segment is not replantable, parts of the tissue may be salvageable. For example, an amputated ear may have severe soft tissue damage, but the underlying cartilage framework may be usable. In children, the amputated segment may be too small to be revascularized but may be reattachable as a composite graft with reasonable results. Additionally, nonreplantable skin can still be useful for wound closure. For example, the skin from an amputated fingertip can be defatted and used as a full thickness skin graft to cover the open wound.

Replantation is usually performed as soon as possible after injury. However, the more muscle that is present in the severed tissue the shorter the amount of ischemia time tolerated. An amputation at the wrist has a 12-hour upper limit of acceptable cool ischemia time, but replanation of a digit can be performed even 24 hours after cool ischemia. The scalp can tolerate significant delay in replantation with reports of successful replantation after 21 hours of warm ischemia time.

There are several steps the general surgeon can do to aid the plastic surgeon in preparing the patient for replantation:

WHAT TO DO

1) Administer intraFvenous fluids—normal saline or Ringer's lactate should be given to keep the patient hydrated. The patient should be receiving nothing by mouth (NPO) except required medications while waiting for surgery.

2) Administer aspirin—the dose is 80–160 mg, which is equivalent to one baby aspirin or one-half of an adult aspirin. It can be given by mouth or as a rectal suppository. Aspirin has antiplatelet properties and may help prevent the vessels from clotting after revascularization has been completed. Do not substitute acetaminophen for aspirin.

3) Administer intravenous antibiotics—a first generation cephalosporin is usually appropriate.

4) Administer pain medications—intravenous hydromorphone or morphine is usually appropriate. Nerve blocks of the affected area should only be performed if it is approved by the plastic surgeon.

5) Clean and dress the wound—saline-moistened gauze (damp but not soaking wet) should be used directly on the wound, and then wrap the wound lightly with dry gauze to control oozing and to keep the wound clean.

SUGGESTED READINGS

Green DP, Hotchkiss RN, Pederson WC, eds. Green's Operative Hand Surgery 4th Ed. New York: Churchill Livingstone, 1999:1139–1157.

Kecheng, J, Kaixiang C, Su Z, et al. Microsurgical replanation of the avulsed scalp: report of 20 cases. Plast Reconstr Surg 1996;97:1099–1106.

DO NOT ALLOW A TRAUMATICALLY AMPUTATED TISSUE SEGMENT TO BECOME IMMERSED UNPROTECTED IN ICE/COLD SALINE

NADINE SEMER, MD

All amputated tissue should be considered potentially replantable until evaluated by a qualified microsurgeon. Minimizing damage during the period of ischemia is vital in increasing the chance for successful replantation. Cooling the amputated segment is important to help preserve the tissue. However, care must be taken to avoid inadvertently freezing the amputated tissue. The proper care of the amputated segment is detailed below:

WHAT TO DO

1) Remove only debris that can be separated easily from the tissue. Do not cut away embedded foreign material or vigorously irrigate as important microstructures may be injured. The definitive debridement will be done in the operating room by the operating surgeon.
2) Clean the amputated segment with sterile saline and wrap the tissue in a saline-moistened gauze. The gauze should be moist but not soaking wet.
3) Place the wrapped amputated segment in a clean plastic bag and seal it.
4) Place the plastic bag containing the tissue in a container of ice mixed with saline (slush). Never place the amputated part or the bag directly on ice.

These steps will help achieve the overall goal to optimally cool the tissue without freezing it.

SUGGESTED READING

Merle M, Dautel G. Advances in digital replantation. Clin Plast Surg 1997;24: 87–105.

COUNSEL THE PATIENT TO STOP SMOKING WHEN TREATING A HAND INJURY, SOFT TISSUE INJURY, OR FRACTURE

NADINE SEMER, MD

Virtually everyone is familiar with the ill effects of tobacco on the pulmonary and cardiovascular systems. The increased risk of head and neck cancer among people who use tobacco products is also well known. What many health professionals and the general public may not be aware of are the deleterious effects of tobacco on wound and fracture healing. It is important to counsel all patients on the dangers of smoking, but this must be reinforced with patients with wounds (both acute and chronic), hand injuries, and fractures.

WATCH OUT FOR

Oxygen delivery to injured tissues and an intact immune response are vital for normal healing. Many of the compounds in tobacco smoke, particularly nicotine, carbon monoxide, and hydrogen cyanide, are harmful to these processes. Nicotine causes decreased blood and oxygen flow to tissues through vasoconstriction. This is particularly important in the hand and fingers as replant success is markedly decreased in smokers. Carbon monoxide and hydrogen cyanide interfere with oxygen transport on the molecular level. Other toxins found in tobacco have damaging effects on leukocyte function. This leads to an abnormal immune response, which further interferes with normal wound healing.

One of the first questions to ask a patient when evaluating a hand or wound injury or fracture is: "Do you smoke cigarettes?" If the answer is yes, to optimize healing and outcome, inform them that they have just smoked their last one.

SUGGESTED READINGS

Krueger JK, Rohrich RJ. Clearing the smoke: the scientific rationale for tobacco abstention with plastic surgery. Plast Reconstr Surg 2001;108:1063–1073.

Mosley LH, Finseth F, Goody M. Cigarette smoking: impairment of digital blood flow and wound healing in the hand. Hand 1977;9:97.

ELEVATE AN INJURED OR INFECTED HAND

NADINE SEMER, MD

WHAT TO DO

One of the most dramatic physical signs of a hand injury or infection is swelling of the hand. This swelling has a deleterious effect on outcome as it limits motion, causes pain, and delays healing. Diffuse swelling can also mask the presence of an underlying abscess. To counter the effects of tissue swelling, the patient should keep the injured hand elevated at all times, with the hand higher than the heart for best effect. However, the use of an arm sling should be avoided because this may lead to shoulder stiffness that can be difficult to correct. A better strategy is to prop the arm and hand on blankets or pillows placed to side of the patient. With a hand infection, when the diffuse swelling starts to resolve, an abscess pocket may become evident. Incision and drainage then should be performed.

WHAT TO DO NEXT

A second measure to facilitate resolution of pain and swelling is to splint the injured hand. Even if there is a soft tissue infection without bony or ligamentous injury, a splint is quite useful. Unless there is a known tendon injury or fracture, it is usually safe to splint the hand in the neutral position (finger joints at 0°, metacarpophalangeal joints at 70° and slight extension of the wrist.) The hand should stay splinted until the pain and swelling improve, and then gentle range-of-motion exercises may begin.

One final note is that all significant hand injuries and infections should prompt consultation with an experienced hand surgeon.

SUGGESTED READINGS

Coppard BM, Lohman H, eds. Introduction to Splinting: A Critical-Thinking and Problem-Solving Approach. St. Louis: Mosby, 1996.

Falkenstein N, Weiss-Lessard S, eds. Hand Rehabilitation: A Quick Reference Guide and Review. St. Louis: Mosby, 1999.

Green DP, Hotchkiss RN, Pederson WC, eds. Green's Operative Hand Surgery. 4th Ed. New York: Churchill Livingstone, 1999:1033.

ADMIT A PATIENT WITH SECOND DEGREE BURNS TO THE DORSUM OF THE FOOT

NADINE SEMER, MD

NADINE SEMER, MD

WATCH OUT FOR

The extensor tendons of the foot are integral for proper gait. They lie in a superficial position on the dorsal surface of the foot. A seemingly non-serious second degree burn (through the epidermis and into the dermis, see *Figure 21.1*) in this area can rapidly deteriorate into a third degree burn (full-thickness dermal injury) if the wound is neglected. Third degree burns of the dorsal foot can lead to exposure of these tendons with possible loss of the vascular peritenon. A skin graft can not be used to cover exposed tendons if the peritenon is not present. Definitive treatment in this situation may require an extensive reconstructive procedure; therefore, even superficial burns to the dorsal foot must be treated as a serious injury.

WHAT TO DO

All patients who present with burns to the dorsum of the foot must be carefully examined with the shoes and socks removed from both feet. The affected areas should be gently cleansed with saline and a topical antibiotic ointment should be applied. The patient should be queried for sulfa allergy before applying the commonly used silver sulfadiazine (Silvadene). The burn area should be wrapped loosely with clean gauze with removal of wrapping and close inspection of the burn once or twice daily. The patient should stay off of his or her feet as much as possible and use a walker or crutches when ambulating. To decrease edema, elevation of the injured foot is vital. No shoes or socks should be worn until the burn has completely healed.

All of these measures are designed to decrease the possibility of having a partial-thickness burn deteriorate into a full-thickness burn. As it is difficult to comply with the necessary treatment plan or to monitor compliance if the patient is discharged to home, hospital admission for these patients may is warranted.

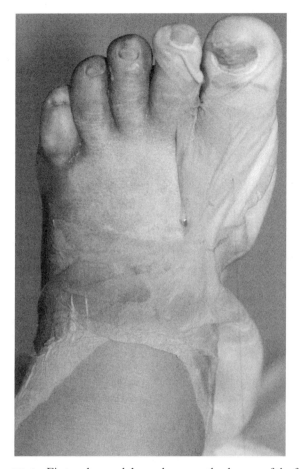

FIGURE 21.1. First and second degree burns on the dorsum of the foot.

SUGGESTED READING

Smith JW, Aston SJ, eds. Grabb and Smith's Plastic Surgery. 4th Ed. Boston: Little Brown, 1991:714.

22

STRONGLY CONSIDER ELECTIVELY INTUBATING A PATIENT WHO HAS SUFFERED INHALATION BURN INJURIES OR SIGNIFICANT BURN INJURIES TO THE FACE OR MOUTH

MICHAEL J. MORITZ, MD

Inhalation burn injury is a complex phenomenon with varying degrees and types of injuries to the respiratory tract. Importantly, inhalation injury results in a higher mortality for a given burn injury. Inhalation burn injuries occur most commonly in the upper respiratory tract due to the ability of the upper airway mucosa to function as a heat sink and the presence of laryngeal reflexes that protect the lower airway. The exception to this is a steam burn, which has a high enough specific heat to cause thermal injury to the lower airway.

SIGNS AND SYMPTOMS

The diagnosis of inhilational burn injury must be suspected based on assessment of risk factors (e.g., closed space fire or exposure to steam), physical evidence such as singed nares or carbonaceous sputum, and laboratory studies including elevated carboxyhemoglobin or cyanide level. The absence of hypoxia or abnormalities on the chest radiograph cannot be used to exclude inhalational burn injury as these are later developments in the disease process.

The physiologic abnormalities that develop as a consequence of the toxicity of inhaled smoke are varied and include increased fluid resuscitation requirements, mucosal edema with airway compromise, bronchospasm, intrapulmonary shunting, temporary loss of alveoli, increased susceptibility to bacterial infection, and respiratory failure (which can progress to multiorgan failure). The diagnosis is usually made bronchoscopically, although radioisotope pulmonary scans can be helpful. The clinical course is highly variable and findings on early bronchoscopy may not correlate with the subsequent course. The lag between injury and the development of pulmonary dysfunction can be quite long, extending up to 72 hours. There is no specific treatment for inhalation injury—only supportive care. However, because of its impact on resuscitation and on prognosis, suspicion of inhalation injury is an indication for transfer to a burn center.

Early intubation is important in management of inhalation injury. First, for the patient requiring transfer, intubation provides a safe airway. In-transit intubation without assistance, suction, etc. can be a disaster with an injured airway. Second, it provides safe, protected access for early diagnostic bronchoscopy and, if warranted, subsequent therapeutic bronchoscopy for aspiration of secretions, sloughed mucosa, and the like. Third, the onset of pulmonary dysfunction is unpredictable in time course, and early airway control and ventilatory support will allow proactive ventilation measures to be started.

SUGGESTED READINGS

American Burn Association. Inhalation injury: diagnosis. J Am Coll Surg 2003;196: 307–312.

Dries D. More than smoke with fire. Crit Care Med 2002;30:2159–2160.

Holm C, Tegeler J, Mayr M, et al. Effect of crystalloid resuscitation and inhalation injury on extravascular lung water: clinical implications. Chest 2002;121: 1956–1962.

Murakami K, Bjertnaes L, Schmalstieg FC, et al. A novel animal model of sepsis after acute lung injury in sheep Crit Care Med 2002;30:2083–2090.

MAKE SURE TETANUS PROPHYLAXIS IS UP-TO-DATE WITH STAB AND GUNSHOT WOUNDS, BURNS, FROSTBITE, CORNEAL INJURY WITH METALLIC IMPLANTS, AND BITE WOUNDS

JAMES KIRKPATRICK, MD

Tetanus is essentially a preventable disease. Adequate immunization programs in developed countries have decreased the incidence to as low as 0.16 per 1 million population per year. This is largely due to the fact that tetanus immunization is part of the recommended childhood vaccination protocol. A series of three doses of tetanus toxoid are given during infancy in concert with diphtheria toxoid and pertussis (DPT, DTaP, or DTwP, where "a" refers to acellular and "w" refers to whole-cell pertussis antigen). A fourth dose of DTP is recommended between ages 2 and 5 (required by most school districts prior to beginning primary school). A fifth dose at age 11 or 12 in combination with diphtheria toxoid (Dt or Td) virtually guarantees immunization. Boosters are given as tetanus toxoid alone (TT).

In the United States, tetanus has a mortality rate of 20%. Most cases occur following an open injury including puncture wounds, open lacerations, wounds with devitalized tissue, frostbite, body piercing, or drug abuse. Following contamination of a wound with spores of *Clostridium tetani*, wounds with an anaerobic environment allow germination of the spores and consequent production of the toxin (it is unusual for *C. tetani* to germinate in normal tissue). The toxin then travels through the peripheral motor neurons by retrograde intraneuronal transport. After migrating across the neuronal synapse, the toxin blocks release of inhibitory neurotransmitters; the resulting increase in firing of alpha motor neurons creates rigidity, such as trismus (lockjaw), risus sardonicus (sardonic smile), opisthotonus, and dysphagia.

WHAT TO DO

Understanding the indications for booster shots (TT) and tetanus immune globulin (TIG) is important. The indications for TT and TIG are based on the history of vaccination and the type of wound. In brief, for clean minor wounds, patients with a history of three or more TT immunizations need no further antitetanus treatment if it has been less than ten years since their last booster. Those with fewer than three (or unknown) vaccinations require a booster. In clean wounds, TIG is not indicated. For tetanus-prone wounds (which include all the risk factors above), patients with three or more TT vaccinations may benefit from a booster (if more than 5 years have elapsed) but don't require TIG, whereas those with fewer than three (or unknown) vaccinations require both a booster and TIG. Remember that some wounds are particularly tetanus prone and require greater attention, including burns, frostbite, corneal injury with metallic debris, bite wounds, and wounds contaminated with feces or soil (think of farming-related injuries).

SUGGESTED READINGS

National Immunization Program, Centers for Disease Control and Prevention. Recommended childhood and adolescent immunization schedule. Available at: http://www.cdc.gov/nip/. Accessed July 16, 2005.

Talan DA, Abrahamian FM, Moran GJ, et al. Tetanus immunity and physician compliance with tetanus prophylaxis practices among emergency department patients presenting with wounds. Ann Emerg Med 2004;43:305–314.

24

DO NOT DEBRIDE TISSUE ON INITIAL EVALUATION IN A PATIENT WITH A FROSTBITE INJURY UNLESS THERE ARE SIGNS OF SURROUNDING INFECTION

NADINE SEMER, MD

Prolonged exposure to cold temperature leads to frostbite. Ice crystals form within the cells and the microscopic blood vessels of the affected tissues. These crystals cause vascular occlusion that may result in tissue ischemia and loss.

WHAT NOT TO DO

When a patient presents with an acute frostbite injury, most surgeons use a multipronged treatment regimen. The one thing that should not be done is early debridement of injured tissue unless there is active infection or wet gangrene present. In frostbite injuries, tissue that initially looks nonviable may ultimately heal, so debridement is usually delayed (sometimes up to several months) until the tissue has "declared itself" and the dead areas are clearly demarcated from the surrounding viable tissue.

The following treatment regimen can be used when evaluating and treating frostbite:

WHAT TO DO

■ Rapidly rewarm the tissue by immersion of the affected part in warm water (104°F–108°F or 40°C–42°C). The use of hotter water can lead to a burn injury. It may take 20 to 30 minutes to completely rewarm the tissues.

■ Check tetanus immunization status, and give a tetanus toxoid booster if appropriate.

■ Offer pain medication—rapid rewarming hurts. Intravenous hydromorphone (Dilaudid) is an acceptable choice.

■ Do not massage the tissues.

Once the tissue has been rewarmed (or if the patient presents for treatment days or weeks after the initial frostbite injury), the following is suggested:

WHAT TO DO NEXT

■ Blisters that are blood-filled should not be disturbed. Blisters containing clear fluid should be unroofed.

- Apply aloe vera (silver sulfadiazene can be used if aloe vera is not available) to the affected areas and cover with a sterile gauze fluff dressing. The dressings should be changed at least once daily.
- To decrease swelling in the tissues, gently elevate the affected area.
- Ibuprofen should be given every 12 hours to reduce inflammation.
- Encourage gentle active and passive range-of-motion exercises to prevent joint stiffness.
- Only administer antibiotics if there are signs of infection.

SUGGESTED READINGS

Green DP, Hotchkiss RN, Pederson WC, eds. Green's Operative Hand Surgery. 4th Ed. New York: Churchill Livingstone, 1999:2061–2067.

Murphy JV, Banwell PE, Roberts, AH, et al. Frostbite: pathogenesis and treatment. J Trauma, 2000;48:171–178.

25

COVER EYELID LACERATIONS PROMPTLY WITH A DAMP DRESSING WHILE WAITING FOR THE OPHTHALMOLOGIC OR PLASTIC SURGEON TO EVALUATE THE PATIENT

MICHAEL J. MORITZ, MD

Ophthalmologic trauma is complicated to evaluate and treat due to the complexity of the anatomy of the globe, the adnexal structures, the supporting skeletal structures, and the emotional response of patients and health care professionals (*Figure 25.1*). Vision-threatening eye injury is common in patients with major facial trauma and lacerations. While definitive management belongs to the specialist, it is incumbent upon the initial treating personnel to first do no harm and then to preserve the vitality of injured structures.

In addition to evaluating the eye, the general condition of the patient must be assessed, including mental status and other associated trauma. After the patient has been stabilized, initial assessment of vision and integrity of the ocular structures is performed before attention is directed to accessory structures such as the eyelids. Intraocular injuries take precedence over injuries to associated structures. In both intra- and extraocular injuries, the exam should be performed expeditiously because of the propensity of these injuries to develop significant edema. Involvement of the globe, particularly laceration or disruption of the globe, mandates emergency ophthamologic consultation and usually surgery.

Eyelid lacerations are common, but the anatomy is somewhat intimidating to the nonophthalmologist. Briefly, the layers of the eyelid include (from superficial to deep): the orbicularis oculi muscle that closes the eye (innervated by cranial nerve VII); the orbital septum; the preaponeurotic fat pockets (and, laterally, the lacrimal gland); the levator palpebrae muscle that opens the eye (innervated by the cranial nerve III) and the levator aponeurosis that inserts into the tarsal plate; the smooth muscles that are accessory lid retractors (innervated by the sympathetic nerves); the medial and lateral canthal tendons; and the deep lamella. Also present in the lid is the lacrimal drainage system (the canalicular system) and the nasolacrimal duct in the lower lid.

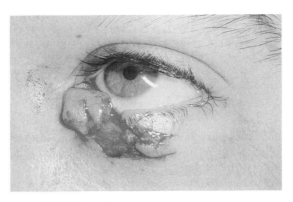

FIGURE 25.1. Eyelid laceration.

WHAT NOT TO DO	Once the eye area has been examined, gauze pads soaked in saline to maintain moistness should be applied. Although,

the postrepair application of gentle pressure dressings is widespread, the use of a pressure dressing before complete evaluation and repair is to be avoided. Applying even gentle pressure to a traumatized globe can worsen the injury.

Although ocular injuries are usually surgical emergencies, injuries to the structures accessory to the globe, such as the eyelids, are not emergencies. Instead, the emphasis is on obtaining as perfect a repair as possible the first time. As secondary repairs are proportionately more difficult, a delay of 24 to 48 hours may be acceptable in some circumstances to optimize the repair on the initial attempt.

In the current medicolegal climate, several points need to be considered when treating patients with ocular adnexal trauma:

- For animal bites, there may be local legal requirements to report the animal to the animal control authorities. Rabies prophylaxis and immunization or animal quarantine may be indicated and required.
- In cases of eye trauma in children, the examining physician must be vigilant for signs of child abuse. Ocular trauma can be the presenting sign of this malicious problem. *Suspicion* (not proof) of child abuse requires legal notification.
- Domestic violence may also present with ocular trauma and many states require notification of the authorities.
- Tetanus immunization should be brought up to date.

One final note is that, like most similar trauma situations, foreign bodies protruding from the eye should be left in place and covered with a moist gauze until definitive evaluation and treatment by a specialist can be obtained.

SUGGESTED READINGS

Long J, Tann T. Adnexal trauma. Ophthalmol Clin North Am 2002;15:179–184.
Poon A, McCluskey PJ, Hill DA. Eye injuries in patients with major trauma.
    J Trauma 1999;46:494–499.
Yanoff M, Duker JS, eds. Ophthalmology. Philadelphia: Mosby, 1999;13.1–13.8.

BE ALERT FOR DUCT AND FACIAL NERVE INJURY IN FACIAL AND CHEEK LACERATIONS

JUSTIN YOUNG, MD, DMD

Injuries to the lateral face (often seen in trauma in young men) require careful evaluation for involvement of the facial nerve, as well as damage to the parotid gland and duct. Superiorly, the parotid gland extends to the zygomatic process of the maxilla and is pyramidal in shape as it overlies the masseter muscle. Inferiorly, it extends down to and frequently wraps around the inferior border and angle of the mandible to extend into the retromandibular and parapharyngeal spaces. The duct courses from the gland anteriorly across the masseter muscle to its anterior border, where it turns abruptly to enter the oral cavity by piercing the buccinator muscle. Its entry into the oral cavity is denoted by a small papilla at or slightly higher than the occlusal level and adjacent to the first or second maxillary molar. The duct is 4 to 7 cm in length and approximately 5 mm in diameter.

To evaluate injury and plan for treatment, the parotid duct may be divided into anatomic sections. These three discrete regions are: posterior to the masseter, or intraglandular (site A); overlying the masseter (site B); and anterior to the masseter (site C). Before repair of a facial laceration, facial films should be obtained to rule out concomitant facial fractures. Definitive repair of a deep facial laceration with duct injury should be done in the operating room as follows:

WHAT TO DO

Site A. Injuries to the intraglandular parotid duct can infrequently be repaired and usually require ligation.

Site B. The duct overlying the masseter muscle is the most common area of injury and also the most amenable to primary repair. The edges of the duct should be debrided and repaired over a Silastic stent using fine (8-0 or 9-0) resorbable interrupted sutures. Care should be taken to place the knots on the outside of the duct to avoid microinflammatory processes that may occlude the lumen. The stent is left in place for 2 to 3 weeks before removal from the oral cavity.

Site C. Injuries in the distal duct may be repaired by freeing up the cut end of the lumen and doing a primary anastomosis to the intraoral papilla using an 8-0 or 9-0 resorbable suture. If the length of the duct is insufficient to do this, a new entrance in the oral cavity can be fashioned with the duct anastomosed to this.

WHAT TO DO

The facial nerve, after exiting the stylomastoid foramen, divides in a variable manner to pierce the substance of the parotid gland. The branches of the facial nerve divide the gland into arbitrary, superficial, and deep lobes. The parotid duct is often adjacent to one of the branches of the nerve and to branches of the transverse facial artery. Arterial bleeding from a lateral facial wound should be assumed to be emanating from this vessel and ligation should be undertaken cautiously to avoid injury to these adjacent critical structures. If branches of the facial nerve have been transected, they should be repaired at the initial surgery if possible with 8-0 to 10-0 nylon sutures. If repair cannot be accomplished, the ends may be tagged for subsequent repair after a period of healing.

WHAT TO DO NEXT

After the duct and nerve injury has been addressed, the facial laceration should be closed in a tension-free manner with medium-fine nonresorbable sutures (e.g., 6-0). For best cosmetic results, closure of the deeper layers with buried or inverted sutures is contraindicated. Use of drains is controversial and may result in a higher risk of wound infection, but they can be used if there is concern of a postrepair duct leak. When closing the wound, branches of the facial nerve (especially the buccal branch) should be carefully identified and protected. A disposable nerve stimulator can aid in visualizing nerve tissue. Postoperative pressure dressings should be used to reduce the risk of salivary leakage and edema. Superficial facial sutures should be removed as soon as possible to minimize scarring. Prophylactic antibiotics should be administered as intraoral bacterial counts are high. Amoxicillin with clavulinic acid (Augmentin) is the drug of choice with doxycycline as the second choice in penicillin allergy. Use of anticholinergics may be helpful both pre- and postoperatively, although side effects can be troublesome.

One final note is that in deep facial lacerations, consultation with an experienced otolaryngologist or oral surgeon should be strongly considered before repair is undertaken. These repairs are technically difficult and should only be attempted once other life-threatening injuries have been addressed.

SUGGESTED READINGS

Abrahamson M. Treatment of parotid duct injuries. Laryngoscope 1973;83(11): 1764–1768.

DeVylder J, Carlo J, Stratigos GT. Early recognition and treatment of the traumatically transected parotid duct: report of a case. J Oral Surg 1978;36: 43–44.

Fonseca RJ,, Walker RV, eds. Oral and Maxillofacial Trauma. Philadelphia: W B Saunders, 1997:430–760.

Revis DR, Seagel M. Parotid duct injuries. Available at: http://www.emedicine.com. Accessed July 18, 2005.

27

REMEMBER TO ACCOUNT FOR ALL MISSING TEETH AFTER MAXILLOFACIAL TRAUMA

JUSTIN YOUNG, MD, DMD

Loose or missing teeth are commonly encountered after maxillofacial trauma. This is frequently overlooked in the initial phases of trauma resuscitation; but on secondary survey, when maxillofacial injuries are often detected, it is important to account for missing teeth. If a tooth has been dislodged and is unaccounted for (i.e., it can not be placed in the palm and counted), it is vital to ascertain that it has not been aspirated. Aspirated teeth that are not removed promptly commonly result in pneumonia (given the accompanying aspirated mouth flora) and bronchial obstruction and erosion.

WATCH OUT FOR

Aspirated teeth usually lodge in one of the three anatomic sites (common to all aspirated foreign bodies): the larynx, trachea, or bronchus (80% to 90% of all aspirations). In adults, teeth tend to lodge in the right main bronchus (*Figure 27.1*) because of its lesser angle of convergence compared to the left main bronchus and because of the location of the carina left of the midline. Larger objects tend to lodge in the larynx or trachea. In children, the anatomic relationships are different; thus, aspirations are equally found in left and right bronchi.

WHAT TO DO

The diagnosis of aspiration is made radiographically. Do not rely on lack of symptoms of aspiration to rule this out. Obtundation seen in trauma patients often precludes the choking, wheezing, gagging, and coughing seen in the initial stages of aspiration. In addition, if there is incomplete blockage, the object may not cause symptoms. To locate the obstruction anatomically, a three-dimensional perspective must be obtained. Initially this is done with high-penetration, anterior-posterior, and lateral chest radiographs. Air trapping and hyperinflation are usually seen distal to the obstruction and the tooth always appears radiopaque. Dislodged dental restorations, with few exceptions, also appear radiopaque. Fluoroscopy is occasionally required if chest radiographs fail to localize a peripheral, obstructing foreign body.

Removal of the foreign body is accomplished with bronchoscopy under general anesthesia as soon as possible. Rarely, thoracotomy may be required if bronchoscopy is unsuccessful. After successful

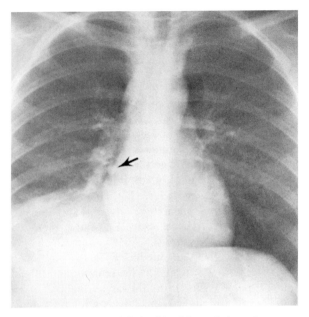

FIGURE 27.1. Aspirated tooth lodged in right main bronchus.

and timely retrieval of the tooth, antibiotics are not necessary unless signs or symptoms of a lobar pneumonia (e.g., infiltration on radiograph, fever, productive sputum, leukocytosis) are present.

SUGGESTED READING

Holinger LD. Management of sharp and penetrating foreign bodies of the upper aerodigestive tract. Ann Otol Rhinol Laryngol 1990;99:684–688.

28

COMPLETELY UNDRESS A PATIENT WHEN EXAMINING THEM FOR TRAUMATIC INJURY

MICHAEL J. MORITZ, MD

A personal vignette from the author: As the only surgeon at a small community hospital, I was called to the emergency room to examine a patient who had been shot in the head. He had a normal pulse and blood pressure, agonal respirations, and was unresponsive. After intubating him, I could not find any wounds on several successive examinations. Finally, when I opened his eyelids, I could barely detect the entry wound of a small caliber bullet through the cornea. This illustrates quite decidedly that all trauma patients, whether injured from blunt or penetrating trauma, must be *completely* examined. Missed injuries due to the patient's modesty or the lack of imagination of the hospital personnel are legendary.

A complete examination of a patient means undressing them, and undressing a patient usually mandates cutting off the clothing. Unless the cervical spine has been cleared, do not allow the patient to sit up and disrobe. Initially open the front of all garments; when the patient is rolled to examine the back, the clothing is removed. Clothing must be retained by security for numerous reasons including the presence of weapons, money, and for forensic evidence. Do not be swayed by patient modesty regardless of age or presumed station in life. The number of times a patient's gender has changed when clothing is removed is the stuff of emergency room lore.

WHAT TO DO

It must be assumed that penetrating trauma patients have an unknown number of entry/exit sites regardless of the supposed history. Complete examination includes likely locations (e.g., rolling the patient to look at his or her back) and unlikely locations. This list must not be given short shrift. Very carefully examine the head and neck. The eyes (the corneas and sclerae), the ears, the nose, and of course, the mouth often attract the attention of the gun muzzle or knife. Look at the palate and under the tongue. Hair can hide a multitude of findings. The axillary and inguinal areas require a careful look amongst the skin folds. Similarly, the perineum, labia, scrotum and buttocks can be the target in a lovers' triangle, or simply an unlikely entry or exit site, and must be carefully inspected. Blood at the anus or vaginal introitus warrant the appropriate internal examinations.

Blunt trauma patients require a similar examination, although the search is for somewhat different findings. The close examination of the face is more concerned with its stability and the possibility of fractures. The ears and nose are examined for cerebrospinal fluid otorrhea or rhinorrhea. The perineum is examined with an eye towards pelvic fractures, and the internal examinations look for blood, bony fragments, prostate displacement (in men), and signs of sexual assault. Sexual assault (that may be a result of domestic violence or child abuse) may become apparent during the examination. If sexual assault is a possibility, based either on the history or signs of perineal trauma, defined protocols for obtaining the necessary forensic evidence must be followed. The appropriate chaperoned internal examinations are vital.

One final note is that after the patient has been completely undressed and examined, the patient should be covered quickly with warm blankets to prevent hypothermia.

29

DO NOT NASOTRACHEALLY INTUBATE OR PLACE A NASOGASTRIC TUBE IN A PATIENT WHO HAS OR MAY HAVE FACIAL OR SKULL FRACTURES

MICHAEL J. MORITZ, MD

The roof of the nasal cavity is formed by the cribiform plate of the ethmoid bone, which is thin and perforated by nerves of the olfactory bulb and the anterior ethmoid nerve. In the midline, the bone is thicker (the crista galli) but just off the midline it becomes quite thin and fragile. The cribiform plate is the thinnest bone of the floor of the skull (including anterior, middle, and posterior cranial fossae). With fractures of the cribiform plate, blind placement of a nasotracheal or nasogastric tube has uncommonly resulted in the tube passing into the cranial vault. As correct technique for both tubes involves passage of the tube along the floor of the nose (perpendicular to the plane of the face) and away from the roof of the nasal cavity, it has been assumed that intracranial placement requires both cribiform fracture and improper technique, but this is impossible to prove.

WATCH OUT FOR

Facial fractures or skull base fractures with cribiform fracture may be subtle in presentation. Rhinorrhea is commonly present but may be disguised early in the course of the traumatized patient by the presence of blood and other secretions. Accordingly, with suspected facial or skull fractures, obtaining control of the airway with an orotracheal tube (in the inhospital setting) is preferred. In the prehospital setting, nasotracheal intubation is no longer in common use, and the safer (if imperfect) laryngeal mask airway (LMA) or cricothyroidotomy avoids this potentially risky technique. Once the airway is controlled, stomach decompression can follow with placement of an orogastric tube.

When inserting either of the nasally placed tubes, significant force is routinely applied to the posterior wall of the nasal cavity where the tube takes its almost 90° bend as it passes from naso- to oropharynx. Here the nasal cavity is separated from the cranial vault by the body of the sphenoid bone, which lies posterior to the ethmoid bone and is a thick, strong bony structure. However, major skull-base fractures involving the sphenoid often disrupt the sphenoid sinus and may also fracture the floor of the hypophyseal fossa and allow unintended passage of a nasogastric tube into the cranial vault (a nasotracheal tube would be too big to pass). This is the same route used surgically for the transsphenoidal hypophysectomy. Significant force is required for this type of major skull-base fracture, and the degree of trauma will be obvious to the treating team. Blind placement of any tube into the blood pooling posteriorly in the naso- or oropharynx is counterintuitive.

SUGGESTED READINGS

Goodisson DW, Shaw GM, Snape L. Intracranial intubation in patients with maxillofacial injuries associated with base of skull fractures? J Trauma 2001;50: 363–366.
Rosen CL, Wolfe RE, Chew SE, Branney SW, Roe EJ. Blind nasotracheal intubation in the presence of facial trauma. J Emerg Med 1997;15:141–145.

30

DO NOT BLAME HYPOTENSION ON AN INTRACRANIAL INJURY IN A TRAUMA SETTING UNLESS ALL OTHER CAUSES HAVE BEEN RULED OUT

X. D. DONG, MD

SIGNS AND SYMPTOMS

Hypotension in trauma may be an ominous sign of impending cardiovascular collapse. Signs of impending shock include diaphoresis, peripheral vasoconstriction, and altered mental status. Tachycardia or hypotension appear only with more severe volume loss, as vital signs are insensitive indicators of hypovolemia. Vital signs are particularly unreliable indicators of perfusion in children, the elderly, and pregnant women.

In the polytrauma patient, neurologic injuries may complicate initial attempts to diagnose and manage the cause of hypotension. Because higher central venous pressure can raise intracranial pressure that can aggravate traumatic brain injuries, some clinicians are cautious in utilizing vigorous isotonic fluid resuscitation of patients who may have brain injury. Nonhemorrhagic causes of shock (such as cardiogenic shock, neurogenic hypotension, spinal shock, and cardiac tamponade) also require aggressive fluid administration. Despite these other causes of hypotension, clinicians caring for trauma patients should assume that shock stems from hemorrhagic causes until a thorough search has excluded external and internal blood loss. Data from the Trauma Coma Data Bank indicate the consequences of secondary brain injury from hypoperfusion outweigh the risks of overresuscitation. Management of trauma patients requires establishment of adequate tissue perfusion via restoration of intravascular volume first, followed by assessment and management of potential head injuries.

Up to 75% of patients with traumatic brain injuries will have serious extracranial injuries for which fluid resuscitation is vital. Further assessment of brain injury by computed tomography (CT) scanning is essential, but it is hazardous for the patient to leave the trauma bay for a relatively inaccessible CT scanner until the patient has been stabilized via adequate volume restoration. Do not be distracted or misled by traumatic brain injury—adequately volume resuscitate the patient first.

The traumatized brain is vulnerable to secondary injury from inadequate cerebral perfusion and hypoxia. Based on data from the

Trauma Coma Data Bank, Chesnut and colleagues reported four determinants as risk factors for poor neurological outcome in traumatic brain injury: early hypotension (time of injury to resuscitation); late hypotension (intensive care unit period); intracranial diagnosis; and advanced age. Hypotension, defined as a systolic blood pressure below 90 mm Hg, remains the most readily correctable factor by the trauma surgeon. Early hypotension translates into a 15-fold excess relative risk and late hypotension translates into an 11-fold excess relative risk of unfavorable outcome for patients with traumatic brain injuries. Prevention of even one episode of hypotension is critical to improve the final outcome.

WHAT TO DO

Restoration of blood pressure requires controlling the source of hemorrhage while simultaneously restoring adequate intravascular volume, with biotonic or hypertonic saline, to an aim serum sodium of 145 to 150 meq/dL. Shock, regardless of etiology, results in the common final pathway of inadequate tissue perfusion. Effective early management of patients with closed head injury concentrates on the goal of maintaining cerebral perfusion pressure greater than 70 mm Hg rather than minimization of cerebral edema. Note that the end point of volume resuscitation is not always clear—adequate tissue perfusion may be better assessed by urine output or normalization of serum lactate and base deficit than by vital signs alone.

To summarize, a useful maxim might be that head injuries do not cause hypotension, but hypotension can significantly worsen a head injury.

Suggested Readings

Chesnut RM. Avoidance of hypotension: condition sine qua non of successful severe head-injury management. J Trauma 1997;42:S4–S9.

Chesnut RM, Gautille T, Blunt BA, et al. Neurogenic hypotension in patients with severe head injuries. J Trauma 1998;44:958–964.

Manley G, Knudson MM, Morabito D, et al. Hypotension, hypoxia, and head injury: frequency, duration and consequences. Arch Surg 2001;136:1118–1123.

Schreiber MA, Aoki N, Scott BG, Beck JR. Determinants of mortality in patients with severe blunt head injury. Arch Surg 2002;137:285–290.

York J, Arrillaga A, Graham R, Miller R. Fluid resuscitation of patients with multiple injuries and severe closed head injury: experience with an aggressive fluid resuscitation strategy. J Trauma 2000;48:376–380.

31

Obtain a Chest Radiograph, Pelvic Radiograph, and Lateral, Anterior-Posterior, and Open Mouth Cervical-Spine Films (or the Computed Tomography Equivalents) in Blunt Trauma or a Fall

Michael Moritz, MD

WHAT TO DO

Blunt trauma to the chest can result in a multitude of injuries to vital structures, including the heart with the associated great vessels, the tracheobronchial tree and the lungs, and the esophagus. The brunt of the force occurs against the supporting structures, including the chest wall, ribs, sternum, cervical and thoracic spine, and diaphragm. In addition, injuries outside the thorax are present in three-quarters of patients with significant thoracic trauma. After completion of the primary and secondary surveys, the supine anterior-posterior (AP) chest radiograph (CXR) should be one of the first diagnostic studies obtained. The supine CXR is 58% sensitive for chest pathology; the upright CXR is 79% sensitive.

The CXR is important in the diagnosis of a variety of disorders requiring early diagnosis and treatment, but the detection of thoracic aortic injury is primary. Of patients with thoracic aortic injury who survive to the emergency room, 30% will die within 6 hours and another 20% within 24 hours without prompt diagnosis and treatment. More than 90% of thoracic aortic injuries occur just distal to the origin of the left subclavian artery at the ligamentum arteriosum. The sensitivity of the CXR for detecting aortic injury by a widened mediastinum (defined as >8 cm at the aortic knob on the supine AP view) is 50% to 92%.

SIGNS AND SYMPTOMS

The other major findings on the CXR that are suggestive of aortic injury include: obliteration of the aortic knob, tracheal deviation to the right, left apical cap (i.e., hematoma outside the left pleural space), elevation and right deviation of the right mainstem bronchus, downward deviation of the left mainstem bronchus, displacement of the nasogastric tube to the right, left hemithorax, and other more obscure findings. A patient with any of the above findings on CXR *or* the appropriate mechanism of injury (significant deceleration, as with a fall from a height or head-on motor vehicle accident) should undergo further testing to look for thoracic aortic injury.

WHAT TO DO NEXT

In addition to CXR, there are three complementary imaging modalities that are effective in seeking evidence of possible thoracic aortic injury, and local availability and expertise often determine which can be obtained quickly. Helical computed tomography (CT) scan, transesophageal echocardiography (TEE), and aortography all have reasonably good sensitivity and specificity in making the diagnosis. CT provides images of the entire thorax, which can provide other diagnostic information but requires patient transport and the use of contrast. TEE does not require patient transport but is often not available rapidly. Also, TEE requires the integrity of the cervicalspine and esophagus be established and is operator dependent, but it provides excellent visualization of the descending aorta in the area usually in question. Aortography is the standard but, as with CT, requires transport and dye.

Other injuries for which the CXR is the primary screen include hemo- and pneumothorax, pneumomediastinum, pneumopericardium, diaphragmatic hernia, pulmonary contusion, sternal fracture, and rib fractures. The findings of pulmonary contusion may not appear for 4 to 6 hours after the injury. The most common finding of diaphragmatic hernia is an elevated hemidiaphragm, but 15% of such injuries will not be detected by CXR.

In addition to throacic injuries, the competent surgeon must be alert for pelvic injuries. The pelvic ring is a strong construct of the sacrum and the two innominate bones plus the supporting ligaments, and it takes a substantial force to disrupt it. Pelvic fractures (see *Figure 31.1*) that occur in only one place in the ring are relatively stable (allowing early weight bearing), have fewer associated injuries, and have lower morbidity and mortality. Fractures that occur in two places in the ring destabilize the ring and have more associated injuries, higher morbidity and mortality, and a longer rehabilitation.

The standard pelvic radiographs are the AP view and an inlet view at 40° from the vertical directed inferiorly. Films are read with two different themes. First, films are read anatomically. The anterior components (symphysis pubis and the four pubic rami) are examined, followed by the posterior components (sacrum, sacroiliac joints, ilia), and then by the acetabula. Second, films are read mechanistically. There are three mechanisms of fracture and fractures can occur in one or two places in the ring. Anterior-posterior compression forces tend

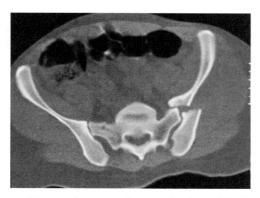

FIGURE 31.1. Computed tomography scan showing pelvic disruption.

to cause vertical pubic rami fractures or greater than 2.5 cm of diastasis of the symphysis anteriorly, sacroiliac joint disruption posteriorly, and, in about 50% of such patients, acetabular fractures. Lateral compression forces tend to cause horizontal pubic rami fractures, crush fractures of the sacrum or sacroiliac diastasis, and acetabular fractures or hip dislocations. Finally, vertical shear forces (fall from a height) tend to result in severe posterior disruption (sacroiliac joint disruption, vertical sacral fracture, or iliac wing fracture) and pubic rami fractures or symphysis pubis disruption.

Bleeding from pelvic fractures can be extensive. The optimal treatment for this is angiography and appropriate vascular embolization. However, intra-abdominal hemorrhage from other sources must be excluded before proceeding to angiography. In patients hemodynamically stable enough, CT scan of the abdomen and pelvis is the appropriate diagnostic test to distinguish intra-abdominal from pelvic hemorrhage.

Please see Chapter 32 for a discussion of cervical-spine films.

SUGGESTED READING

Ferrera PC, Colucciello SA, Gibbs MA, eds. Trauma Management: An Emergency Medicine Approach. St. Louis: Mosby, 2001:232–258, 330–343.

DO NOT CLEAR A NECK BASED ON LACK OF TENDERNESS IF PATIENT HAS DISTRACTING PAIN OR IS INTOXICATED

RICHARD PUCCI, DO

Neck trauma is common in the United States with 10,000 to 14,000 spinal cord injuries occurring annually. Knowing the appropriate workup is the key to providing efficient, cost-effective care that does not risk missing an injury that can lead to catastrophic sequelae for the patient.

In the ideal setting, a patient who does not have neck pain or tenderness can have clinical clearance of his or her neck using the Canadian C-spine Rule (CCR) as detailed below. This setting requires the following parameters: (1) the patient is awake and cooperative (Glasgow Coma Score of 15) and is not under the influence of drugs or alcohol; (2) the patient has stable vital signs; and (3) the patient is without other injuries that distract the patient and influence the accuracy of the history and physical examination.

The CCR has been shown to accurately identify patients who are at such low risk of injury that radiography of the cervical (C) spine is not necessary. The CCR has three parts:

WATCH OUT FOR

1) Is there a high risk factor that mandates radiography (i.e., age 65 years and older, dangerous mechanism of injury, or extremity paresthesias)? Dangerous mechanism of injury includes a fall of 1 meter or more or of 5 or more stairs, axial load to the head (e.g., diving accident), high speed motor vehicle accident (MVA), rollover MVA, ejection from vehicle, bicycle accidents, and off-road vehicle accidents. If any of these mechanisms are present, then C-spine radiography is indicated.

2) Is there a low risk factor present that can be evaluated with range of motion tests? These factors include straightforward rear-end MVA, sitting position in the emergency room, ambulatory at any time since the trauma, delayed (not immediate) onset of neck pain, or absence of midline C-spine tenderness. A straightforward rear-end MVA excludes being pushed into traffic, hit by bus or truck, hit by high-speed vehicle, or a rollover.

3) Can the patient actively rotate the neck 45° both left and right? If the patient can do this, the neck is cleared, and radiography is not

indicated. If the patient cannot rotate the neck in the setting of a low risk factor, then radiographic tests are required.

WHAT TO DO

If clinical assessment is unreliable and the CCR is not applicable, the cervical spine must be immobilized in a cervical collar and clearance obtained radiologically. Radiologic clearance requires that the cervical spine be seen from the skull base to the top of the T1 vertebral body. Routine C-spine films for trauma consist of three radiographs: cross-table lateral; anterior-posterior (AP); and odontoid views. A complete C-spine plain x-ray series has a high sensitivity (99%) for C-spine injury, particularly fractures and dislocations. When the top of T1 cannot be visualized (which occurs in approximately 20% of C-spine series), the next step is to obtain a swimmer's view. If the top of T1 still cannot be seen, then a computed tomography (CT) scan should be obtained.

In addition to inability to visualize the complete cervical spine, indications for obtaining a CT scan include abnormal plain films (for better visualization of a fracture or dislocation) and normal plain films when the physician's clinical suspicion of a C-spine injury is high—for example, with persistent neck pain or neurological dysfunction. Ligamentous injuries that cause spinal instability will not be visualized on plain radiographs but may be seen on flexion and extension films, magnetic resonance imaging (MRI), or CT scan.

WHAT TO DO NEXT

For patients with neurologic deficits or deteriorating neurological conditions, an MRI of the spinal cord should be arranged after the patient's hemodynamic stability has been assured. Similarly, suspicion of ligamentous or intervertebral disk injuries should prompt consideration of an MRI. In children in particular, the spinal cord may be injured without evidence of plain x-ray or CT abnormalities. Termed SCIWORA (spinal cord injury without radiologic abnormality), such injuries are best visualized by MRI.

There are several types of injuries that have an association with C-spine fractures and that warrant extra consideration. Facial fractures are associated with a variety of significant injuries, particularly intracranial bleeds and contusions (in almost 50% of instances), but 5% to 10% of patients with facial fractures will also have cervical spine injuries. Noncervical spinal fractures also have a 5% to 10% association with C-spine fractures. Motor vehicle accident victims with head injury or a Glasgow Coma Score less than 8 upon initial evaluation have at least a 10% incidence of significant C–spine injury. In addition, many experienced trauma surgeons will evaluate the carotid arteries for injury in a significant C–spine injury.

SUGGESTED READINGS

Alvi A, Doherty T, Lewen G. Facial fractures and concomitant injuries in trauma patients. Laryngoscope 2003;113:102–106.

Frohna WJ. Emergency department evaluation and treatment of neck and cervical spine injuries. Emer Med Clin North Am 1999;17:739–791.

Marx JA, Hockberger RS, Walls RM, eds. Rosen's Emergency Medicine: Concepts and Clinical Practice. 5th Ed. Philadelphia: Mosby, 2002:330–364.

Mower WR, Hoffman JR, Pollack CV, et al. Use of plain radiography to screen for cervical spine injuries. Ann Emerg Med 2001;38:1–7.

Stiell IG, Wells GA, Vandemheen KL, et al. The Canadian c–spine rule for radiography in alert and stable trauma patients. JAMA 2001;286:1841–1848.

OBTAIN LUMBAR SPINE RADIOGRAPHS IN PATIENTS WITH A POSITIVE SEAT BELT SIGN

LISA MARCUCCI, MD

The use of two-point restraint rear seat belts, particularly in children, can cause a constellation of injuries in motor vehicle accidents via a mechanism of sudden mechanical compression of intra-abdominal contents and forced flexion/distraction of the lumbar spine. Any patient with the above history (especially if there is abdominal pain) or with transverse ecchymosis (abdominal wall bruising; the seat belt sign [transverse abdominal or diagonal chest well ecchymosis caused by contact with seat belt when patient is thrown forward]) must have a careful and thorough evaluation for the following injuries:

Intestinal perforation—small bowel perforation is most common, but partial transection of the stomach and colon have been reported and carry a higher mortality than small bowel injury. The likely mechanism is sudden and severe mechanical compression of the hollow viscus against the rigid spine causing rupture. Cases of delayed rupture occurring more than six days after injury have been reported. Signs and symptoms include abdominal pain and tenderness, peritonitis (although children often do not develop frank peritonitis until later in the course), hypotension, free air, air in the retroperitoneum, fluid in the pelvis or abdomen, leukocytosis, and positive diagnostic peritoneal lavage. Imaging studies used for evaluation include abdominal radiograph, FAST (Focused Abdominal Sonogram for Trauma) exam, and computed tomography (CT).

Mesenteric vascular injury—sudden compression of intra-abdominal contents can result in shearing of the mesenteric vessels, causing mesenteric hematomas and frank intraperitoneal bleeding. This injury can occur in the absence of other associated injuries and may manifest itself several days after injury. Signs and symptoms include abdominal distention, falling hemoglobin, and profound hypotension. Imaging studies used for evaluation include FAST exam, CT, and angiography.

Abdominal wall injury—transverse tears and traumatic hernia in the rectus muscle are often overlooked on initial exam and even may be missed on laparotomy. Adding to the diagnostic difficulty is that bruising associated with these injuries is sometimes attributed to external contact with the seat belt. Signs and symptoms include pain, swelling and ecchymosis, drop in hemoglobin, and a palpable defect. Studies used in evaluation include CT, ultrasound and magnetic resonance imaging. A high index of suspicion is needed to correctly diagnose this injury.

SIGNS AND SYMPTOMS

Lumbar spine injury—the most common injury is a lumbar fracture dislocation at L1 or L2 (Chance fracture); somewhat less common is a posterior ligamentous disruption. Presence of a Chance fracture is highly associated with intestinal perforation, with one study reporting 6 of 7 patients with a Chance fracture also having intestinal perforation. Signs and symptoms are back pain, palpable spine deformity, kyphosis, and neurological deficits in the lower extremities. Regardless of the presence of these findings, all patients should receive a lumbar spine series including anterior-posterior and lateral views to look for this injury if the patient has mechanism or abdominal wall ecchymosis. It is important to note lumbar spine injury can be missed on the abdominal computed tomography that is often obtained to evaluate for intra-abdominal injury. If a ligamentous injury is suspected, magnetic resonance imaging should be obtained.

SUGGESTED READINGS

Anderson PA, Rivara FP, Maier RV, et al. The epidemiology of seatbelt-associated injuries. J Trauma 1991;31:60–67.

Eltahir EM, Hamilton D. Seat belt injuries and sigmoid colon trauma. J Accident Emerg Med 1997;14:338–339.

Thompson NS, Date R, Charlwood AP, et al. Seat-belt syndrome revisited. Int J Clin Prac 2001;55:573–575.

Winton DL, Girotti MJ, Manley PN, et al. Delayed intestinal perforation after nonpenetrating abdominal trauma. 1985;28:437–439.

34

DO A RECTAL EXAM BEFORE INSERTING A URINARY CATHETER IN MALE TRAUMA

MICHAEL MORITZ, MD

Posterior urethral injury is an injury with potentially devastating long-term consequences. Because failure to recognize this injury or inappropriate initial treatment can worsen the injury, recognition and initial treatment is crucial.

The male urethra has two portions separated by the urogenital diaphragm: the anterior urethra (bulbous and pendulous segments) and the posterior urethra (membranous and prostatic segments), in retrograde order. The posterior urethra is fixed to the pelvis in two locations: the membranous urethra pierces the urogenital diaphragm, which is attached to the ischiopubic rami, and the prostatic urethra is fixed with the prostate to the pubic symphysis. Injuries to the anterior urethra are usually due to external blunt or saddle-type injuries, whereas the posterior urethra is susceptible to injuries in major pelvic fractures.

WATCH OUT FOR

The incidence of posterior urethral injury has been reported at 4% to 6% for males with less severe pelvic fractures and 10% to 25% in major pelvic fractures that disrupt the pelvic ring. The fractures with the greatest likelihood of causing these injuries are Malgaigne fractures—namely concomitant anterior (pubic rami or symphysis pubis) and posterior (sacrum, sacroiliac joints, or ilium) pelvic fractures. Straddle fractures involving all four of the pubic rami are also likely to injure the urethra. In general, posterior urethral injuries can be thought of as due to shear or distraction separating the prostate and prostatic urethra from the more distal segments. Such injuries will almost always be accompanied by a substantial pelvic hematoma. There are three general types of posterior urethral injuries: stretch (about 25% of injuries), partial disruption (about 25%), or complete disruption (about 50%).

SIGNS AND SYMPTOMS

The diagnosis is not difficult—the typical presentation is a male with pelvic fractures who cannot void or who has blood at the meatus. Patients with partial tears of the posterior urethra may still be able to void but will have gross hematuria. On

examination, the flanks, scrotum, and perineum are inspected for ecchymoses, swelling, and frank blood as evidence of a pelvic fracture.
Other suggestive findings include leg length discrepancy and asymmetry. The pelvis is manually examined for pain and instability. The
meatus is examined for the presence of blood, and a digital rectal examination is performed.

In the trauma setting, the rectal examination assesses anal
sphincter tone, the position and feel of the prostate, and the
presence of blood or bone fragments in the rectum. The usefulness
of the rectal examination in making these diagnoses has been
questioned. The most common finding on rectal examination in
the presence of posterior urethral injury is a boggy mass from
the pelvic hematoma, which may hide the prostate. In addition,
if the prostate is displaced superiorly (high-riding prostate),
unusually mobile, not palpable, or if there is blood at the meatus, then a urethral injury must be assumed, and a retrograde urethrogram must be performed.

WHAT TO DO

Retrograde urethrogram is the cornerstone of diagnosis. To perform this study, the penis is stretched
perpendicular to the femur. About 20 mL of diluted
water-soluble contrast is instilled into the urethra via the meatus, and
a radiograph is obtained as the instillation is finished. Fluoroscopy is
preferred but often unavailable. Diagnosis by inability to pass a
urinary catheter risks worsening the injury. Both the force of passing
the catheter and inflating the balloon may convert a partial urethral
tear into a complete disruption. If urethral disruption is diagnosed,
urologic consultation is essential. In the rare critical situation, suprapubic cystostomy can be used, but the pelvic hematoma that is present makes placement more difficult. The three major long-term
complications of urethral disruption are stricture, incontinence, and
impotence. Early treatment can decrease the incidence of long-term
complications. Broadly speaking, there are two modes of treatment:
(1) realignment of the urethra using endoscopic techniques to place a
urinary catheter to stent the injury, and (2) open surgical reapproximation of the disrupted urethra.

One final note is that in women, the urethra is shorter and more
mobile, hence less susceptible to shear and distraction injury. Laceration from bony fragments is the most common mechanism of injury.
Labial edema may be due to urinary extravasation. Urethrography is
not as accurate; urethroscopy may be preferred. Emergent consultation with a urologist should be obtained if this injury is suspected.

SUGGESTED READINGS

Brandes S, Borrelli J Jr. Pelvic fracture and associated urologic injuries. World J Surg 2001;25:1578–1587.

Dreitlein DA, Suner S, Basler, J. Genitourinary trauma. Emerg Med Clin North Am 2001;19:569–590.

Koraitim MM. Pelvic fracture urethral injuries: the unresolved controversy. J Urol 1999;161:1433–1441.

Koraitim MM, Marzouk ME, Atta MA, et al. Risk factors and mechanism of urethral injury in pelvic fractures. Br J Urol 1996;77:876–880.

Do not rule out intra-abdominal trauma by clinical exam if the patient is intoxicated or has altered sensorium

Michael Silber, DO

A common diagnostic problem encountered in the trauma bay is a patient with significant soft tissue and/or bony injury, significant mechanism for intra-abdominal trauma, and an altered sensorium from intoxication or neurological injury. In this setting, rapid and accurate diagnosis of intra-abdominal trauma is needed to insure proper management and to minimize morbidity and mortality. The physical exam is the initial and least expensive diagnostic tool. Although unable to diagnose the exact location of intra-abdominal injuries, the physical exam (including vital signs) alone is sufficient to rule in significant intra-abdominal trauma in altered sensorium, but is never sufficient to rule out significant trauma.

The best tests to use to rule out intra-abdominal trauma in the patient with altered sensorium are the focused abdominal sonogram for trauma (FAST), high speed/high resolution computed tomography (CT) scan, and laparoscopy. The exact protocols for use of these diagnostic tools are a popular topic in the trauma community and indications for their use are constantly being revised. However, in virtually all major trauma centers, at least one of these modalities is used in lieu of the physical exam in patients with altered sensorium.

SUGGESTED READING

American College of Surgeons Committee on Trauma. Advanced Trauma Life Support. 7th Ed. Chicago: American College of Surgeons, 2002.

Cushing BM, Clark DE, Cobean R, Schenarts PJ, Rutstein LA. Blunt and penetrating trauma—has anything changed? Surg Clin North Am 1997;77: 1321–1332.

Mattox KL, Feliciano DV, Moore EE, eds. Trauma. 4th ed. New York: McGraw-Hill, 2000:583–602.

BE AWARE THAT IT IS POSSIBLE TO BLEED TO DEATH FROM A SCALP WOUND

X.D. DONG, MD

Any seasoned trauma physician can relate a story of a patient who presented only with a scalp laceration and signs of shock. Scalp lacerations may be underestimated and go unattended because they are hidden behind rolls of bandages or do not appear to be sufficiently long or deep to have caused significant blood loss in the field. With the good intention of seeking and controlling more urgent, life-threatening causes of shock such as pneumo- and/or hemothorax, pericardial tamponade or abdominal hemorrhage, scalp lacerations may be ignored during the diagnostic search for other sources of shock. It is imperative that the trauma survey include an examination of the scalp and, when appropriate, apply temporary, expedient control of the bleeding from scalp lacerations.

WHAT TO DO

Temporary control of a bleeding scalp laceration is usually obtained by compression of the scalp against the underlying skull. Direct finger pressure over bleeding areas will effectively stop bleeding until more definitive means can be accomplished. Lack of enough hands to provide sustained, continuous compression and fracture of the underlying skull are common reasons to use a temporary hemostatic device such as Rainey clips. These are spring-loaded clips designed to provide hemostasis from scalp flaps raised during craniotomies and are effective at hemostasis. Akin to binder clips found in office supply stores, Rainey clips temporarily compress the skin edges and can provide hemostasis until definitive repair can be accomplished. If Rainey clips are not available, approximating the laceration edges with a running, locked, baseball stitch using a silk suture usually will slow the bleeding significantly. If time is critical, the scalp edges can be reapproximated and stapled. Some scalp lacerations may be difficult to control in the emergency room and require a trip to the operating room. If scalp lacerations are particularly deep or particularly long (*Figure 36.1*) or if the patient is hemodynamically compromised, treatment should be managed in the operating room. Lacerations associated with an underlying fracture or that define an open skull fracture must also be managed in the operating room.

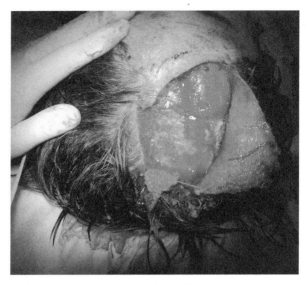

FIGURE 36.1. Complex scalp laceration with laterally based flap.

One final note is that the serum hemoglobin level is not a reliable indicator of blood loss in the field and can not be used to classify a scalp laceration as non-life threatening.

SUGGESTED READINGS

Coleman RJ, Rocko JM. Rapid control of hemorrhage of the scalp in the patient with trauma. Surg Gynecol Obstet 1988;166:165–166.

Lemos MJ, Clark DE. Scalp lacerations resulting in hemorrhagic shock: case reports and recommended management. J Emerg Med 1988;6:377–379.

Turnage B, Maull KI. Scalp lacerations: an obvious 'occult' cause of shock. South Med J 2000;93:265–266.

37

CLOSE THE GALEA AS A SEPARATE LAYER WHEN REPAIRING A FULL-THICKNESS LACERATION TO THE SCALP

NADINE SEMER, MD

The scalp has five tissue layers. SCALP is the acronym for these layers. From superficial to deep they are: skin, subcutaneous tissue, galea aponeurosis, loose connective tissue, and periosteum (also called pericranium) overlying the skull. A laceration that goes through all layers down to the bone is considered a full-thickness scalp laceration. The layers that require repair are the galea and the skin. The galea closure is important for two reasons. First, it often controls the brisk bleeding associated with scalp wounds (it is possible to bleed to death from a scalp wound). Second, by closing the galea you close off access to the loose connective tissue underneath. If the galea is not closed and the wound becomes infected, the infection has access to the entire undersurface of the scalp through the loose subgaleal areolar space. The spread of infection in this plane can lead to a significant soft tissue loss and may require a major reconstructive procedure to treat.

WHAT TO DO

In adults, the galea should be closed as a distinct layer with a long-lasting absorbable suture material, such as Vicryl, Monocryl, or PDS. The skin can be closed with staples or any type of absorbable or nonabsorbable suture material (usually size 3-0 or 4-0). If nonabsorbable sutures are used, a color distinct from the patient's hair color should be used (e.g., Prolene in a brunette, nylon in a blonde). The tails of the sutures should be left sufficiently long to facilitate easy suture removal.

Unlike the eyebrow area, it is acceptable to shave the hair surrounding a scalp laceration to help fully delineate the wound. Slathering the hair with sterile, water-soluble lubricant (e.g., Surgilube) that can be mixed with a small amount of Betadine if desired can help expose the wound and decrease the amount of hair that needs shaving. The area underneath clotted blood and matted hair should be checked carefully to insure no occult lacerations are missed. Postrepair, the patient should wash their hair with gentle shampoo (e.g., baby shampoo) daily, starting 1 to 2 days later.

One final note is that in children it is acceptable to close a full-thickness scalp wound with a single full-thickness suture bite that includes the galeal layer.

SUGGESTED READING

Smith JW, Aston, SJ, eds. Grabb and Smith's Plastic Surgery. 4th Ed. Boston: Little Brown & Company, 1991:397–400.

DO NOT REMOVE A KNIFE THAT IS PENETRATING TISSUE UNLESS YOU HAVE DIRECT INTRAOPERATIVE VISION AND CONTROL

JAMES HERRINGTON, MD

One of the tenets of trauma surgery is that penetrating foreign objects are not removed until the patient is in the operating room and the surgeon can visualize the penetrating tract. When a patient comes to the trauma bay with a knife protruding from any part of the body, leave the knife in place, follow Advanced Trauma Life Support (ATLS) protocol, and proceed to the operating room. Before removal, large bore IV access must be obtained. Depending on the vascular structures at risk, an appropriate amount of blood should be typed and crossed.

Potential vascular injuries may be anticipated by the location of the knife and wound and by physical examination of distal pulses (although presence of pulses does not rule out vascular injury). Once in the operating room, direct visualization of the knife tract and tip is important as the knife may be acting to tamponade bleeding from a vessel that has been perforated, lacerated, or transected. Removing the knife prior to being in a position to control hemorrhage from the injured vessel and repair the vascular injury can lead to substantial bleeding. Unanticipated bleeding will sully the field, increase the difficulty of exposure, and increase the risk of injuring neighboring structures, thus compromising the repair and increasing the risk of intraoperative and postoperative problems.

Proximal and distal control of potentially injured vessels should be obtained before removing the knife. After this is done, lacerated vessels should be repaired. This is usually possible because there is little tissue damage except where the knife has penetrated and vessel length loss is usually slight. If direct repair is not possible, a repair with autologous vein is preferred. Synthetic material should only be used in unusual circumstances because the wound is, by definition, contaminated.

SUGGESTED READING

Mattox KL, Feliciano DV, Moore EE, eds. Trauma. 4th Ed. New York: McGraw-Hill, 2000:146.

EXPLORE AN EXPANDING RETROPERITONEAL HEMATOMA CAUSED BY TRAUMA

X.D. DONG, MD

Retroperitoneal vascular injury remains a frequent cause of death following abdominal trauma, and this injury often presents as an expanding hematoma. Retroperitoneal hematomas are classified by their location as central or zone 1 (both supra and inframesocolic), lateral or zone 2 (pericolic gutters), and pelvic or zone 3 (beginning at the sacral promontory and encompassing the pelvis). Within the trauma literature, there is some controversy regarding the management of these hematomas.

Zone 1—Zone 1 supramesocolic hematomas extend superiorly from the transverse mesocolon and contain vital vascular structures. The arteries in zone 1 include the suprarenal abdominal aorta, celiac axis, and proximal superior mesenteric artery. The veins in zone 1 include the infrahepatic, inferior vena cava, portal vein, and the proximal superior mesenteric vein. Traditionally, zone 1 injuries discovered during a laparotomy require exploration regardless of whether they are expanding because of the potential for serious underlying injury. Arterial injuries in this zone are best approached through a left-sided medial visceral rotation; that is, by opening the avascular line of Toldt of the left colon and lateral splenic attachments, and then rotating the left colon, spleen, tail and body of the pancreas, and stomach medially. Central inframesocolic hematomas (below the transverse mesocolon) are usually approached by opening the small bowel mesentery on the left and reflecting the small bowel superiorly and to the right. This exposes the infrarenal aorta from the left renal vein to the bifurcation, the inferior vena cava, and the proximal renal arteries. For injuries to the inferior vena cava, superior mesenteric vein, or portal vein, right visceral rotation (mobilizing the cecum, right colon, and duodenum) provides exposure.

Zone 2—Nonexpanding lateral or perirenal hematomas caused by blunt trauma should not be explored if there is renal function because the retroperitoneum has a general tamponade effect. Expanding hematomas or hematomas caused by penetrating trauma, however, should be explored. Of interest to the surgeon is that expanding zone 2 injuries due to renal artery injuries require exploration to salvage the kidney; conversely, if the injury is due to renal parenchymal injury, exploration increases the risk of loss of the kidney.

Zone 3—Nonexpanding hematomas caused by blunt trauma can be closely observed. There is controversy over the management of expanding blunt and penetrating zone 3 hematomas. Expanding zone 3 hematomas are particularly difficult to manage if entered because of the difficulty in identifying and managing arterial and venous bleeding that is secondary to pelvic fractures. Zone 3 hematomas secondary to penetrating trauma are best approached by displacing the small bowel superiorly, the cecum and ascending colon or the sigmoid medially, opening the retroperitoneum, and obtaining proximal control of the common iliac arteries at the level of the aortic bifurcation. Distal control of the external iliac artery is obtained at the level of the inguinal ligament. If control remains elusive after entering a hematoma, packing may provide enough tamponade to temporize the situation until the patient can be further resuscitated and additional diagnostic and management options begun. Although the standard surgical dictum is that expanding hematomas should be explored, if the surgeon opts not to do so, then a clear plan to diagnose and manage the bleeding site must be in place. Typically, interventional radiologic techniques such as angiography and embolization of arterial bleeding sites are used to manage expanding zone 3 injuries from pelvic fractures.

Expanding hematomas can be difficult to manage without proper vascular control. Where feasible, the vascular pedicle should be isolated prior to opening the hematoma to control bleeding, as for perinephric hematomas. In other instances, such as pelvic hematomas, obtaining vascular control is impossible due to the widespread venous bleeding, which underscores the gravity of the decision to open the hematoma. In the presence of diffuse bleeding, a "damage control" procedure can be performed to temporize the situation until the patient can be further resuscitated and additional diagnostic and management options undertaken. Regardless of the location, control of the vascular inflow and outflow will minimize the bleeding seen upon opening an expanding hematoma.

One final note is that the first and most important goal in trauma is control of bleeding. If the patient arrives profoundly hypotensive or experiences cardiopulmonary arrest in the operating room, an emergent left anterolateral thoracotomy with aortic cross-clamping may be warranted. When the patient arrives with some degree of hemodynamic stability but decompensates during laparotomy, the abdominal aorta can be controlled at the aortic hiatus digitally, by the use of an aortic compressor, or by placement of a vascular clamp. Obtaining exposure to cross-clamp in this area is difficult because the supraceliac aorta is posterior to the esophagus and surrounded by the crura of the diaphragm.

SUGGESTED READINGS

Costa M, Robbs JV. Management of retroperitoneal haematoma following penetrating trauma. Br J Surg 1985;72:662–664.

Falcone RA, Luchette FA, Choe A., et al. Zone I retroperitoneal hematoma identified by computed tomography scan as an indicator of significant abdominal injury. Surgery 1999;126:608–615.

Feliciano DV. Management of traumatic retroperitoneal hematoma. Ann Surg 1990;211:109–123.

Goins WA, Rodriguez A, Lewis J, et al. Retroperitoneal hematoma after blunt trauma. Surg Gynecol Obstet 1992;174:281–290.

Henao F, Aldrete JS. Retroperitoneal hematomas of traumatic origin. Surg Gynecol Obstet 1985;161:106–116.

DO NOT GIVE DISULFIRAM (ANTABUSE) OR METRONIDAZOLE (FLAGYL) TO A PATIENT WHO HAS ALCOHOL IN HIS OR HER SYSTEM

MICHAEL J. MORITZ, MD

Disulfiram (Antabuse) is a once-a-day oral medication used as part of the treatment of chronic alcoholism. Upon taking disulfiram, very unpleasant effects occur to an individual when even small amounts of alcohol (ethanol) are consumed. These effects include facial flushing, headache, nausea, vomiting, chest pain, weakness, blurred vision, mental confusion, sweating, choking, breathing difficulty, and anxiety. These effects begin about 10 minutes after ethanol ingestion and last for an hour or more. The flushing, nausea, and vomiting are the most consistent effects and the source of its deterrence. Disulfiram is not a cure for alcoholism but can discourage drinking.

WHAT NOT TO DO

Accordingly, one should not give disulfiram to a patient who is intoxicated, nor should it be administered without the patient's full onset and knowledge. The patient should not take disulfiram for at least 12 hours after drinking any alcohol to insure that the alcohol has been eliminated from the system. Because of the long half-life of disulfiram, a reaction may occur for up to 2 weeks after disulfiram has been stopped if alcohol is ingested.

It is commonly stated in compendia of drugs and drug reactions that the combination of metronidazole and ethanol will produce a disulfiram-like reaction. For example, the description of metronidazole drug interactions with ethanol in ePocrates (updated July 31, 2003) specifies "avoid combination during and for 72 hours after metronidazole treatment: combination may result in alcohol-disulfiram-like reaction (aldehyde dehydrogenase inhibited)." A variety of case reports have noted disulfiram-like reactions, including fatal reactions, in patients taking metronidazole with ethanol ingestion. Two reports from the 1960s claimed that metronidazole could substitute for disulfiram in discouraging ethanol ingestion due to this effect.

More recently, a review and a small scientific study have reopened the question of this metronidazole-ethanol effect. A double-blind, placebo-controlled study of 12 healthy male volunteers showed no subjective or objective effects nor an increase in blood acetaldehyde concentrations in individuals ingesting metronidazole plus ethanol. Both reports suggested that metronidazole lacks predictable, reproducible disulfiram-like effects but that disulfiram-like reactions may occur in some subgroups of susceptible individuals. As ethanol is not a vital nutrient, it seems appropriate to warn patients prescribed metronidazole to avoid ethanol during their antibiotic course. Similarly, it seems prudent to prescribe other anaerobic coverage for patients seen in the emergency room with recent ethanol ingestion.

SUGGESTED READINGS

Cina SJ, Russell RA, Conradi SE. Sudden death due to metronidazole/ethanol interaction. Am J Forensic Med Pathol 1996;17:343–346.

Visapaa JP, Tillonen JS, Kaihovaara PS, Salaspuro MP. Lack of disulfiram-like reaction with metronidazole and ethanol. Ann Pharmacother 2002;36:971–974.

Williams CS, Woodcock KR. Do ethanol and metronidazole interact to produce a disulfiram-like reaction? Ann Pharmacother 2000;34:255–7.

HAVE AN EXTREMELY LOW THRESHOLD FOR MECHANICAL CONTROL OF THE AIRWAY IN LUDWIG'S ANGINA

LISA MARCUCCI, MD

Ludwig's angina is decreasing in frequency and, in large medical centers, is more commonly the purview of otolaryngologists or oral surgeons. However, in many communities, general surgeons receive the initial consult from emergency room and primary care physicians; therefore an understanding of the underlying pathology and correct treatment paradigm is key to preventing progression to a life-threatening condition.

SIGNS AND SYMPTOMS

Ludwig's angina is a bacterial infection of the fascial planes of the oral cavity. Causative bacteria are most commonly *Staphylococcus* and *Streptococcus*, but *Haemophilus* and anaerobic bacteria have also been reported. Ludwig's angina presents with neck swelling and erythema, submandibular swelling, fever, boardlike rigidity in the floor of the mouth, elevation and posterior displacement of the tongue, and difficulty swallowing. Less common signs and symptoms are earache, confusion and mental status changes, drooling, and fatigue. Other serious complications of Ludwig's angina include mediastinitis, thoracic empyema, pericarditis, pericardial tamponade, and sepsis. Its etiology is most closely associated with a dental infection such as an abscess in the tooth roots or severe gingivitis, but it can be seen in immunocompromised states such as HIV/AIDS.

WHAT TO DO

The urgent concern on initial evaluation of a patient with Ludwig's angina is the potential for rapid and complete airway obstruction. Many experienced clinicians will intubate the patient if there is any degree of tongue displacement or if the patient has even the slightest symptoms of airway obstruction such as stridor or any subjective complaints of respiratory distress. This allows the intubation to be done on a more planned basis (e.g., with availability of a fiberoptic scope) by an experienced airway professional (preferably an anesthesiologist) and eliminates the possibility of a later, truly emergent tracheostomy (previously a mainstay of treatment). If intubation is attempted, a surgeon capable of performing cricothyroidotomy should be on hand to intervene if necessary. If the patient is not intubated, close observation in a monitored setting is mandatory.

WHAT TO DO NEXT

In addition to mechanical control of the airway extremely early in the disease course, broad spectrum antibiotics (e.g., high-dose penicillin G or clindamycin with metronidazole) should be instituted after mouth and blood cultures have been obtained, with coverage narrowed as results become available. Patients should be continued on antibiotics as long as cultures are positive or empirically for 4 to 6 weeks if cultures are negative. Computed tomography (CT) of the head and neck with thin cuts should be obtained, but the patient should never be sent to the CT suite unescorted by a physician with an uncontrolled airway. Surgical incision and drainage (in the operating room if necessary) should be done for any accessible fluid collections. Definitive dental treatment must be effected before antibiotics can be stopped if this was the underlying etiology.

To reiterate, it cannot be stated too strongly that the key to preventing catastrophic progression of this disease is extremely early mechanical control of the airway. At the risk of being flippant—if the surgeon even considers whether the patient needs airway control, the patient probably should receive it.

SUGGESTED READINGS

Allen D, Loughnan TE, Ord RA. A re-evaluation of the role of tracheostomy in Ludwig's angina. J Oral Maxillofac Surg 1985; 43:436–439.

Doldo G, Alabanese I, Macheda S, Caminiti, G. Ludwig angina: a disease of the past century. Minerva Anestesiol 2001;67:811–814.

Honrado CP, Lam SM, Karen M. Bilateral submandibular gland infection presenting as Ludwig's angina: first report of a case. Ear Nose Throat J 2001; 80:217–218, 222–223.

Srirompotong S, Art-Smart T. Ludwig's angina: a clinical review. Eur Arch Otorhinolaryngol 2003:260:401–403.

TREAT MYOGLOBINURIA WITH COPIOUS INTRAVENOUS SALINE FLUID

RACHAEL A. CALLCUT, MD

Myoglobinuria occurs when skeletal muscle fibers are destroyed (rhabdomyolysis) and serum myoglobin levels exceed 1500 ng/mL (normal serum values of myoglobin are < 85 ng/mL). Normally, small elevations of circulating myoglobin are bound to haptoglobin and safely cleared by the reticuloendothelial system. Excessive myoglobinemia results in an overload on the reticuloendothelial system and myoglobin being filtered by the kidney. There are many etiologies of myoglobinuria, including:

Burns—electrical and thermal
Crush injury
Ischemia—arterial compromise or venous thrombosis
Infectious—*Salmonella, Staphylococcus, Clostridia, Streptococcus,*
Snake bites—cobra, coral, viper, rattlesnake
Exercise-induced—military training, extreme athletic training
Drugs—amiodarone, Amicar, statins, isoniazid, propofol, lithium

The most common etiology of rhabdomyolysis in the United States is unconsciousness associated with drug or alcohol overdosage that results in prolonged muscle compression and ischemia (a more subtle crush-type injury). By the same mechanism, improper positioning in the operating room or excessively long surgery (often in combination with obesity) can result in rhabdomyolysis.

SIGNS AND SYMPTOMS

The most common clinical sign of myoglobinuria is dark or tea-colored urine, although the degree of darkness does not accurately reflect the extent of underlying muscle destruction. Urinalysis showing a positive dipstick for blood but with the absence of red blood cells on the microscopic analysis is a rapid and inexpensive way to make the diagnosis, although hemoglobinuria will produce the same results. The most useful lab measurement in diagnosing and managing rhabdomyolysis is serum creatine kinase (CK), which has a rapid, relatively inexpensive, and universally available assay (unlike myoglobin). Rhabdomyolysis that is sufficient to cause myoglobinuria will be accompanied by the cellular release of CK.

Serum CK levels roughly correlate with the extent of muscle injury and severity of rhabdomyolysis. An increased CK can also be used to distinguish myoglobinuria from hemoglobinuria. Other signs and symptoms seen with rhabdomyolysis/myoglobinuria include fever, leukocytosis, proximal muscle weakness, and muscle pain.

Acute renal failure occurs in 4% to 33% of cases of rhabdomyolysis, with a mortality of 3% to 50%. The pathology of acute renal failure in myoglobinuria is multifactorial and may include initial hypovolemia (and vasoconstriction), precipitation of myoglobin in the renal tubules with direct tubular toxicity, and mechanical obstruction of tubules from myoglobin casts. Precipitation of myoglobin protein in the renal tubules can be lessened by crystalloid administration in copious quantities to force a solute diuresis. Some experienced clinicians strive for 1.5–2 mL/kg/hr of urine. In vitro, acidic pH promotes myoglobin precipitation so alkalinization of the urine (to a pH >6.5) with sodium bicarbonate added to the intravenous solution is sometimes used. Conclusive evidence in vivo showing the benefit of alkalinizing the urine in preventing renal failure is spotty. Use of mannitol to increase the diuresis is sometimes advocated (without supporting data). Mannitol has several distinct disadvantages, including hyperosmolarity, electrolyte derangements, and volume overload (if diuresis is unsuccessful), and must be used carefully.

With crush injuries, the muscle ischemia and reperfusion mechanism causes sequestration of fluid and calcium in the injured site. Along with initial resuscitation with large volumes of intravenous crystalloid, monitoring of calcium with replacement is usually required. Other intracellular constituents that are released during rhabdomyolysis and that require monitoring and intervention include hyperkalemia (which can reach cardiotoxic levels early postcrush injury), hyperphosphatemia (which worsens hypocalcemia), and tissue thromboplastin (causing disseminated intravascular coagulation, or DIC).

The prompt diagnosis and institution of therapy with intravenous saline (perhaps augmented with sodium bicarbonate) to force a diuresis can prevent acute renal failure despite early oliguria from myoglobinuria.

SUGGESTED READINGS

http://www.neuro.wustl.edu/neuromuscular/msys/myoglob.html. September 2004.

Arnold WC. Myoglobinuria. Available at: http://www.emedicine.com/PED/topic1535.htm. Accessed July 19, 2005.

Malinoski DJ, Slater MS, Mullins RJ. Crush injury and rhabdomyolysis. Crit Care Clin 2004;20:171–192.

43

CONSIDER AND EXCLUDE THE HIGHLY LETHAL DIAGNOSIS OF MIDGUT VOLVULUS IN AN INFANT WITH BILIOUS VOMITING

MICHAEL J. MORITZ, MD

Intestinal malrotation, more accurately incomplete rotation of the midgut, leaves the jejunum, ileum, and right colon attached posteriorly only by the narrow vascular pedicle of the superior mesenteric vessels (without the broad attachments to the retroperitoneal aspect of the small bowel mesentery and right colon). Rotation or torsion of the midgut about the vascular pedicle defines volvulus of the midgut and causes two events: (1) obstruction of the distal duodenum with bilious vomiting; and (2) occlusion of the superior mesenteric vein and artery, causing intestinal ischemia and progressing to intestinal necrosis.

SIGNS AND SYMPTOMS

More than 50% of cases of midgut volvulus present within the first month of life as an acute event. The child most commonly presents with bilious vomiting and abdominal pain (crying). The abdominal examination may be normal, or abdominal distention without tenderness may be present. As the intestine becomes progressively more ischemic, increased abdominal distention, abdominal pain, and peritonitis develop. With bowel infarction fever, peritoneal signs and shock will occur. Without prompt surgery, the entire midgut necroses. Early surgery to untwist the volvulus and restore circulation to the midgut is potentially lifesaving. Mortality with the acute presentation is reported as 2.5% to 25% and is a function of the amount of intestinal necrosis, younger age at presentation, and the presence of associated anomalies.

WHAT TO DO

The diagnosis can be made preoperatively by radiograph. Abdominal films may reveal a "double bubble" sign from the air bubbles in the distended stomach and duodenum (as with duodenal atresia) but may also be normal. The gold standard for the diagnosis of anomalies of intestinal rotation is an upper gastrointestinal (UGI) contrast study and must be obtained on an emergency basis. Computed tomograph (CT) scan and ultrasound can also be helpful in making the diagnosis.

Slightly fewer than 50% of cases present after the first month of life. With increasing age, the acute presentation becomes less common. Instead, one of two chronic presentations can be seen. The child may have recurrent abdominal pain and bilious vomiting. The pathophysiology is the same—midgut volvulus with proximal small bowel obstruction—but instead of the bowel continuing to rotate with worsening vascular and intestinal obstructions, the process spontaneously reverts. These children have episodes of severe abdominal pain, often accompanied by bilious vomiting, yet between episodes appear fine, with appropriate appetite and bowel movements. The second chronic presentation consists of feeding intolerance and failure to thrive related to partial chronic bowel obstruction. UGI in both instances makes the diagnosis.

Other diagnoses in the differential of bilious vomiting include pyloric stenosis (nonbilious vomiting, longer duration of symptoms, dehydration, a hungry child), incarcerated hernia (abdominal distention, diagnosed with a careful exam), duodenal or ileal atresia (usually diagnosed in the newborn nursery, infant not usually ill-appearing), necrotizing enterocolitis (rare in term neonates), meconium ileus (abdominal distention, "ground glass" sign on abdominal film), intestinal hematoma (from child abuse), and (more rarely) congenital adrenal hyperplasia or Hirschsprung's disease. The diagnosis of acute gastroenteritis should be made with great caution in infants and only after excluding diagnoses requiring surgery.

Because of the mortality and devastating consequences of midgut necrosis associated with the acute presentation of midgut volvulus and the ability of emergency surgery to rescue the ischemic intestine, the following principle must be followed: any infant presenting with bilious vomiting *must* have midgut volvulus considered first in the differential diagnosis and the possibility of intestinal malrotation excluded by an emergency UGI contrast study.

SUGGESTED READINGS

Kimura K, Loening-Baucke V. Bilious vomiting in the newborn: rapid diagnosis of intestinal obstruction. Am Fam Physician 2000;61:2791–2798.

Millar AJ, Rode H, Cywes S. Malrotation and volvulus in infancy and childhood. Semin Pediatr Surg 2003;12:229–236.

Okada PF, Hicks B. Neonatal surgical emergencies. Clinical Pediatric Emergency Medicine 2002;3:3–13.

44

Consider the Possibility of an Underlying Malignancy When Treating a Woman with Breast Inflammation or Abscess

Michael J. Moritz, MD

Inflammatory breast conditions should prompt consideration of an underlying malignant condition. Breast cancer may occur separately from a benign inflammatory breast disorder or may be a part of the inflammatory process. Regardless, with any breast disorder or complaint and given the incidence and mortality of breast cancer, it is incumbent upon the physician to look for malignancy.

Benign Inflammatory Breast Disorders

Mastitis and Lactation Abscess. Mastitis is uncommonly seen in pregnant women and is marked by tenderness, erythema, fever, and malaise and rarely progresses to abscess formation. Because this disorder is uncommon in pregnancy, further workup to exclude inflammatory carcinoma is essential. In contrast, in nursing mothers, mastitis and abscess are quite common with up to one-quarter of nursing mothers developing at least one episode of mastitis. Mastitis in the lactating woman is an ascending infection from the nipple spreading proximally via the lactiferous ducts in a susceptible breast, presumably from milk stasis. The appropriate treatment is increased fluids, local measures (use of a breast pump on the affected side, warm compresses), analgesics, and when needed, oral antibiotics to cover *Staphylococcus,* the most common pathogen (less often coagulase negative staphylococci or streptococci). Some cases continue to progress with worsening pain and tenderness and the appearance of a tender mass, representing an acute breast abscess or a lactation abscess. The diagnosis of an abscess can be confirmed by ultrasound, although ultrasound may not be able to ascertain the fluid-filled center. Abscesses are treated with operative incision and drainage under general anesthesia—the abscess will often be significantly deeper than initially assumed. Alternative treatments of daily aspiration and catheter drainage have been successful in very small series. Breast-feeding or a breast pump should be continued.

The presence of a purulent collection does not completely exclude the possibility of malignancy, as necrotic tumors rarely can become infected. Mastitis and breast abscess rarely occur in women who are not nursing, thus the presence of this condition in a non-lactating woman increases the likelihood of an underlying malignancy.

Recurring Subareolar Abscess, Mammary Duct Ectasia, Plasma Cell Mastitis. This multiple-named condition is sometimes considered a spectrum of one disease, but this is probably an oversimplification because of the bimodal age distribution. The pathophysiologic features common to the disorder are: the development in one or more of the subareolar ducts of squamous metaplasia (normal lactiferous ducts have columnar epithelium) with chronic or recurring duct obstruction within the nipple-areolar complex; upstream duct inflammation; rupture; or destruction. Nipple discharge is common in this disorder. Cigarette smoking is associated with an increased risk of this condition.

In younger women (20–40 years of age) there is no relation to pregnancy or lactation. It typically begins as a small inflammatory area in the subareolar area which progresses to form a small subareolar abscess. The abscess drains, spontaneously or with appropriate surgery, but recurs as a draining sinus or recurrent abscess. This disorder may be associated with congenital nipple inversion. Treatment is incision and drainage, but if it continues to recur, then cure requires resection of the chronically inflamed space plus removal of the affected duct into the nipple which can become a substantial procedure.

In older women (usually over age 65), the subareolar inflammation can produce a mass-effect difficult to distinguish from breast cancer. Similarly, the inflammatory process can cause nipple retraction, another sign of malignancy. A yellowish or brownish nipple discharge can appear. Patients have clinical signs of inflammation, including pain, tenderness, an indurated mass, and intermittent erythema, but abscess development is more indolent and less common than in younger women. As with any inflammatory disease of the breast, excluding the possibility of breast cancer is essential.

Mondor's Disease. This is an uncommon disorder of superficial thrombophlebitis involving the veins of the breast, usually the thoracoepigastric or lateral thoracic vein. The tender, erythematous, indurated mass will have a cord-like configuration. Appropriate treatment is nonsteroidal anti-inflammatories, warm compresses, and support. The question of whether an underlying breast malignancy is present, causing the initiation of thrombophlebitis, should be addressed as soon as the acute inflammatory process has improved.

Miscellaneous Benign Inflammatory Conditions. In the United States, tuberculosis, sarcoidosis, and syphillis rarely involve the breast. Each has a spectrum of chronic inflammatory changes and each can produce a mass that may mimic breast cancer.

MALIGNANT INFLAMMATORY BREAST DISORDERS

Some inflammatory breast carcinomas can be difficult to distinguish from breast infections and benign breast inflammation, particularly when the inflammatory component is more prominent than the underlying malignant mass. Inflammatory carcinoma of the breast causes a significant area of breast skin to develop erythema, warmth, edema, and peau d'orange changes of edematous skin with retraction. Peau d'orange—meaning orange peel—refers to the dimpled appearance of an orange peel which is caused by lymphedema of breast skin and tethering of the skin to the connective tissue of the breast. The etiology of the inflammatory changes is not infection; rather diffuse involvement of intradermal lymphatics with tumor results in the inflammatory changes and lymphedema of the breast skin. A skin biopsy is essential (a simple punch biopsy may be adequate) in excluding inflammatory carcinoma if the physician's level of concern warrants it or if treatment for a benign condition does not promptly and substantially improve the skin changes.

The coexistence of a benign inflammatory breast condition and a separate breast cancer has been mentioned above, and the possibility must be sought. Similarly, infection involving a necrotic portion of a breast cancer can mimic breast abscess, and for this reason, incision and drainage of breast abscesses should be accompanied by a biopsy of the cavity wall to search for malignancy. This pathophysiology has been reported to occur in squamous cell carcinoma of the breast, a rare tumor. The contents of a necrotic tumor may be viscid, yellowish fluid indistinguishable from an abscess. Inflammatory carcinoma in a lactating patient is rare—biopsy of the underlying mass or of the overlying skin is important to exclude this diagnosis.

Because inflammatory breast carcinoma often occurs in younger patients, is rapidly progressive, has an overall poorer prognosis than most breast cancers, and because the diagnosis can be substantially delayed by several courses of antibiotics for presumed benign breast disease, it is vital to exclude the diagnosis of malignancy when treating a woman for presumed benign breast disease.

To briefly summarize, breast abscess is usually not associated with cancer but inflammatory breast cancer is easily confused with breast cellulitis. If breast redness does not completely resolve with two weeks of antibiotics, then biopsy is warranted.

SUGGESTED READINGS

Clark RM, Reid J. Carcinoma of the breast in pregnancy and lactation. Int Radiat Oncol Biol Phys 1978;4:693–698.

Marchant DJ. Inflammation of the breast. Obstet and Gynecol Clin 2002;29:89–102.

Strombeck JO, Rosato FE, eds. Surgery of the breast: diagnosis and treatment of breast diseases. New York: Thieme, 1986:48–52.

WEAR GLOVES WHEN EXAMINING A PATIENT IN THE EMERGENCY ROOM

MICHAEL J. MORITZ, MD

Some surgeons feel gloves should be worn anytime a patient is touched in any clinical setting. This seems extreme to other surgeons (e.g., the use of gloves when shaking hands?) who feel the risk of contracting a disease from a patient is quite low and have adopted lesser degrees of glove protection when interacting with patients. A commonsense compromise to these philosophies would suggest the use of gloves should be adopted by all surgeons when examining anyone whose skin is not intact. This includes virtually every inpatient whose skin has been punctured with recent surgery, an intravenous (IV) catheter, or recent percutaneous procedure. Most body fluids (blood, cerebrospinal fluid, and synovial, pleural, peritoneal, and pleural fluids) are potentially infectious, as are other fluids when contaminated with blood (e.g., urine, sputum, etc.). While many bloodborne infections are potentially transmissible, the major infections of concern are hepatitis C virus (HCV), hepatitis B virus (HBV), and human immunodeficiency virus (HIV) in descending order of prevalence in the United States. HBV and HIV transmission via blood contamination of the nonintact skin of an uninfected individual has been well documented (e.g., a blood splash onto a cut on a surgeon's hand).

WATCH OUT FOR

In particular, care must be taken to wear gloves when examining patients in the emergency room (ER). Patient populations in the ER have a higher prevalence of HCV, HBV, and HIV than the general population, as high as 18%, 5%, and 6% respectively (as reported for eastern U.S. inner city ERs). Although no patient can be assumed to be infection-free, there are higher risk groups. The prevalence of HCV is higher in IV drug abusers, dialysis patients, transplant recipients (kidney and liver in particular), patients with cirrhosis, and patients from certain countries (Saudi Arabia, Egypt, Zaire, and others). The prevalence of HBV is higher in homosexual men, heterosexuals with multiple partners, IV drug abusers, and patients from particular areas of the world (highest risk includes China, sub-Saharan Africa, and southeast Asia; intermediate risk includes Mediterranean countries,

TABLE 45.1	OCCUPATIONAL TRANSMISSION OF THE THREE MAJOR BLOODBORNE PATHOGENS.			
VIRUS*	PREVALENCE IN U.S. POPULATION	CHRONICALLY INFECTED IN THE U.S.	EASY-TO-REMEMBER NEEDLE STICK INJURY RISK	TRANS-MISSION VIA OTHER ROUTES
HBV	0.5%	1–1.25 million	30%	Yes; various
HCV	1.5%	3.9 million	3%	Conjunctiva
HIV	0.2%	~500,000	0.3%	Nonintact skin; mucous membrane

*HBV, hepatitis B virus; HCV, hepatitis C virus; HIV, human immunodeficiency virus.

Japan, India, and Singapore). The prevalence of HIV is higher in IV drug abusers, homosexual men, hemophiliacs, and individuals from sub-Saharan Africa.

The risk of acquiring a bloodborne infection via an occupational exposure (*Table 45.1*) has many variables. The inoculum varies with the instrument involved (hollow needles deliver a larger volume than solid needles, such as suture needles) and the depth of penetration. The route of contamination is also important. Although skin contamination has been estimated to be one-thirtieth the risk of a needlestick, this risk is multiplied by the need for the surgeon's skin to touch the skin of virtually every patient he or she is asked to see. The concentration of pathogen is also important and varies with the involved fluid (typically pathogen concentrations are higher in blood than other body fluids) and with prior treatment of the infected patient (e.g., lamivudine, interferon, and antiretroviral therapy). The response to any occupational exposure must include assessment of both the source and the injured party for the relevant potential pathogens. As there are a variety of studies available (antibody tests, antigen tests, polymerase chain reaction tests), appropriate expert consultation is essential.

One final note is that the integrity of disposable gloves is imperfect and leakage/breakage will increase with duration of wear and performance. In high risk situations or patients, consideration should be taken to double glove to further reduce (but not eliminate) the risk of exposure.

SUGGESTED READINGS

Fahey BJ, Koziol DE, Banks SM, Henderson, DK. Frequency of nonparenteral occupational exposures to blood and body fluids before and after universal precautions training. Am J Med 1991;90:145–153.

Ippolito G, Puro V, De Carli G. The risk of occupational human immunodeficiency virus infection in health care workers. Italian multicenter study. Arch Intern Med 1993;153:1451–1458.

Kelen GD, Green GB, Purcell RH, et al. Hepatitis B and hepatitis C in emergency department patients. N Engl J Med 1992;21:1399–1404.

PROMPTLY DISPOSE OF YOUR OWN SHARPS AFTER DOING A BEDSIDE OR EMERGENCY ROOM PROCEDURE

MICHAEL MORITZ, MD

Bedside procedures generate an assortment of sharps. Common procedures where needles and scalpels are used include phlebotomy, insertion of arterial and venous catheters and lines, lumbar puncture, thoracentesis, paracentesis, and repair of lacerations. More critical situations, such as trauma resuscitations and codes will generate a larger number of sharps with more individuals at the bedside (in a usually more chaotic situation). In all of the situations above, the person performing the procedure is best able to adequately track the use of sharps and where they have been stashed and placed. It is vital to the safety of the health care team that the sharps are properly disposed of and not left amongst the debris surrounding the patient, in the bed, on the stretcher, with the bed linen, or in the trash. Failure to do so will inevitably result in accidental needlesticks to other health care workers and custodial personnel.

Accidental needlesticks are demoralizing and dangerous for the injured. At the very least, time is lost for the trip to the emergency room, employee health, or other designated area for testing and risk counseling. More seriously for the surgeon is that in specific circumstances, it may be recommended that the injured take post exposure prophylaxis to prevent viral transmission. Then follows a period of anxiety until the relative risk to the injured has been ascertained, with perhaps a longer time before the possibility of transmission is excluded. This possibility of viral transmission may have deleterious effects on the personal and family life of the injured.

Therefore, regardless of the situation and the seniority of the person performing the procedure, the individual who actually uses the sharps must take responsibility for properly disposing of them. This is true in all nonoperating room situations including the bedside, trauma bay, and following a code. Delegating this task to someone junior (a medical student, intern, nurse, or other personnel) is inappropriate, unprofessional, and unfair.

One final note is that sharps should never be dropped onto the floor after they have been used. Although this removes them from the procedure field, very few people approaching the procedure area will be looking at the floor. Sharps on the floor can be inadvertently kicked into another provider's ankle or foot (especially if the provider is wearing the popular type of clogs with ventilation ports) and are a hazard for custodial personnel. After using them, sharps (including broken glass from a lidocaine vial with a pop top) should be grouped together so they can be easily retrieved and disposed of.

Suggested Readings

APIC. Position paper: prevention of device-mediated bloodborne infections to health care workers. Association for Professionals in Infection Control and Epidemiology, Inc. Am J Infect Control 1998;26:578–580.

Moloughney BW. Transmission and postexposure management of bloodborne virus infections in the health care setting: where are we now? CMAJ 2001;165:445–451.

EMERGENCY DEPARTMENT

OPERATING ROOM

MEDICATIONS

LINES, DRAINS, AND TUBES

WOUNDS

BLEEDING

GASTROINTESTINAL TRACT

WARDS

INTENSIVE CARE UNIT

LABORATORY

Institute Deep Vein Thrombosis Prophylaxis Before the Induction of Anesthesia

Diane Ferrara, RN, PA
Michael J. Moritz, MD

Given the high prevalence of postoperative deep vein thrombosis (DVT), prophylaxis should be considered for all surgical patients. DVT is often clinically silent and the first manifestation can be a life-threatening PE. DVT can lead to long-term morbidity from the post-phlebitic syndrome and puts patients at higher risk of recurrent venous thromboembolism. The use of effective, safe methods of prophylaxis to prevent DVT is both excellent medical care and cost-effective care. Despite this, a recent study of U.S. patients showed that only one third of general surgery patients actually receive prophylaxis despite the presence of multiple risk factors for venous thromboembolism. *Asymptomatic* DVT occurs in about 25% of patients after a general surgical procedure of moderate severity without perioperative antithrombotic prophylaxis.

Clinically significant DVT affects more than 2.5 million people in this country annually, and PE leads to, or contributes to, between 50,000 and 200,000 deaths annually. The risk of *symptomatic* DVT or PE is related to the type of surgery being performed (orthopedic surgery of the hip and knee and intercranial surgery have the highest incidences), the degree of postoperative immobilization, the use of prophylaxis, and the presence of other risk factors. Risk factors that increase the perioperative risk include: trauma (especially fractures of the pelvis, hip, and leg), increasing age, malignancy, paralysis from stroke or spinal cord injury, previous DVT, pregnancy, oral contraceptive or estrogen use, obesity, nephrotic syndrome, varicose veins, cardiac dysfunction, indwelling central venous catheters, and inflammatory bowel disease. Congenital and acquired thrombophilic disorders (hypercoagulable states) also increase the thromboembolic risk and include: activated protein C resistance (factor V Leiden); prothrombin variant 20210A; antiphospholipid antibodies (lupus anticoagulant and anticardiolipin antibody); deficiency or dysfunction of antithrombin III, protein C, or protein S; decreased levels of plasminogen and plasminogen activators; heparin-induced thrombocytopenia; hyperhomocystinemia; and myeloproliferative disorders such as polycythemia vera and essential thrombocytosis.

Intermittent compression devices, which are pneumatically driven sleeves or stockings that intermittently compress the calves. They have been found to reduce the likelihood of clots developing in the lower extremities following orthopedic, general, prostatic, and neurosurgery at rates similar to pharmacological prophylaxis. These devices increase venous return and may increase fibrinolytic activity. They are also useful for patients who have a higher risk of bleeding and in whom pharmacological prophylaxis is undesirable. *To be effective, intermittent compression devices must be in place and operating prior to induction of anesthesia.*

The chief effect of pharmacologic DVT prophylaxis is that it alters a portion of the coagulation cascade without causing hemorrhage. Low-dose heparin prophylaxis uses 5,000 units of heparin given subcutaneously at least one hour prior to induction of anesthesia, and then 2 to 3 times daily. Such low doses of heparin work by enhancing the inhibition of activated factor X (Xa) by antithrombin III. Measured PT and PTT values usually remain normal. Low-dose heparin has been shown to reduce PT by 50% pulmonary emboli and DVT by 60% in general surgery, but it is not as effective for prophylaxis following orthopedic surgery or trauma. Low-dose heparin does not increase the rate of major hemorrhage but does increase minor complications, such as wound hematomas, in up to 2% of patients. Heparin-induced thrombocytopenia occurs in 0.4% of patients.

Compared to standard heparin, low–molecular-weight heparin (LMWH) has an increased affinity for factor Xa and lower inhibition of thrombin. The result is increased bioavailability, longer half-life, increased antithrombotic activity, and a potentially lower rate of bleeding complications compared to unfractionated heparin. The incidence of heparin-induced thrombocytopenia is lower in patients treated with LMWH. Low-dose unfractionated heparin and LMWH appear equally efficacious in preventing DVT in general surgery patients, but unfractionated heparin is the more economical choice. LMWH should be considered for higher risk patients. There are three LMWHs that are approved by the U.S. Food and Drug Administration, and a fourth, the pentasaccharide fondaparinux, is called a very-LMWH. Aspirin and warfarin (Coumadin) are both less effective and have higher risk of hemorrhage as compared to heparins for prophylaxis.

For DVT prophylaxis, it is generally recommended that all surgery patients receive either low-dose heparin or intermittent compression devices, while higher risk patients should receive LMWH with or without compression devices. As prophylaxis is initiated at least 1 hour preoperatively, caution in using the heparins is needed when spinal or epidural catheters are to be placed perioperatively, and consultation with the anesthesiologist is *mandatory* before administering preoperative or postoperative heparin or LMWH.

To reemphasize—critical to the efficacy of all of the above methods of prophylaxis is initiation before the induction of general anesthesia. Thinking about and instituting DVT prophylaxis afterwards is not nearly as effective.

SUGGESTED READINGS

Clagett GP. Prevention of postoperative venous thromboembolism: an update. Am J Surg 1994;168:515–522.

Geerts WH, Heit JA, Clagett GP, et al. Prevention of venous thromboembolism. Chest 2001;119:132S–175S.

Kaboli P, Henderson MC, White RH. DVT prophylaxis and anticoagulation in the surgical patient. Med Clin North Am 2003;87:77–110.

Ryan MG, Westrich GH, Potter HG, et al. Effect of mechanical compression on the prevalence of proximal deep vein thrombosis as assessed by magnetic resonance venography. J Bone Joint Surg Am 2002;84:1998–2004.

Thromboembolic Risk Factors (THRIFT) Consensus Group. Risk of and prophylaxis for venous thromboembolism in hospital patients. BMJ 1992;305:567–574.

DO NOT USE CHLORHEXIDINE TO PREP THE FACE (TO AVOID CORNEAL AND MIDDLE EAR INJURY)

SUE-MI CHA, MD

Hibiclens is an antiseptic agent used commonly as a preoperative preparation in surgery. This solution, available in the United States since 1976, consists of the antiseptic 4% chlorhexidine solution and detergent. Chlorhexidine is useful in that it has microbiocidal activity against both Gram-positive and Gram-negative bacteria and yeast. In dilute amounts, corneal contact with chlorhexidine appears to be safe. In fact, in concentrations of 0.005%, chlorhexidine has been used as a preservative for soft and gas-permeable contact lens solutions. In addition, a nontoxic concentration of chlorhexidine (0.02%) has been used in combination with propamidine to treat *Acanthamoeba* keratitis.

However, corneal injuries after contact with 4% chlorhexidine cause injuries ranging from transient epithelial defects to chronic ulcers. The toxic effects to the cornea appear to be amplified by the presence of detergent, which increases the permeability of the epithelium. The histopathologic findings have demonstrated corneal epithelial cell death and desquamation. In addition, chlorhexidine is cytotoxic to fibroblasts and results in delay of wound healing. Other symptoms associated with Hibiclens toxicity are conjunctival hyperemia, chemosis, hypotony, anterior chamber flare, corneal pannus, and corneal edema. Several patients with more concentrated chlorhexidine exposure have required corneal transplantation. Equally as serious as the corneal damage that can be cause by contact, chlorhexidine instilled in the middle ear may cause progressive sensorineural deafness—it must not be used in or near the ear if there is a possibility that the tympanic membrane is not intact.

In light of the associated risks of Hibiclens when used on the face, iodine-based solutions should be considered as an alternative. If the use of Hibiclens cannot be avoided, extreme care must be used in its application. If Hibiclens comes in contact with the ocular surface or the ear canal, one should copiously irrigate and consult an ophthalmologist or otolaryngologist.

SUGGESTED READINGS

Hamed LM, Ellis FD, Boudreault G, Wilson FM 2nd, Helveston EM. Hibiclens keratitis. Am J Ophthalmol 1987;104:50–56.

Murthy S, Hawksworth NR, Cree I. Progressive ulcerative keratitis related to the use of topical chlorhexidine gluconate (0.02%). Cornea 2002;21:237–239.

Phinney RB, Mondino BJ, Hofbauer, JD et al. Corneal edema related to accidental Hibiclens exposure. Am J Ophthalmol 1988;106:210–215.

Tabor E, Bostwick DC, Evans CC. Corneal damage due to eye contact with chlorhexidine gluconate. JAMA 1989;261:557–558.

Varley GA, Meisler DM, Benes SC, et al. Hibiclens keratopathy: a clinicopathological case report. Cornea 1990;9:341–346.

49

PREP AND DRAPE BOTH LEGS TO THE MIDFOOT WHEN DOING VASCULAR PROCEDURE ON AN EXTREMITY

MICHAEL MORITZ, MD

The need for autologous vein for the repair or reconstruction of vessels should be considered not only in vascular surgery, but in traumatic, oncologic, and other surgeries as well. The conduit of choice for most arterial reconstructions is saphenous vein (coronary bypasses excluded). A classic example requiring vein conduit repair is a combined arterial and venous injury in the lower extremity, where autologous contralateral vein is the best conduit for the arterial repair because the deep venous system has been jeopardized as well. Contralateral saphenous vein is the optimal conduit. Failure to plan ahead for the above situations can compromise the outcome. Sterilely prepping and draping the other leg for vein harvest is most easily done as part of prepping and draping the principal operative field. Performing this in midcase is awkward, jeopardizes the sterility of the operative field, and compromises the sterility of the vein harvest field.

WHAT TO DO
When a significant vein repair is required, consideration must be given to being able to procure adequate length and quality of saphenous vein. The groin to midfoot should be prepped, ensuring that the saphenofemoral junction proximally is included in the operative field and the full length of the vein will be available. Both legs should be included in the operative field as the ipsilateral saphenous vein may not be adequate when performing femoral to distal arterial (infrageniculate popliteal artery or below) bypasses.

If the legs have not been prepped and draped preoperatively and the surgeon opts not to prep and drape for a vein harvest in midcase, then an alternative, less preferable conduit must be chosen. For an arterial reconstruction, upper extremity vein (usually cephalic vein) can be used, but it is thinner walled, harder to work with, and more prone to aneurysm formation than saphenous vein. Alternatively, prosthetic graft material can be used but it has a higher infectious risk than autologous vessel and a patency that may approach that of autologous vessel, but never exceeds it, depending on the involved vessel. Nonprosthetic, nonautologous conduits exist but must be ordered beforehand (e.g., glutaraldehyde-treated umbilical vein, cryopreserved human saphenous and superficial femoral vein) and also have issues of cost, patency, immunogenicity, infection, and late aneurysm formation.

One final note is that consideration should be given to prepping the legs in some oncologic procedures. For example, preoperative planning for an extremity sarcoma resection should include the potential need for arterial and venous replacement conduits. The same preoperative consideration would be appropriate for intra-abdominal and pelvic tumors close to vital vessels, such as the superior mesenteric artery, where reconstruction with a suboptimal conduit may not be appropriate.

50

USE METICULOUS ATTENTION TO CORRECT POSITIONING WHEN PLACING A PATIENT IN THE LATERAL DECUBITUS POSITION

ASHRAF OSMAN, MD

The scenario is all too familiar. A patient has surgery, anesthesia is uneventful, and the procedure goes well. Later that evening the patient complains of numbness, weakness, or pain, and a neurological deficit is found.

Peripheral neuropathy occurring during anesthesia is a significant source of morbidity and an extremely common source of professional liability in anesthesia practice. The anesthesiology literature and texts are replete with how to properly position patients in the operating room. In contrast, surgical literature and texts cover the topic tersely and without detail. However, the surgeon must be cognizant of correct positioning technique to minimize the risk of position-related neuropathy (and its attendant medical liability). Listed below are details on how to properly position a patient in one high-risk position, the lateral decubitus position, and how to minimize or prevent neurologic injury.

The lateral decubitus position is an inherently unstable position and places the relaxed, anesthetized patient at significant risk for pressure and stretch damage to the brachial plexus and more distal nerves.

The following are general rules and recommendations (nerve[s] at risk are given in parentheses):

- Avoid shoulder girdle compression (brachial plexus).
- Avoid abduction of the extremity greater than 90° (brachial plexus).
- Avoid lateral rotation of the arm (brachial plexus).
- Avoid full elbow extension (ulnar nerve).
- Avoid lateral flexion of the patient's head (brachial plexus).

Specific details are as follows:

_____ The patient is turned to the lateral position with padding or use of a "beanbag" in the upper torso region to help provide secureness.

_____ If the shoulder and arm are allowed to remain directly under the rib cage after turning the patient into the lateral position, the brachial plexus can be compressed leading to injury.

_____ A padded roll (axillary or chest roll) under the dependent chest decreases the pressure on the neurovascular supply of the dependent arm. However, be careful because the roll itself becomes a compressive force if it becomes displaced superiorly into the axilla.

_____ Pressure points are padded to prevent pressure necrosis.

_____ The extremities are positioned and secured in a manner that avoids excessive stretch. Complete extension of joints should be avoided; aim for neutral position.

_____ Supination of the forearm (palm anterior) produces the least amount of pressure at the ulnar groove, pronation produces the most, and neutral forearm position results in intermediate pressure.

_____ Intermittent inflation of the sequential compression devices (SCDs) on the lower extremities not only decreases the risk of deep vein thrombosis, but also shifts the pressure points and may aid in the prevention of lower extremity pressure- or stretch-induced nerve injuries.

_____ The dependent leg is flexed at the hip and the knee, a pillow is placed between the legs, and the upper leg is relatively straight or slightly flexed (avoid knee hyperextension).

_____ Padding and pillows are required at all bony prominences and also between the extremities to prevent nerve compression or the development of painful cutaneous pressure points and to facilitate venous drainage.

_____ The neck is positioned in the neutral position.

_____ After positioning is relatively complete, additional table adjustments are made (e.g., lateral extension of the spine by "breaking" the table, raising the kidney rest, etc.). The entire sequence of positioning and checking the padding is then repeated, step-by-step and site-by-site.

_____ Only then is the patient secured in position. If a beanbag is used, suction is applied at this time. The hips are secured to the table by wide adhesive tape.

_____ Two arm boards may be used to stabilize the upper extremity in the lateral position. The elbows should not be in full extension.

_____ Make sure the patient is stable (does not move) if the table is rotated side to side or tilted into Trendelenburg or reverse Trendelenburg position.

SUGGESTED READINGS

Caplan RA. Will we ever understand perioperative neuropathy? A fresh approach offers hope and insight. Anesthesiology. 1999;91:335–336.

Coppieters MW, De Velde MV, Stappaerts KH. Positioning in anesthesiology: toward a better understanding of stretch-induced perioperative neuropathies. Anesthesiology 2002;97:75–81.

Dawson DM, Krarup C. Perioperative nerve lesions. Arch Neurol 1989;46: 1355–1360.

Prielipp RC, Morell RC, Walker FO, et al. Ulnar nerve pressure: influence of arm position and relationship to somatosensory evoked potentials. Anesthesiology 1999;91:345–354.

51

DO NOT INJECT ANY SUBSTANCE INTO A PATIENT IN THE OPERATING ROOM WITHOUT FIRST INFORMING THE ANESTHESIOLOGIST

CATHERINE MARCUCCI, MD

A variety of substances may be injected into patients in the operating room by the surgical team. A partial list includes local anesthetics (with or without epinephrine), papaverine, isosulfan blue (lymphocyte mapping dye), heparin (porcine and bovine), cholangiogram dye, and intravenous (IV) contrast dye. Before any injection the anesthesiologist should be informed what substance is being injected, why it is being injected, and the site where it is being injected. Unfortunately, it is not rare for a patient to experience an allergic reaction or hemodynamic instability as a result of an injection. Having to brief the anesthesia provider as to the possible etiology of acute adverse event squanders precious seconds that could be used in beginning treatment.

WATCH OUT FOR

There are several possible ways problematic events can occur post injection. First, omission or error in checking for a known allergy or initial presentation of an unknown allergy can contribute to an adverse event after injection. Second, the infiltrative doses of some drugs given by surgeons are additive with the IV dose that may have been given by the anesthesia provider and the maximum dose may be exceeded. Third, local anesthetics may be prepackaged with epinephrine which may exacerbate a preexisting tachycardia or hypertension. This last mechanism is significant because control of intraoperative heart rate is increasingly recognized as important in decreasing perioperative morbidity and mortality. Alerting the anesthesia provider before injecting a drug mixed with epinephrine allows the provider to review the vital signs before giving permission for the injection.

The site of an injection is also significant, particularly for the local anesthetics. If an injection is in a visceral structure in the chest, abdomen, pelvic or perineal areas an adult (or anywhere in a child), significant bradycardia or tachycardia can occur. In addition, unintentional intra-arterial injections can result in seizures, especially if they occur in the neck. Unintentional injections into the chest cavity can result in pneumothorax (e.g., local injection or localization needle placement for breast biopsy). Finally, patients can have significant responses to injections that broach major nerve structures, such as spinal nerve roots and the brachial plexus.

SUGGESTED READINGS

Cimmino VM, Brown AC, Szocik JF, et al. Allergic reactions to isosulfan blue during sentinel node biopsy—a common event. Surgery 2001;130:439–442.

Kaye AD, Eatom WM, Jahr JS, Nossman BD, Youngberg, JA. Local anesthesia infiltration as a cause of intraoperative tension pneumothorax in a young healthy woman undergoing breast augmentation with general anesthesia. J Clin Anesth 1995;7:422–424.

52

DO NOT MOVE AN INTUBATED PATIENT (ESPECIALLY THE PATIENT'S HEAD AND NECK) WITHOUT FIRST OBTAINING PERMISSION FROM THE ANESTHESIA STAFF

CATHERINE MARCUCCI, MD

Surgical personnel should not move or reposition an intubated patient without first consulting with the anesthesia provider. The are several reasons for this. First, doing so may cause dislodgement or displacement of the endotracheal tube or laryngeal mask airway. Unintentionally extubated patients can be surprisingly difficult to reintubate, especially if the patient has been repositioned from the original intubating position. If the patient has been receiving an inhalational anesthetic with a significant concentration of nitrous oxide, there may be as little as 30 to 60 seconds to diagnose the dislodgement and regain control of the airway before significant arterial desaturation occurs. Secondly, moving the patient can cause a disconnection in the breathing circuit, which is usually (but not always) at the elbow or Y-piece in the circuit. This can be difficult to find and fix, especially if a significant portion of the breathing circuit is under the drapes. Thirdly, moving a patient who is breathing spontaneously with an unsecured airway (as in a sedation case) can result in coughing and laryngospasm.

WATCH OUT FOR

Of all the body parts that are positioned in surgery, moving the head or neck in a patient under anesthesia is particularly dangerous. Intubation and the ongoing presence of an endotracheal airway in the glottis is one of the most stimulating procedures to the autonomic nervous system known in medicine. Stimulation by the endotracheal tube can cause powerful responses from both the sympathetic and parasympathetic nervous systems, depending on the patient's age and other medical conditions. Before the head is moved with consequent stimulation of the trachea by the endotracheal tube, the anesthesiologist may prefer to further secure the endotracheal tube, deepen the level of anesthesia, raise or lower the heart rate, or institute neuromuscular blockade. In addition, flexing the neck can easily cause the endotracheal tube to slip into a mainstem bronchus which can cause increased airway pressures, wheezing, desaturation, and atelectasis of the nonventilated lung. By far, the safest practice when the head needs to be repositioned is to request assistance from the anesthesia provider. This will allow the anesthesia provider to evaluate the patient, personally disconnect the circuit, and support the head during repositioning.

53

REPAIR A COMMON BILE DUCT INJURY AS CLOSE TO THE HILAR PLATE AS POSSIBLE

ADRIAN LATA, MD

Expert repair of bile duct injuries requires knowledge of bile duct anatomy and its attendant structures. The blood supply to the extrahepatic biliary tree is inconstant but does follow certain patterns that define the anatomic basis for performing biliary reconstruction procedures. The extrahepatic bile duct receives its blood supply via paired 3-o'clock- and 9-o'clock-position arteries. These two vessels receive most (60%) of their inflow inferiorly from the superior pancreaticoduodenal and retroduodenal arteries. A smaller inflow contribution to the paired arteries arises superiorly at the hilum of the liver, usually from branches of the right hepatic artery or from the generous arterial supply to the intrahepatic biliary tree. Only 2% of the arterial blood supply to the extrahepatic biliary tree is segmental, arising from the right hepatic artery. In two-thirds of individuals, interruption of the 3-o'clock- and 9-o'clock-position arteries results in ischemia of the duct superior to the injury. In the other one-third of individuals, the superiorly derived blood supply to the bile duct superior to the injury is adequate. The paired arteries are small (typically 0.3 mm in diameter), vulnerable, and easily damaged.

WATCH OUT FOR

If the common bile duct is divided, clipped, or thermally injured, the 3-o'clock- and 9-o'clock-position arteries will be interrupted. Given the absence of a segmental arterial supply, injuries to the midcommon duct are likely to result in ischemia to the cut end(s) of the transected duct. Accordingly, repair at this level, whether end-to-end reconstruction or choledochojejunostomy, has a high failure rate as a result of stricture formation. This relative ischemia of the midcommon duct is best avoided if the anastomosis is performed superior to the injury. In addition, the blood supply from the end of the bile duct superiorly should always be checked (looking for arterial backbleeding) prior to creating an anastomosis. However, duct ischemia may not be fully appreciated at the time of injury or may progress postinjury (particularly with cautery or clip injury), decreasing the likelihood of success with repair at the time of injury.

In general after duct transection or resection, biliary reconstruction should be performed with a hepaticojejunostomy to the most

117

superior portion of the extrahepatic biliary tree, usually at the level of the bifurcation of the bile duct or optimally extending superiorly onto the left hepatic duct. This upper segment is likely to be well vascularized because it is quite close to the relatively well-perfused intrahepatic biliary tree. When transection of the common duct and biliary reconstruction is required in an operative procedure (e.g., liver transplantation or pancreaticoduodenectomy), the bile duct should be divided and anastomosed at a level well superior to the cystic duct entry and close to the hilum. A long common hepatic duct has a greater risk of ischemia inferiorly, with increased chance for anastomotic breakdown or late stricture formation.

WHAT TO DO The best strategy of dealing with common bile duct injuries is to avoid them. To briefly review, to minimize the risk of common duct injury: (1) during cholecystectomy, retract the infundibulum of the gallbladder laterally at a 90° angle to the common duct (not superiorly and parallel to the common duct) to most clearly define it; (2) ligate the cystic artery close to the gallbladder and away from the common duct to avoid injury to the arteries of the common duct; (3) protect the 3-o'clock- and 9-o'clock-position arteries from injury (whether sharp, crush, or electrocautery injury) by not stripping the main bile duct of surrounding tissue during surgical exposure or during retrieval for transplantation; and (4) for a common duct exploration, open the common duct longitudinally through the relatively avascular area anteriorly. When repairing a biliary injury, perform the anastomosis to well-vascularized duct superiorly, the further superiorly the better.

One final note is that if the surgeon is not experienced with hepatobiliary surgery and common bile duct injuries, consideration should be given to widely draining the area, marking the duct with a clip, and referring it urgently to a center with experience repairing these injuries.

SUGGESTED READINGS

Adkins RB Jr, Chapman WC, Reddy VS. Embryology, anatomy, and surgical applications of the extrahepatic biliary system. Surg Clin North Am 2000;80: 363–379.

Al Ghnaniem R, Benjamin IS. Long-term outcome of hepaticojejunostomy with routine access loop formation following iatrogenic bile duct injury. Br J Surg 2002;89:1118–1124.

Jarnagin WR, Blumgart LH. Operative repair of bile duct injuries involving the hepatic duct confluence. Arch Surg 1999;134:769–775.

Terblanche J, Allison HF, Northover JM. An ischemic basis for biliary stricture. Surgery 1983;94:52–57.

54

REMEMBER THAT THE PRINGLE MANEUVER (THE USE OF WHICH IN HEPATIC TRAUMA IS LESS SUCCESSFUL THAN GENERALLY THOUGHT) WILL NOT CONTROL A REPLACED OR ACCESSORY LEFT HEPATIC ARTERY OR CONTROL HEPATIC VENOUS BLEEDING

MICHAEL J. MORITZ, MD

The management of trauma to the liver, particularly blunt trauma, recently has undergone considerable change. Improved resuscitation with prevention of hypothermia, earlier diagnosis and staging by computed tomography (CT) scan, nonoperative management (i.e., embolization) in appropriate cases, and alterations in operative management have led to a decrease in mortality for grade III and IV injuries. The grading of blunt liver trauma is as follows:

Grade I—Subcapsular hematoma, less than 10% surface area or laceration less than 1 cm deep

Grade II—Subcapsular hematoma, 10% to 50% surface area or laceration 1 to 3 cm deep and less than 10 cm long

Grade III—Subcapsular hematoma, greater than 50% surface area or expanding or laceration greater than 3 cm deep

Grade IV—Parenchymal disruption, 25% to 75% of one lobe or 1 to 3 Couinaud segments

Grade V—Parenchymal disruption, 75% of one lobe or greater than 3 Couinaud segments or juxtahepatic vein injuries (i.e., involving the retrohepatic cava or hepatic veins)

Surgery for liver trauma is fraught with peril and is best accomplished via a midline incision with a table-mounted retractor. The indication for surgery in liver trauma is almost always bleeding, and at least partial control must be very rapidly obtained. Otherwise, release of the tamponade effect by laparotomy in addition to the hypothermic effect of general anesthesia, the operating room below normal body temperature, and the administration of cold blood products can lead to the development of hypothermia, acidosis, and coagulopathy with worsening bleeding and potential mortality. The other critical factor to remember in liver trauma surgery is the three different sources of liver parenchymal bleeding—from branches of the hepatic artery, the portal vein, and the hepatic veins. Fortunately, while a strategy is being devised to investigate those three sources, most parenchymal venous bleeding can be initially controlled with manual compression of the parenchyma with one or two hands (while avoiding having the fingers further violate the parenchyma).

WHAT TO DO

In general, bleeding (especially from grade III and IV injuries) should be approached stepwise. First, the hilum should be isolated and surrounded with a large loop such as a Penrose drain and cross-clamped with a noncrushing vascular clamp (i.e., the Pringle maneuver). This temporarily interrupts the proper hepatic artery, replaced or accessory right hepatic arteries, the portal vein, and arterial collaterals around the bile duct. Total portal vein flow varies with time, meals, etc. but is generally about 20% to 30% of cardiac output, or about 800 to 1200 mL/minute in a resting adult. Hepatic arterial flow is about one-quarter of portal flow. In a hemodynamically stable, well-oxygenated patient on no vasopressors, the hilum can remain clamped for more than 30 minutes without ill effect. In the hypovolemic bleeding patient with liver trauma, it is difficult to prescribe a safe duration of hilar clamping, but clearly shorter is better; also, the clamp can be intermittently released with partial control of bleeding maintained manually or by packing.

There are several disadvantages of the Pringle maneuver in liver trauma surgery. The Pringle maneuver does nothing to lessen hepatic vein bleeding. Normal flow through the inferior vena cava is 2 to 3 L/minute, so backbleeding via injured hepatic veins can be torrential. Also, even when a cross clamp is correctly applied to the hepatic hilum, a replaced or accessory left hepatic artery will not be occluded because these arteries approach the liver via the lesser hepatic omentum far from the hilum, accompanying the vagal fibers to enter the liver at the umbilical fissure. This anomaly is present in about 10% of humans. However, flow through this branch will be less than 200 mL/minute, and arterial bleeding from disrupted liver parenchyma is typically easier to identify and control.

SUGGESTED READINGS

Gao JM, Du DY, Zhao XJ, et al. Liver trauma: experience in 348 cases. World J Surg 2003;27:703–708.

Kim YI, Ishii T, Aramaki M, et al. The Pringle maneuver induces only partial ischemia of the liver. Hepato-Gastroenterol 1995;42:169–171.

Man K, Fan ST, Ng IO, et al. Prospective evaluation of Pringle maneuver in hepatectomy for liver tumors by a randomized study. Ann Surg 1997;226: 704–711.

Pachter HL, Feliciano DV. Complex hepatic injuries. Surg Clin North Am 1996;76: 763–782.

55

DO NOT ALLOW A PATIENT TO BLEED TO DEATH FROM A LIVER INJURY

MICHAEL J. MORITZ, MD

Because of its large size, the liver is the most frequently injured abdominal solid organ secondary to both blunt and penetrating trauma. It also can be damaged during cholecystectomy and other right upper quadrant surgeries. The principles of surgical management of liver injury are the same regardless of the severity or mechanism of injury. They are: (1) control of bleeding; (2) removal of devitalized tissue; and (3) adequate drainage.

WHAT TO DO

Most liver injuries are minor (grades I and II) and can be managed with simple procedures such as direct pressure, electrocautery, argon beam coagulation, topical agents, or simple suture and stapling. However, control of profuse bleeding from deep hepatic lacerations is a formidable problem, with a substantial risk of mortality. These severe liver injuries draw the surgeon into more complex procedures to control bleeding which usually involves opening the liver wound and directly approaching the bleeding vessels in an attempt to ligate them. However, opening the liver creates more bleeding, devitalizes more tissue, and is time–consuming. The degree of venous bleeding is always underappreciated by the surgeon and hypovolemia, shock, and hypothermia can develop quickly. Temporary packing that provides reasonable control of bleeding may be preferable to longer, drawn out explorations that provide better hemostasis at the cost of more transfusions, hypothermia, and so on.

Packing of the liver is quick and relatively easy to perform. Whether portal venous or hepatic venous, most liver bleeding is venous, and is consequently low pressure and controllable with packing. In most circumstances, packing around the liver to compress the liver injury upon itself is effective, although in some circumstances a small pack or conglomeration of topical hemostatic agents placed in the injury prior to packing around the liver can be helpful. Generally, packing is fairly effective for parenchymal bleeding and may be less effective for retrohepatic vena caval or arterial bleeding.

If packing is found to reasonably control the bleeding from the liver, the patient is closed, closed suction drains are placed, and the patient is taken to the intensive care unit postoperatively for rewarming and resuscitation. Postoperative care focuses on promotion and preservation of homeostasis by providing adequate tissue oxygenation, normovolemia, and avoidance of pressors. The goal is to avoid further ischemia to the liver, allowing recovery of hepatocyte function and appropriate hepatocyte regeneration. Prophylactic antibiotics should be given. Blood products should be available and administered liberally. Re-exploration is performed within 48 to 72 hours after the initial operation, sooner if bleeding accelerates rather than slows. Continued bleeding may be an indication for arteriography to locate and selectively embolize arterial bleeding, which is very helpful before re-exploration. At re-exploration, packs are removed, hemostasis is achieved with the least manipulation possible, and closed-suction drains are placed.

If the surgeon does not wish to pack and elects instead to try to control bleeding at the time of initial surgery and the bleeding continues despite directly ligating vessels, the Pringle maneuver can be tried. The Pringle maneuver consists of surrounding and temporarily occluding the entire porta hepatis. However, the Pringle maneuver is not often successful—hepatic venous bleeding is unaffected, and replaced or accessory left hepatic arteries do not enter the porta hepatis. (They enter at the umbilical fissure and are not controlled with the Pringle maneuver.) If bleeding stops after clamping the portal triad, it can be assumed to be from portal venous or hepatic arterial branches. If bleeding continues despite clamping the portal triad, then the hepatic veins or the retrohepatic vena cava are injured. The portal triad also can be intermittently clamped to allow visualization during placement of sutures as parenchymal vessels are ligated. If a Pringle maneuver is applied, caution regarding the duration of inflow occlusion is necessary.

Ligation of the *common* hepatic artery is also an alternative for continued bleeding but is seldom required. It should be reserved for the occasional penetrating injury or deep laceration with apparent arterial bleeding for which exposure of the wound's depths will require extensive opening of the liver. Test clamping before ligation is sensible. The *proper* hepatic artery should not be ligated; common hepatic artery ligation preserves a small amount of antegrade arterial flow via gastroduodenal artery collaterals. Proper hepatic artery ligation may result in liver infarction, particularly if associated with portal vein injury or biliary strictures. Packing and selective (distal) arterial embolization are better alternatives to hepatic artery ligation.

Placement and use of drains in an abdominal cavity packed for bleeding varies. Generally if the skin or fascia has been closed the drains are placed to suction to help estimate amount of residual bleeding and to prevent buildup of volume and possible abdominal compartment syndrome. If the drain output is copious and outgoing, they can be taken off suction to facilitate partial tamponade while plans for a return to the OR are being devised.

One final note is that surgeons should have a low threshold for requesting assistance from an experienced trauma or liver surgeon in cases of major liver injury. Although some may take it as a blow to professional pride, liver injuries have a significant risk of on-table and early postoperative deaths related to exsanguination; therefore, it is a wise surgeon who considers packing, seeks assistance from other surgeons, and controls bleeding well enough to continue the battle another day.

SUGGESTED READINGS

Juhl JH, Crummy AB, Kuhlman JE, eds. Paul and Juhl's Essentials of Radiologic Imaging. 7th Ed. Philadelphia: Lippincott-Raven, 1999:511–512.

Mrksic MB, Farkas E, Cabafi Z, et al. Kkomplikacije laparoskopske holecistektomije [Complications in laparoscopic cholecystectomy]. Medicinski Pregled 1999;52:253–257.

Richardson DJ, Franklin GA, Lukan JK, et al. Evolution in the management of hepatic trauma: a 25–year perspective. Ann Surg 2000;232:324–330.

Townsend CM, Beauchamp RD, Evers BM, eds. Sabiston Textbook of Surgery: The Biological Basis of Modern Surgical Practice. 16th Ed. Philadelphia: W.B. Saunders, 2001:336–338.

56

HAVE A LOW THRESHOLD FOR CONVERTING A LAPAROSCOPIC CHOLECYSTECTOMY TO AN OPEN CHOLECYSTECTOMY

MICHAEL SILBER, DO

Laparoscopic cholecystectomy is one of the most common general surgerical procedures performed and has become the gold standard for treatment of symptomatic cholelithiasis. Large series have shown both the effectiveness and relative safety of this procedure compared to open cholecystectomy. In fact, almost all patients undergoing evaluation for cholecystectomy should be considered for a minimally invasive approach. The few remaining contraindications for attempting a laparoscopic cholecystectomy include: contraindication to an open procedure given the risk of conversion from a laparoscopic procedure; inability to tolerate pneumoperitoneum; pregnancy (although more from a medicolegal aspect than from a technical aspect, since no long-term study has shown the effect of pneumoperitoneum on the fetus); and an inexperienced surgeon.

The last contraindication, the experience level of the surgeon, is low. Currently, most surgeons have participated in vigorous educational programs or completed residency training that included formal laparoscopic and minimally invasive training. However, even the most skillful laparoscopic surgeon today must realize when his or her level of expertise has been reached and recognize when to convert a laparoscopic cholecystectomy to an open one. Although less than 5% of elective laparoscopic cholecystectomies are converted to open procedures today, several considerations discussed below should be reviewed by the surgeon when deciding whether to convert to an open operation.

WATCH OUT FOR

First, good visualization of the right upper quadrant, specifically the structures of the triangle of Calot, is of paramount importance for the successful completion of a laparoscopic procedure. If the patient has dense adhesions from previous upper abdominal surgeries or if severe inflammation is present from acute cholecystitis, visualization of the right upper quadrant can be extremely difficult. Use of a 30° camera may aid the surgeon in identifying structures. If the anatomy is uncertain, open conversion should take place. Second, time for dissection should take less than 120 minutes. If, at two hours, little or no steady progress has occurred, conversion to an open procedure is recommended. Thirdly, excessive bleeding is an obvious indication for conversion of a laparoscopic procedure to an open one. Reportedly, the majority of complications associated with bleeding are due to avulsion of the cystic artery or excessive bleeding from the liver bed. Although both of these occurrences could be corrected laparoscopically, it is important to remember that poor visualization and difficulty controlling the source of bleeding may in fact lead to further, more severe injury. The surgeon should never place clips blindly into a blood-filled field. Conversion to an open operation should be performed early if control of bleeding is not rapidly obtained. Major vascular injuries to the right hepatic artery or portal vein are uncommon but mandate prompt laparotomy if they occur.

The purpose of timely conversion from a laproscopic to an open approach is the prevention of biliary injury, which is the major complication of laparoscopic cholecystectomy. Most reports suggest that the incidence of major bile duct injury is between 0.3% and 0.6% when performed laparoscopically, compared to 0.10% to 0.13% for an open procedure (i.e., three- to fourfold higher). Review of laparoscopic biliary injuries reveals that many injuries occur in the setting of the surgeon having noted some small difficulty in defining the anatomy, followed by transection, clip, or cautery injury to the common hepatic duct, after which the possibility of biliary injury is first entertained. However, a substantial proportion of injuries are not suspected intraoperatively and come to light postoperatively. If a biliary injury is diagnosed or even suspected, conversion is almost always indicated. If an injury is recognized laparoscopically, the damage should be thoroughly assessed in the open procedure because the actual damage is usually more extensive than can be assessed via the laparoscopic view. If a bile duct injury does occur, it would be prudent to obtain an intraoperative consultation with an experienced biliary surgeon. If this is not feasible, an appropriate next step is to place tubes in biliary structures with adjacent drains to help identify anatomy and prevent sepsis, followed by transfer to a referral center for definitive care. In all regards, the recovery from an open cholecystectomy is less problematic than from an injury to the biliary or portal system and its often complex repair and attendant problems.

Suggested Readings

Cameron JL, ed. Current Surgical Therapy. 7th ed. Philadelphia: Mosby, 2001;441–445,1369–1376.

Gadacz TR. Update on laparoscopic cholecystectomy, including a clinical pathway. Surg Clin North Am 2000;80:1127–1149.

Hannah EL, Imperato PJ, Nenner RP, et al. Laparoscopic and open cholecystectomy in New York State: mortality, complications, and choice of procedure. Surgery 1999;125:223–231.

Strasberg SM. Laparoscopic biliary surgery. Gastroenterol Clin North Am 1999;28:117–1362.

KNOW THE THREE PLACES WHERE SMALL BOWEL ANTIMESENTERIC FAT IS FOUND WHEN "LOST" AMONG LOOPS OF BOWEL

MICHAEL J. MORITZ, MD

When the surgeon feels lost among loops of bowel in a difficult abdomen, any landmark that helps distinguish small bowel from large bowel is a welcome sign. The presence of antimesenteric fat can be helpful in determining "where you are." Fat on the antimesenteric aspect of the small bowel is not commonly seen, occurring in one normal, one anomalous, and one pathological state (see below). In contrast, fat on the large bowel is commonly found as the greater omentum and the appendices epiploicae. Other distinguishing features of large bowel are the tinea coli and the external sacculations of the large bowel wall, as compared with the smooth external walls of the small bowel.

Normal antimesenteric fat. Small bowel antimesenteric fat is normal only at the terminal ileum. A constantly occurring tissue fold containing fat passes from the lower border of the last three inches of the ileum to the cecum and appendix. If the patient is obese, this fold may contain a considerable amount of fat. In some references, this fold is inaccurately referred to as the fold of Treves (Treves described the transparent fold of peritoneum from the cecum to ileum, not the antimesenteric fat present on the terminal ileum).

Anomalous antimesenteric fat. Meckel's diverticulum is an anomaly that occurs in 2% of individuals, about 2 feet proximal to the junction of the terminal ileum and cecum. There is a male to female ratio of 2:1 (the rule of 2's).

Pathologic antimesenteric fat. Crohn's disease can affect any part of the gastrointestinal tract; 50% of patients have both small and large bowel involvement, 25% have only small bowel involvement, and 25% have only large bowel involvement. Grossly involved small bowel will have a shortened, thickened mesentery with "creeping" of mesenteric fat around the circumference of the bowel, which may reach the antimesenteric aspect. The bowel itself is thickened, indurated, and discolored along a grayish to violaceous spectrum.

SUGGESTED READINGS

Addison C. Ellis's Demonstrations of Anatomy: Being a Guide to the Knowledge of the Human Body by Dissection. 12th Ed. New York, William Wood & Company, 1906:314.

Addison C. On the topographical anatomy of the abdominal viscera in man, especially the gastrointestinal canal, Part III. *J Anat Physiol* 1900–1901;35:166–204.

Miele V, De Cicco ML, Andreoli C, et al. US and CT findings in complicated Meckel diverticulum. Radiologia Medica 2001;101:230–234.

FREE UP THE BOWEL PROXIMALLY AND DISTALLY WHEN REPAIRING AN ENTEROTOMY TO AVOID FISTULA FORMATION

X. D. DONG, MD

Fortunately for both patients and surgeons, the mortality associated with enterocutaneous fistulae has fallen significantly over the past 40 years with improvements in care, particularly the availability of parenteral nutrition. Anastomotic leaks, inadvertent enterotomy, and iatrogenic compromise to the blood supply of the bowel cause a significant proportion of enterocutaneous fistulae with neoplasms, Crohn's disease, and intra-abdominal sepsis accounting for the remainder. With control of infection, nutritional support, and other supportive measures, most enterocutaneous fistulae (about 70% to 90%) can be induced to close spontaneously (i.e., nonoperatively). However, the overall mortality is still approximately 20%; therefore, given this mortality, the formation of fistulae should be assiduously avoided.

WATCH OUT FOR

Prevention of inadvertent enterotomies is crucial in preventing fistulae. Correctly, entering the abdominal cavity and performing division of adhesions requires knowledge of the following principle: adhesions between loops of bowel or between bowel and the abdominal wall can have more strength than the bowel wall itself. Thus, overly blunt maneuvers to find tissue planes can cause inadvertent entry into the bowel lumen. Accordingly, fascial edges should not be distracted excessively until the underlying adherent bowel has been sharply dissected off the fascia to avoid bluntly tearing bowel wall. Unintentional serosal tears of the bowel wall should be promptly repaired with interrupted sutures. Failure to promptly tag or repair such minor injuries often leads to them being forgotten or lost amongst the bowel loops.

In addition to blunt injury to the bowel wall, care must be taken to avoid electrocautery burns to the bowel as well. Although this modality is commonly used to divide adhesions, the cautery mark seen in the operating room notoriously underestimates the amount of tissue that has been thermally injured which may result in necrose over successive days. Cautery injuries to the bowel wall must be carefully repaired as they occur so as not to be overlooked.

WHAT TO DO Proper repair if an enterotomy does occur must include adequate exposure of the injured bowel proximally and distally. The mesentery of the affected bowel segment must be carefully inspected and preserved with any ischemic bowel resected. The bowel distal to the enterotomy should be traced to minimize any risk of bowel obstruction that might compromise the repair. Repair of an enterotomy can be done in a two-layer, hand-sewn fashion if the bowel lumen will not be narrowed from the repair and bowel viability is not in question from ischemia, radiation, or surgical damage. Most surgeons favor a transverse closure of a longitudinal enterotomy to insure that the bowel lumen is not compromised. Resection of defects greater than half of the bowel circumference may be best to prevent formation of strictures and to decrease the risk of breakdown and fistula formation. A "clean" surgical anastomosis may be less risky than closing a ragged enterotomy resulting from traction injury.

SUGGESTED READINGS

Cameron JL, ed. Current Surgical Therapy. 7th Ed. Philadelphia: Mosby, 2001:156–161.

Martinez D, Zibari G, Aultman D, et al. The outcome of intestinal fistulae: the Louisiana State University Medical Center–Shreveport experience. Am Surg 1998;64:252–254.

Pickhardt PJ, Bhalla S, Balfe DM. Acquired gastrointestinal fistulas: classification, etiologies, and imaging evaluation. Radiology 220;224:9–23.

59

MAKE SURE THAT THE RED RUBBER CATHETER IN A WITZEL JEJUNOSTOMY IS GOING DISTALLY IN THE SMALL BOWEL LUMEN

MICHAEL J. MORITZ, MD

Surgical placement of a feeding tube in the stomach or jejunum was never an "easy" case, but this procedure has become more difficult in recent years as the frequency and indications for placement have changed. Today, fewer patients require surgical feeding tube placement because endoscopic techniques have become successful and widespread. Small caliber feeding tubes placed via the nose into the stomach and distally are well tolerated by patients and can be repositioned endoscopically if they become dislodged. The few remaining indications for a surgically placed tube include extensive intraabdominal adhesions (from prior surgery, radiation therapy, or malignancy) likelihood of a progressive upper gastrointestinal obstruction, need for laparotomy, obesity, and inability of the bowel to be endoscopically manipulated anteriorly to the abdominal wall.

WHAT TO DO

Because the Witzel jejunostomy is such a "small" procedure, the expectation on all sides is that the incision will be concordantly small. This may tempt the surgeon into a situation with improper lighting or exposure that can increase the difficulty of the case. However, an incision large enough for adequate exposure must be made. The small bowel in the left upper quadrant inferior to the transverse colon should be identified (omentum may need to be mobilized or divided to define the transverse colon). Proximal and distal bowel should be defined by tracing the jejunum to the ligament of Treitz, where the small bowel emerges from the retroperitoneum. It must be remembered that the ligament of Treitz is the *only* reliable marker of proximal versus distal jejunum through the limited exposure of this procedure. Most surgeons place the entry site of the tube about 30 cm distally from the ligament and as the jejunum comes up to the anterior abdominal wall without tension. It is important that the purse string at the enterotomy should encompass as little bowel wall as possible; it does not need to be overly constricting. The Witzel tunnel should be fashioned using as little of the serosa as possible to preserve the maximal bowel lumen, especially at the ends. The jejunum is tacked to the parietal peritoneum anteriorly over a long length, at least 5 cm proximal and distal to where the tube enters the Witzel tunnel (with sufficient length between the ligament of Treitz and the enterotomy to allow for this distance). The feeding tube is brought through the abdominal wall tangentially and placed into the enterotomy and directed distally for more than 10 cm so that it cannot flip around inside the lumen and point proximally. As many patients with feeding tubes suffer from altered mental status and are inclined to dislodge tubes, the tube must be securely and *redundantly* fixed at the exit site (0-polypropylene sutures are a good choice) and the patient's hands must be kept from the tube with an abdominal binder. If the tube should come out before the serosal tunnel has fully formed (10 to 14 days), the tube should not be reinserted and reoperation is generally required.

Four other considerations with surgically placed feeding tubes are as follows:

1) Any tube that is not behaving perfectly or has been manipulated should not be used until a radiograph with contrast through the tube verifies its position within the lumen of the gastrointestinal tract.

2) If the tube is directed improperly in the proximal direction, the tube may ultimately work, but the feeds will enter the jejunum proximal to the surgically manipulated segment of jejunum. The tube feeds will not pass easily in the distal direction for a week or more until edema resolves and motility normalizes. If motility is impaired, the feeds will pool with the potential for hyperosmolar injury to the bowel wall or they will reflux proximally. Consideration should be given to reoperating to replace the tube.

3) The most common major complication of surgical feeding jejunostomy is obstruction, typically from kinking where the bowel is brought to the anterior abdominal wall or from excessive narrowing of the bowel lumen where the tube enters the lumen. If at any time during the procedure the surgeon thinks, "Is this too tight?," consideration should be given to redoing that part of the procedure.

4) What should be done if the tube has been placed in the colon? This has happened to more than one surgeon and is usually detected when the patient develops diarrhea resembling tube feeds. Reoperation is required with primary closure of the colon as feeding colostomy tubes are not effective for nutritional support.

SUGGESTED READINGS

Fontana RJ, Barnett JL. Jejunostomy tube placement in refractory diabetic gastroparesis: a retrospective review. Am J Gastroenterol 1996;91:2174–2178.

Holmes JH 4th, Brundage SI, Yuen P, et al. Complications of surgical feeding jejunostomy in trauma patients. J Trauma 1999;47:1009–1012.

Rosenkranz LG. Nutritional support in the postoperative period. Med Clin North Am 2001;85:1255–1262.

Wakefield SE, Mansell NJ, Baigrie RJ, Dowling BL. Use of a feeding jejunostomy after oesophagogastric surgery. Br J Surg 1995;82:811–813.

AVOID UNDUE TRACTION ON THE LEFT RENAL VEIN WHEN EXPOSING THE NECK OF AN AORTIC ANEURYSM

MICHAEL J. MORITZ, MD

Most students and physicians think of the anatomy of the left renal vein as straightforward, and it is a common subject for intraoperative quizzing of junior residents and medical students. Everyone knows the named branches of the left renal vein: from right to left (from inferior vena cava toward the kidney), adrenal vein superiorly and gonadal vein inferiorly. However, the anatomy is in fact much more complex. Without a clear understanding of the normal variants of this vein, intraoperative injury risk is greatly increased.

WATCH OUT FOR For starters, the left renal vein is single and anterior to the aorta in 90% of individuals. In almost 10%, the vein is circumaortic, meaning that there are two components to the left renal vein: one anterior to the aorta and one posterior to it. If there is a circumaortic left renal vein, the adrenal and gonadal veins will usually drain into the anterior branch. In 1% or fewer cases, the anterior component is absent, with only the retroaortic left renal vein present. The vein may receive other renal branches outside the hilum, most usually polar veins.

On the superior side of the left renal vein, in 75% of cases there is one venous branch consisting of the joined adrenal and inferior phrenic veins. In 25%, there are two or more branches, either separate entrances of the two tributaries, a bifid adrenal vein, or both.

On the inferior side of the renal vein, the gonadal vein empties into the left renal vein approximately 95% of the time. It is usually singular, although it may be bifid. In the other 5%, the gonadal vein or, if bifid, one of its components empties into the adrenal vein or one of the lumbar veins. The gonadal vein usually enters the renal vein lateral to the entrance of the adrenal vein, occasionally at the same level, and rarely medial to the adrenal vein.

However, the greatest misconception regarding renal vein anatomy relates to *posterior* branches. In more than 50% of individuals, there will be at least one branch arising from the lumbar veins that drains into the posterior-inferior aspect of the left renal vein. Most commonly, the L2 vein communicates with the left renal vein, although the L3 or L4 vein also may do so. The position of this tributary is usually quite lateral; it is lateral to the gonadal vein and close to the renal vein's origin from the parenchyma in the hilum of the kidney. It is important to note that the four lumbar veins may, in all or part, be interconnected by the ascending lumbar vein. Additionally, the more superior lumbar veins may be confluent with the origin of the left hemiazygous vein. In summary, these intercommunications ensure that disruption of lumbar vein branches to the left renal vein will produce substantial bleeding. Lumbar communications will always be to the posterior component of the renal vein.

WHAT TO DO
The most common (nontransplant) operation involving the left renal vein is open abdominal aortic aneurysm surgery. During this procedure, the neck of the aneurysm below the renal arteries is exposed; therefore, vital to this exposure is the identification, dissection, and superior mobilization of the left renal vein. The lumbar veins are closely applied to the vertebral bodies and body wall, hence communicating veins between the lumbar veins and the left renal vein will tether the renal vein posteriorly and inferiorly. In performing this maneuver, the surgeon must carefully search for these posterior branches of the left renal vein, as they are not usually visible on preoperative imaging. Finding and dividing these branches under direct vision is the best way to avoid injury to them. The most common technical injury is avulsion, which causes more bleeding and is more difficult to control than a sharp venous injury.

When proper exposure of the aorta is precluded by the left renal vein's location, position, or inability to be adequately mobilized, one alternative is to divide the left renal vein. When this is done between the inferior vena cava to the patient's right and intact adrenal and left gonadal branches, the kidney will generally survive and recover normal or nearly normal function, with its venous drainage through collaterals via the intact gonadal and adrenal veins. Once divided, the left renal vein is not generally reconstructed in this setting. In addition, when the posterior lumbar branch is torn, exposure to control the bleeding will also often require division of the left renal vein. As the lumbar branch usually enters the renal vein near the renal hilum and close to the parenchyma as mentioned above, care must be taken not to interrupt the adrenal and gonadal veins during this maneuver to obtain control of bleeding.

SUGGESTED READINGS

Anson BJ, Cauldwell EW, Pick LW, et al. The anatomy of the pararenal system of veins, with comments on the renal arteries. J Urol 1948;60:714–737.

Anson BJ, Kurth LE. Common variations in the renal blood supply. Surg Gynecol Obstet 1955;100:157–162.

Elsharawy MA, Cheatle TR., Clarke JM, Colin JF. Effect of left renal vein division during aortic surgery on renal function. Ann R Coll Surg Engl 2000;82:417–420.

Mathews R, Smith PA, Fishman EK, Marshall FF. Anomalies of the inferior vena cava and renal veins: embryologic and surgical considerations. Urology 1999;53:873–880.

61

REMEMBER THAT INFERIOR POLAR ARTERIES TO THE RIGHT KIDNEY CROSS THE INFRARENAL INFERIOR VENA CAVA

JAMES HERRINGTON, MD

Vascular anomalies are a reality and all physicians who perform surgery or invasive procedures must be familiar with anatomic variations to avoid inadvertent injury. Accessory renal arteries in humans are found in 15% to 30% of kidneys. Most accessory renal arteries, especially those to the hilum or upper pole, arise from the lateral aspect of the aorta, as do classic renal arteries. However, accessory lower polar arteries have an increased tendency (10% of patients) to arise from the anterior aspect of the aorta. This violates the old surgical dictum that no major vascular structures cross the infrarenal inferior vena cava (IVC).

WATCH OUT FOR

Many surgeons operate in the retroperitoneum and must be familiar with arterial anatomy. Gynecologists perform retroperitoneal lymphadenectomy as part of ovarian and uterine cancer treatment. Urologists perform a variety of surgeries on the para-aortic and paracaval lymph nodes and the ureters and kidneys in the retroperitoneum. General surgeons of many areas of expertise perform procedures in the retroperitoneum and need to be aware of this anomaly. This is particularly important when the Cattell-Braasch maneuver is performed, which involves mobilizing the terminal ileum, cecum, ascending colon, and proximal transverse colon. To begin, the white line of Toldt is identified in the right paracolic gutter and represents the entry point to find the avascular plane posterior to the colonic mesentery. This may be incised sharply or with the electrocautery. This maneuver allows mobilization of the cecum superiorly and medially, and the dissection proceeds smoothly up the anterior surface of the IVC. At this point, a lower polar artery to the right kidney is vulnerable to injury. In the case of a trauma laparotomy, the blood suffusing the retroperitoneum can make the artery hard to identify. For a cadaver organ donor, after exsanguination, the lack of color and lack of pulsation increase the vulnerability of this artery. In these and other instances of compromised exposure and haste, only the surgeon's care in excluding the presence of this anomaly can prevent injury. In the elective setting, preoperative determination of the arterial supply to the kidneys can be done with contrast CT scan, angiography, or magnetic resonance imaging. If no preoperative imaging is obtained, the existence of a possible anomalous lower pole artery must be kept in mind to avoid bleeding or vessel damage. Inadvertent injury to this anomalous artery can cause bleeding, which is not difficult to control. However, repair of this small vessel is difficult, and thrombosis will typically occur.

In addition to bleeding and thrombosis, loss of the artery will result in kidney ischemia, possible infarction of the lower pole, and possible hypertension. Aquino et al have reported their results on occluding anomalous arteries with endograft repairs of abdominal aortic aneurysms. Postoperatively, 5 of 24 patients who had accessory renal arteries occluded by an endograft showed evidence of ischemia, with one patient who developed hypertension that required pharmacotherapy. There was one case of late renal failure in a patient who had a normal renal perfusion study—this was attributed to dye toxicity. Similar results were also reported by Kaplan and colleagues.

One final note is that in the setting of a transplant kidney where ureteral and capsular collaterals no longer exist, loss of an inferior polar artery will result in a substantially increased risk of ureteral ischemia and ureteral complications.

SUGGESTED READINGS

Anson BJ, Cauldwell EW, Pick LW, Beaton L. The anatomy of the pararenal system of veins with comments on the renal arteries. J Urol 1948;60:714–737.

Aquino RV, Rhee RY, Muluk SC, et al. Exclusion of accessory renal arteries during endovascular repair of abdominal aortic aneurysm. J Vasc Surg 2001;4:878–884.

Benedetti-Panici P, Maneschi F, Scambia G, et al. Anatomic abnormalities of the retroperitoneum encountered during aortic and pelvic lymphadenectomy. Am J Obstet Gynecol 1994;170:111–116.

Kaplan DD, Kwon CC, Mann MD, Hollier LH. Endovascular repair of abdominal aortic aneurysm in patients with congenital renal vascular anomalies. J Vasc Surg 1999;30:407–516.

Reis RH, Esenther G. Variations in the pattern of renal vessels and their relationship to the type of posterior vena cava in man. Am J Anat 1959;104:295–317.

Skinner DG, Melamud A, Lieskosky G. Complications of thoracoabdominal lymph node dissection. J Urol 1982;127:1107–10.

Use clips for hemostasis sparingly and with care in proximity to where vascular clamps might be used

Michael J. Moritz, MD

Vascular clamps have relatively gentle, springy, noncrushing jaws that hold tissue without injuring it. When a noncompressible object is unintentionally included between the jaws of a vascular clamp, the clamp will become ineffective; the structure intended to be controlled or occluded by the clamp will leak or slip out of the clamp's jaws. The most common noncompressible objects that interfere with the correct function of vascular clamps are surgical clips, the small titanium hemostatic devices that can be very useful in obtaining hemostasis. Clips and vascular clamps are two incompatible instruments and are a bad mix in the same operative field. In planned elective procedures with good exposure, the vigilant surgeon will carefully place vascular clamps with this in mind, avoiding clips and other similar obstacles. In the face of emergency procedures, bleeding, and suboptimal exposure, the temptation to use clips for hemostasis is greater as they can be faster than ties, for example; however, the ability to see all the clips adjacent to a vessel to be clamped is compromised. In this difficult situation, having problems with the vascular clamp because of clips within its jaws only makes the situation worse.

Pertinent examples of this abound. When a hepatic lobectomy is performed with clips used to control the inferior vena caval side of the small hepatic veins, placing a vascular clamp to control major or minor hepatic veins becomes even more difficult and, if there is bleeding, can be hazardous. Similarly, when performing an abdominal aortic aneurysm resection, particularly one that has ruptured, clips to control the periaortic tissue are a real hazard. Also, for an open nephrectomy, clips in the area of the venous clamp are decided obstacles.

A similar parallel issue involves stapling devices used in gastrointestinal and pulmonary surgery. Closing a linear stapler (e.g., a TA or RL) onto a clip will lead to incompletely closed staples and, if unrecognized, a leak through the staple line. A clip in an anastamotic stapler (e.g., a GIA or EEA) will be hard to ignore because the stapler will usually refuse to fire when incompletely closed. In this situation, do not force the stapler—remove it, inspect the situation, and try again. Regardless, carefully inspect the area around any intended staple line to exclude any clips from the device. Ties are not a problem with such instruments and can be used liberally without concern.

63

CHECK THE JAWS OF A VASCULAR CLAMP BEFORE APPLYING

JAMES HERRINGTON, MD

Three true stories:

1) A urologist performing an open right nephrectomy asks for a Satinsky (side-biting) vascular clamp to control the junction of the right renal vein and inferior vena cava (IVC). The scrub nurse, also a specialist in urologic procedures, picks out the appropriately shaped clamp from the vascular instrument set, and the surgeon places it. The vessels are divided and the kidney removed. The clamp then falls off of the IVC, leaving a gaping opening that is controlled only after several units of blood are lost and a passing general surgeon scrubs in to help obtain control. The reason: the clamp was *not* a Satinsky vascular clamp—rather it was a clamp shaped like a Satinsky but lacking the correct jaw configuration. The clamp had smooth jaws that did not touch with the clamp fully closed rather than having fine teeth that intermeshed when the clamp was closed. The smooth-jawed clamp was intended for use only after Silastic boots were applied to the jaws, and its intended use is for occluding vascular grafts, not vessels.

2) A vascular surgeon asks for and receives a pediatric Cooley clamp (a soft, delicate clamp) from a tray of instruments with which he is very familiar and applies it to a fragile vessel. Later, when preparing the vessel for anastamosis, the vessel is dissected further proximally, a second clamp placed, and the first one removed. It was discovered that the first clamp had almost completely transected the vessel wall, crushing the intima and media. Although it had vascular teeth, the clamp was a new replacement for a worn out one, and the hospital had switched instrument suppliers; the new clamp was extremely firm and stiff and inappropriate for the small fragile vessels for which it was ostensibly designed.

3) During a routine peripheral vascular case, a surgeon places a vascular clamp across an artery. Minutes later, bleeding is noted in the area. Inspection reveals bleeding from the vessel at the clamp through the vessel wall, not from the vessel lumen. The vessel is dissected further proximally in the now blood-filled field and control obtained. The first clamp is removed, revealing laceration of the vessel wall. The reason: the clamp was old and loose, and the

jaws, instead of meeting head-on, slipped by one another—what surgeons call scissoring. The "scissoring" jaws did just that, lacerating the side of the artery and making a routine case longer and more involved.

In all three cases, the surgeon had unknowingly placed an inappropriate clamp on a vessel, whether because of unfamiliarity with vascular clamps in general or because of a problem with what was thought to be a familiar clamp.

Vascular clamps belong to a family of clamps called noncrushing clamps. Other noncrushing clamps include those used for bowel and lung. Noncrushing clamps and forceps are different from standard crushing clamps in two distinctive ways: (1) standard clamps are made of stiff, nonyielding steel such that tissue within the jaws will be crushed, whereas vascular instruments are made of softer, springy steel that holds tissue within the jaws firmly but without crushing; and (2) vascular instruments have fine longitudinal rows of teeth within their jaws that are specially designed to hold but not crush. Most vascular instruments have one of two distinct patterns of teeth. DeBakey-style teeth have odd numbers of rows of fine teeth that mesh, providing a firm noncrushing grip, and are very popular for forceps and many vascular clamps (see *Figure 63.1A*). Cooley-style teeth have even numbers of rows of finer teeth that meet head on. Cooley-style teeth are more traumatic than DeBakey-style teeth and so are partnered with softer, springier steel jaws; they are typically used for very fine vascular clamps and pediatric vascular clamps (see *Figure 63.1B*). A newer family of clamps has soft disposable jaw inserts made of rubber, plastic, or fabric and adhere to the same principle of not damaging the vessel wall. A vascular clamp, if too strong or applied incorrectly to a vessel, can lead to late narrowing of the vessel from scarring, referred to as "clamp injury."

WHAT TO DO

Utilizing the above jaw configuration, vascular clamps are available in a dizzying array of sizes and shapes. Many clamps have been designed specifically for particular steps of certain operations. Excluding emergencies, vascular clamps should be selected by the surgeon in advance of their use, inspected by the surgeon for the correctness of the teeth and the alignment of the jaws, and tested for the relative firmness of the steel by applying the clamp to the hypothenar eminence of the hand. These steps insure that the clamp is safe and appropriate to use and help the

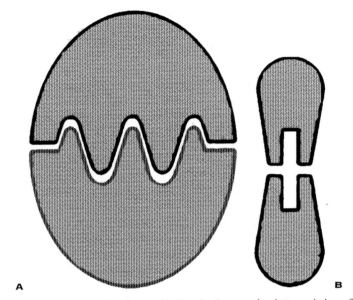

FIGURE 63.1. Vascular clamps. Both styles have each edge consisting of a row of tiny teeth. **A:** DeBakey-style teeth in their interdigitating configuration shown as three rows into two rows (smaller clamps and forceps are often two rows into one row). **B:** Cooley-style teeth are opposed head-on.

surgeon assess the force that will be applied to the vessel, with the aim being to apply just enough force to occlude the vessel without damaging it.

SUGGESTED READINGS

Margovsky AI, Chambers AJ, Lord RS. The effect of increasing clamping forces on endothelial and arterial wall damage: an experimental study in sheep. Cardiovasc Surg 1999;7:457–463.
Rutherford RB, ed. Vascular Surgery. 5th Ed. Philadelphia: W.B. Saunders, 2000:477–478.

64

Obtain Proximal and Distal Control Before Exploring a Vascular Wound

Michael J. Moritz, MD

Management of traumatic vascular injuries is one of the most challenging aspects of surgery. Unlike elective surgery, the surgeon is faced with an injury and a hematoma without time for extensive reoperative studies and planning. Before entering a hematoma, it is imperative to obtain both proximal and distal *vascular* control so that excessive bleeding and compromise of exposure will not occur. Directly entering a hematoma without control usually provokes bleeding—the tamponade effect of the hematoma is lost, and bleeding will accelerate or, if previously stopped, will restart. Digital pressure will usually provide reasonable control of bleeding but handicaps the surgeon or assistant whose digit is now occupied. In addition, a finger in the surgical field presents an obstacle to better exposure, vascular control, and precise repair. To successfully repair a traumatic injury, the surgeon must know critical maneuvers for each vessel, know the anatomy for adequate exposure, and understand the anatomy of associated structures (e.g., veins and nerves) that need to be protected.

WATCH OUT FOR

Classic structures susceptible to injury when arterial repair is undertaken include the nerves adjacent to the brachial artery, which have a complex anatomy along the artery's course. The proximal brachial artery lateral to the axilla is covered anteriorly by the lateral and medial cords of the brachial plexus proximally, which branch into the median nerve (anterior to the artery) and the ulnar and musculocutaneous nerves posteriorly. A hematoma in the upper arm with potential injury to the proximal brachial artery must not be entered directly; to do so is likely to add an iatrogenic component to any nerve injury already present. Rather, formal proximal and distal control of the brachial artery before entering the hematoma is much safer.

Another common example of traumatic vascular injury is bleeding into the groin after angiographic access via the femoral artery. As most patients tolerate these procedures without a problem, the patient that bleeds is usually somehow "different," often from a coagulopathy, a diseased artery unable to physiologically contract, puncture at an unintended site or of a different artery, an anatomic anomaly, or

145

a more extensive injury than a simple puncture. Numerous types of injuries are encountered in this seemingly simple situation and include unintended profunda femoris artery puncture, tangential or oblique artery laceration, transection of a branch artery, arterial dissection, and combined arterial and venous injury. When any of these occur at or superior to the inguinal ligament, a component of the bleeding will be retroperitoneal, and the degree of preoperative blood loss may be grossly underestimated. Regardless, as the vessels are relatively anterior and the scope of injury limited, proximal exposure inferior to the inguinal ligament is usually adequate. In contrast, a penetrating knife or gunshot injury to the groin has a much greater range of potential injuries and should be accorded much greater respect for the potential severity of injury, with greater exposure obtained prior to entering the hematoma. In this example, proximal control will likely require exposure of the suprainguinal external iliac artery, and full distal control is desirable as well.

One final note is that interventional radiologic techniques can be utilized to help with vascular control. A radiologically placed occlusion balloon can be used as proximal control for an injury requiring surgical repair. Interventional placement of covered stents, metallic stents sheathed with vascular fabric (Dacron or Gore-Tex) can be used to cover short-segment arterial wall defects that are causing bleeding or feeding a pseudoaneurysm. Nonessential bleeding vessels can be embolized. Standard technique for management of femoral artery pseudoaneurysms (usually iatrogenic in nature) is no longer primarily surgical and includes ultrasound-guided compression and percutaneous injection of thrombin, both of which have high success rates and low complication rates.

SUGGESTED READINGS

Hoyt DB, Coimbra R, Potenza BM, Rappold JF. Anatomic exposure for vascular injuries. Surg Clin North Am 2001;81:6.

Radonic V, Baric D, Giunio L, et al. War injuries of the femoral artery and vein: a report on 67 cases. Cardiovasc Surg 1997;5:641–647.

Scalea T, Sclafani S. Interventional techniques in vascular trauma. Surg Clin North Am 2001;81:1281–1297.

Steinsapir ES, Coley BD, Fellmeth BD, Roberts AC, Hye RJ. Selective management of iatrogenic femoral artery injuries. J Surg Res 1993;55:109–113.

65

DO NOT USE A PERMANENTLY NON-ABSORBABLE SUTURE ON THE BLADDER OR URETER

MICHAEL J. MORITZ, MD

Permanent sutures in the urinary tract are at risk to become a nidus for stone formation. Presumably most permanent sutures become covered with urothelium (or epithelium in bowel); however, if they do protrude into the urinary stream, they can become a site where stones can begin to form.

WHAT TO DO

In years past, the use of absorbable sutures was a major problem because chromic gut was the longest-lasting absorbable suture, with strength lasting only 14 days under good circumstances and less in the presence of infected urine. Use of permanent sutures, either monofilament or braided, to avoid the high leak rate associated with chromic gut urinary anastamoses led to an increased incidence of late urinary stone formation. The availability of longer-lasting absorbable monofilament sutures (e.g., PDS and Maxon) quickly led to the abandonment of chromic gut for urinary anastamoses and their use yielded a lower leak rate from such anastamoses. Thus permanent suture is no longer necessary or used in urinary anastamoses.

The advent and popularity of staplers for gastrointestinal anastamoses has led to their use in urinary conduits. If this is the case, staples can protrude into the intestinal lumen where they are exposed to the urinary stream and, again, are a potential nidus for stone formation. Oversewing the staple line with absorbable suture will generally isolate the staple line from the urinary stream. In one report, more extensive laparoscopic urologic procedures, such as bladder augmentation, utilize staple lines within the urinary tract and only long-term follow up can determine the risk of stone formation in such patients.

The increasing use of laparoscopic techniques provides yet another scenario for stone formation, as most surgeons performing laparoscopic nephrectomy apply permanent clips to the distal ureter prior to transecting the ureter. To date, no reports have appeared of clip migration into the lumen of the urinary tract or of stone formation on the clip. However, clips used in tubal ligation procedures have rarely migrated into the peritoneal cavity, uterus, bladder, or appendix. In addition, clips used in laparoscopic cholecystectomy have rarely migrated into the common bile duct and also into the lungs via venous embolism.

SUGGESTED READINGS

Besson JM, Vinson RK, Leadbetter GW. Urolithiasis from stapler anastamoses. Am J Surg 1979;137:280–282.

Costello AJ, Johnson DE. Modified autosuture techniques for ileal conduit construction in urinary diversion. Aust N Z J Surg 1984;54:477–482.

Edlich RF, Rodeheaver GT, Thacker JG. Considerations in the choice of sutures for wound closure of the genitourinary tract. J Urol 1987;137:373–379.

Walsh PC, ed. Campbell's Urology. 8th Ed. Philadelphia: W.B. Saunders, 2002;Chapter 107,3791.

66

NEVER ASSUME YOU KNOW WHERE THE BLADDER IS—IT CAN LOOK A LOT LIKE THE COLON

MICHAEL J. MORITZ, MD

WATCH OUT FOR

In a pelvis filled with adherent bowel loops, identifying the bladder wall or avoiding the bladder when searching for other viscera can be a difficult task. One anatomy book truism for the bladder that is commonly of little help in the operating room is the anatomy of the bladder wall. It is classically described as having three muscle layers, which differs from the two-layered bowel wall. These three layers are inner longitudinal, middle circular, and outer longitudinal. However, even in the normal bladder, the three muscle layers become indistinct superiorly and anteriorly and away from the bladder neck. In the bladder altered by prior surgery or radiation, the muscle layers often appear fused and the muscle may be barely recognizable as such. In the atrophic bladder of the long-term dialysis patient, the muscle may not be recognizable at all. Hence, the three muscle layers are not a guide to distinguishing bladder from bowel.

Another example of altered anatomy occurs in prior bladder augmentation surgery (cystoplasty). An extensive variety of procedures are performed that utilize many different hollow lumen structures to enlarge the bladder's capacity, including stomach, small bowel, colon (from the gastrointestinal tract), and dilated ureter. Bowel-cystoplasty of any type will mandate preservation of the mesentery supplying the bowel that is anastamosed to the bladder. Foreknowledge of prior bladder surgery is key, as distinguishing these structures intraoperatively and preserving the blood supply to the augmentation can be exceedingly difficult. Additionally, an augmented bladder will be asymmetric, further increasing the difficulty of distinguishing bowel from bowel-as-part-of-the-bladder and from native bladder.

How then should the surgeon go about locating the bladder? If the retropubic space (anterior to the bladder, between the bladder and the symphysis pubis, eponymously the space of Retzius) has not been previously opened surgically, then this is the most reliable anatomic landmark and will easily define the anterior wall of the bladder. Entering the space of Retzius exposes the avascular space between the symphysis pubis anteriorly and the bladder posteriorly. It should be noted that this space will have been opened for operations anterior to the bladder; for example, suprapubic prostatectomy, suprapubic cystostomy, and renal transplants with a ureteroneocystostomy. If previously opened, the space will have adhesions, but bowel rarely comes between the bladder and the symphysis. Operations on the uterus, including cesearian section, open the space posterior to the bladder between the bladder and the uterus. As a consequence, there may be bowel loops adherent to the bladder's posterior wall, which should be anticipated by the surgeon.

In pelvic procedures where the peritoneal space seems obliterated from prior surgery, inflammation or radiation, minimizing dissection saves time and avoids unintentional surgical entero-, colo-, and cystotomies. Palpating the Foley balloon can be difficult in a scarred field and can be unreliable, but filling the bladder retrograde via the Foley tubing will make it easier to define the bladder. Rather than have a nurse or nursing assistant crawl under the drapes to reach the Foley, consider inserting a three-way catheter before the surgical procedure begins. This will allow the bladder to empty urine as the case proceeds, and then, when appropriate, will allow the bladder to be distended with fluid.

WHAT TO DO

Palpating the bladder as it is filled (and/or emptied) gives a tactile appreciation of the bladder wall and whether bowel loops are adherent to it. Once the bladder is full, it assumes its smooth, ovoid shape, making it much easier to define the bladder wall and dissect other viscera off of it. This technique is useful for defining the superior wall of the bladder, but the bladder will need to be successively deflated to carry the dissection posteriorly. Another useful technique is palpating what is thought to be the bladder as it is filling; observe then if the flow from the fluid bag attached to the three-way Foley catheter stops or slows as the bladder is decompressed and the inflow occluded.

SUGGESTED READINGS

Grant JCB. An Atlas of Anatomy. 6th Ed. Baltimore: Williams & Wilkins, 1972: Figures 203, 236.
Rink RC. Bladder augmentation: options, outcomes, future. Urolog Clin North Am 1999;26:111–123.

67

AVOID INITIALLY GRABBING THE APPENDIX OR TIP OF APPENDIX WHEN DOING A LAPAROSCOPIC APPENDECTOMY

MICHAEL J. MORITZ, MD

Most cases of appendicitis start with obstruction of the appendiceal lumen. This may be from lymphoid hyperplasia, inspissated stool (fecalith), foreign body, or tumor. The mechanism of appendicitis likely follows a pattern of luminal obstruction, continued mucous secretion and bacterial overgrowth causing distention of the lumen, a rise in intraluminal pressure, venous obstruction, and edema. The ensuing acute inflammatory response results in more edema, vascular compromise and ischemia (and translocation of bacteria through the wall). The ischemic appendix then progresses to necrosis and perforation.

WHAT NOT TO DO

The key point of the above described pathophysiology is to understand that the area of compromised wall starts at the point of luminal obstruction and extends towards the tip. Until the entire appendix has been visualized, one cannot know whether or where the wall is compromised. When performing laparoscopic appendectomy, grasping the appendix on initial visualization and pulling anteriorly to expose the appendix and cecum can lead to the appendix coming apart at the point of obstruction, increasing the soilage of the peritoneum, increases the difficulty in visualizing and controlling the base of the appendix, and can require conversion to an open procedure.

The correct technique is to very gently and bluntly maneuver the appendix and surrounding tissues from side to side and up and down (as a kitten bats a ball of yarn between its paws) to separate tissue planes and gradually expose the cecum and appendiceal base. The cecal wall is uninvolved in uncomplicated appendicitis and can be safely grasped and retracted anteriorly. By putting traction on the cecum and continuing gentle blunt dissection, the appendix from the base to the tip can be freed up enough to identify the pathology and determine the plan for controlling the mesoappendix and the appendiceal stump. Once the appendix has been completely freed and inspected, it can then be safely grasped with a minimum of traction placed on it to improve the exposure for the subsequent steps in appendectomy.

The mesoappendix is usually divided first. Numerous methods for division are safe and effective, including bipolar cautery, harmonic scalpel, clips, ties (preformed loops), and the laparoscopic stapler with a vascular cartridge. Next, the appendix is ligated with preformed loops or a stapler with a gastrointestinal staple load. The appendix is removed through a specimen bag or similar device to protect the wound from further contamination. The procedure concludes after the peritoneum is lavaged, hemostasis checked, unintended injury sought, the trocars removed, and the sites closed.

What should the surgeon do if, despite her best intentions, the appendix disrupts from manipulation? One option is to convert to an open procedure, particularly if the avulsion leaves an insufficient stump for reliable control using laparoscopic methods or if visualization is difficult, whether because of body habitus, adhesions, inflammatory changes, and so on. If the cecum can be identified and manipulated to allow exposure of the appendiceal base, then one can proceed with the laparoscopic procedure with the difference that the open appendiceal stump is ligated before the mesoappendix is controlled. If the appendix has been avulsed, it is important not to lose the separate piece of appendix—it must be removed, preferably in a bag to reduce the risk of wound infection. It must be remembered that the distal avulsed segment may have attached mesoappendix that requires control before it can be freed for extraction from the peritoneal cavity. Finally, the abdominal cavity should be lavaged thoroughly as in perforated appendicitis.

SUGGESTED READINGS

Easter DW. The diagnosis and treatment of acute appendicitis with laparoscopic methods. In Hunter JG, Sackier JM, eds. Minimally Invasive Surgery. New York: McGraw-Hill, 1993:171–177. http://www.laparoscopyhospital.com/lap%20app.htm.

Wagner M, Aronsky D, Tschudi J, Metzger A, Klaiber C. Laparoscopic stapler appendectomy: a prospective study of 267 consecutive cases. Surg Endosc 1996;10:895–899.

68

DO NOT INITIALLY CLOSE THE SKIN COMPLETELY AFTER DOING FASCIOTOMY FOR COMPARTMENT SYNDROME

JAMES HERRINGTON, MD

Compartment syndrome is a phenomenon that occurs in enclosed body spaces. It has been described in the abdomen, thorax, orbit, cranial vault, and the extremity compartments. Compartment syndrome pathophysiology is characterized by increased pressure in an enclosed, rigid space that exceeds capillary perfusion pressure, resulting in ischemia of the compartment contents. Intracompartmental damage is directly related to the extent and duration of increased pressure. Complications of a missed diagnosis in an extremity include infection and muscle necrosis with hyperkalemia and myoglobinuria. The tenet of treatment is prompt relief of the pressure in the affected compartment.

Compartment syndrome begins with an initial insult such as trauma (e.g., fractures, crush injuries, electrical injuries, vascular injuries, snakebites, severe overexertion of muscle groups) or extremity ischemia. Nontraumatic etiologies are more varied. Arterial occlusion for greater than six hours with reperfusion of an ischemic extremity results in edema and toxic oxygen radical production that may cause a compartment syndrome. External pressure from bandages or casts can cause compartment syndrome by restricting the inflow and outflow of the extremity. The offending cast/bandage should be removed promptly if there are any signs of hypoperfusion to the distal extremity. Malpositioning of patients on the operating room table can result in excessive pressure on an extremity and subsequent compartment syndrome. Extravasation of medications and blood products from intravenous catheters can rapidly cause a compartment syndrome, as can intracompartmental bleeding from coagulopathy or anticoagulation.

SIGNS AND SYMPTOMS

The diagnosis of compartment syndrome is based on clinical suspicion with the aid of adjunctive tests. Severe pain in the compartment, often out of proportion to the perceived injury, is an early symptom. Excruciating pain upon passive stretch of a muscle in the compartment, such as plantar flexing the great toe to test the anterior compartment of the calf, is a helpful finding. The earliest neurologic findings are tingling and numbness. Paralysis is a late finding. Pulselessness and pallor of the distal extremity are also late findings unless there is a concomitant vascular injury. With the exception of the deep posterior compartment (which cannot be appreciated by palpation), the affected compartment will be firm on palpation.

In addition to clinical exam, compartment pressures in the extremities can be directly measured. A large-bore needle is connected via pressure tubing to a pressure transducer. The needle is inserted into the compartment and a pressure reading obtained. Commercial devices include a product manufactured by Stryker Instruments that uses a side port to measure the pressure, as tissue occlusion of a straight needle's tip will result in an inaccurate reading. Strict numerical parameters for diagnosis as an indication for surgery do not exist. The lowest capillary pressure necessary to perfuse tissue is in the range of 30 mm Hg. In general, normal compartment pressures are less than 20 mm Hg, pressures of 20 to 30 mm Hg are marginal, whereas pressures above 30 mm Hg are abnormal and may be indication for compartment release in the appropriate clinical setting. Many experienced clinicians do not use the compartment pressure alone, but rather calculate the difference between the compartment pressure and the diastolic pressure when deciding on intervention.

For extremity compartments, treatment consists of fasciotomies. The number of compartments varies; the arm has three; the forearm has two; the hand has two plus eight intrinsic compartments; and the thigh has three. The calf is the region most commonly affected by compartment syndrome. The four calf compartments are the anterior, lateral, posterior superficial, and the posterior deep compartments.

WHAT TO DO

Calf fasciotomies are performed via medial and lateral incisions at least 15 cm in length, extending from the upper part of the tibia or fibula to the medial or lateral malleolus. The lateral incision is placed approximately 2 fingerbreadths posterior to the tibia to release the anterior and lateral compartments. The medial incision is placed approximately 2 fingerbreadths posterior to the tibia to open the superficial and deep posterior compartments. Fascial membranes should be incised the entire length of the compartment. Inadequate fasciotomies can result in recurrent compartment syndrome, resulting in a return to the operating room and a trip to the lectern at the morbidity and mortality conference. With the release of pressure, muscle should bulge through the fasciotomy sites. Muscle should be inspected for viability and necrotic tissue debrided. As the goal of fasciotomy is the release of excessive compartment pressure, the fasciotomy skin incisions should never be closed at the initial operation for compartmental release. Often, bulging muscle precludes closure. If the skin is closed, a compartment syndrome can redevelop in the extremity. Frequent dressing changes are employed to reassess muscle viability. To partially reapproximate the skin, the rubber band or vessel loop technique can be employed. At the time of fasciotomy, sterile rubber bands or vessel loops are stapled to the wound edges in a zigzag fashion or in the shape of a rectangle. These can rapidly be released if there is any sign of recurrent compartment syndrome. As the edema subsides, the tension on the rubber bands will bring the wound edges closer together until the rubber bands are lax. They are then stapled in additional places to maintain tension.

Wound closure can be accomplished after the edema subsides. In the last several years, the use of the WoundVac system manufactured by KCI has been employed to reduce swelling of the tissue. Timing of definitive closure is a matter of clinical judgment, based on visual inspection of the wounds, palpation of the compartment, and assessment of the patient's mobilization of edema. The fascia is never reapproximated. If possible, the skin edges are reapproximated with sutures or staples. Skin grafts may be required to cover the wound. If not all skin incisions can be closed, for optimal cosmesis the more visible side should be closed and the less visible one grafted.

SUGGESTED READINGS

Cameron JL, ed. Current Surgical Therapy. 7th Ed. Philadelphia: Mosby, 2001:1140–1144.

Davies MG, Hagen PO. The vascular endothelium. A new horizon. Ann Surg 1993;218:593–609.

Harris KA, Walker PM, Mickle DA, et al. Metabolic response of skeletal muscle to ischemia. Am J Physiol 1986;250:213–220.

Moore RE, Friedman RJ. Current concepts in pathophysiology and diagnosis of compartment syndrome. J Emerg Med 1989;7:657–662.

Rowe VL, Salim A, Lipham J, Asensio JA. Shank vessel injuries. Surg Clin North Am 2002;82:91–104.

Velmahos GC, Toutouzas KG. Vascular trauma and compartment syndromes. Surg Clin North Am 2002;82:125–141.

USE BLUNT DISSECTION WHEN DOING AN EMERGENCY VENOUS CUTDOWN

MICHAEL J. MORITZ, MD

Venous cutdown for venous access is a procedure used less and less often in clinical medicine. Indeed, many recent and current trainees have never seen nor done one. The technique was popularized in the trauma resuscitation protocols of the military during the Vietnam War. During its heyday, cutdown on the saphenous vein at the medial malleolus was a standard procedure for inhospital cardiac arrest/resuscitation and in some trauma centers. The impetus for this was the high complication rate of subclavian vein puncture in patients during cardiac arrest and a general lack of expertise in alternative routes of central venous access. Also, in the trauma setting, a cutdown provided the opportunity for a much larger caliber access than the percutaneous devices then in existence, with correspondingly higher flow rates.

Despite the increasingly infrequent use of the cutdown technique, it can still be useful in select situations. For example, venous cutdown is still a good technique in severely hypovolemic patients with chest injuries where upper torso lines may not be accurately placed. The technique of venous cutdown is reviewed in depth in the first of the Suggested Reading references and many older sources. When performing this procedure, four sites that are quickly accessible include the saphenous vein at the ankle, the saphenous vein at the fossa ovalis (just inferior and superficial to the saphenofemoral junction), the median basilic vein 1 cm from the median epicondyle of the elbow, and the cephalic vein laterally in the antecubital crease. Exposure of the arm veins or the ankle saphenous vein in the emergency situation requires a full thickness skin incision followed by blunt dissection through the subcutaneous tissue using a hemostat or gauze pads *parallel* to the vein. Dissection perpendicular to the vein is likely to directly injure the vein or "twang" it hard enough to send it into vasospasm, making identification and cannulation difficult. Dissection with scissors is discouraged, both for fear of injuring the vein and the risk to the cutaneous (sensory) nerve(s) adjacent to each of the above veins.

WHAT TO DO

As opposed to the more superficial cutdown sites in the arm and ankle, exposure of the saphenous vein in the proximal thigh allows access to the largest superficial vein available for placement of very large cannulas, but this vein is significantly deeper than the other sites and therefore requires more surgical expertise. It is also much closer to the trunk and hence is awkward to access when cardiac compressions, diagnostic peritoneal lavage, or other procedures on the trunk are being performed. The anatomy and technique are rather different than for the other veins described above. The saphenous vein in the thigh lies just superficial to the superficial fascia of the thigh, but is still relatively "deep." The saphenous nerve is in proximity. As it approaches the fossa ovalis, there are at least three or four relatively constant branches radiating superiorly, medially, and laterally, fixing its location and making blunt dissection trickier. With the exception of the superior branch(es), none of the branches will be superficial; they are all in the same plane or deeper. Accordingly, the safest approach is through a longitudinal incision directly over its anticipated course (on a vertical line through the pubic tubercle with the thigh gently abducted and externally rotated and the knee slightly bent to expose the medial thigh). After a full-thickness skin incision, medial and lateral distracting traction with two or three fingers on sponges should part the subcutaneous fat down to the superficial fascia, making it relatively easy to find the proximal saphenous vein. The femoral nerve is much deeper and lateral to the intervening femoral artery. The saphenous nerve is quite close, just medial to the vein, and hard to identify without good lighting.

In an emergency, percutaneous puncture of the femoral vein is faster than a cutdown and not very risky, even with a bleeding diathesis; however, there are two major cautions. First, there must be a palpable femoral artery pulse to safely puncture the femoral vein. Second, the surgeon should not attempt to puncture the femoral vein too far proximally, particularly in a patient with a clotting problem. Once the needle is above the inguinal ligament, any vascular injury will not be detectable, will not be compressed or be compressible manually, and will continue to bleed into the retroperitoneum until manifest by hypovolemia and vascular collapse, pain, or paralytic ileus. Finally, increasing availability of bedside ultrasound for indirect visualization of vessels while being punctured has increased the safety of jugular and femoral venous cannulation. Only the limited availability of the devices and the set-up time restrict ultrasound-guided central venous cannulation from even wider use.

SUGGESTED READINGS

Asheim P, Mostad U, Aadahl P. Ultrasound-guided central venous cannulation in infants and children. Acta Anaesthesiologica Scandinavica 2002;46(4):390–392.
Keenan SP. Use of ultrasound to place central lines. J Crit Care 2002;17:126–137.

Muhm M. Ultrasound guided central venous access: is useful for beginners, in children, and when blind cannulation fails. BMJ 2002;325:1373–1374.

Robert JR II, Hedges JR, eds. Clinical Procedures in Emergency Medicine. 3rd Ed. Philadelphia: W.B. Saunders, 1998:341–351.

Westfall MD, Price KR, Lambert M, et al. Intravenous access in the critically ill trauma patient: a multicentered, prospective, randomized trial of saphenous cutdown and percutaneous femoral access. Ann Emerg Med 1994;23:541–545.

70

MAKE SURE THAT BREAST BIOPSY SITES ARE BONE DRY BEFORE CLOSING

MICHAEL J. MORITZ, MD

Although somewhat being replaced by stereotactic needle biopsy, excisional breast biopsy is still a common procedure for palpable and nonpalpable breast lesions to diagnose or exclude breast cancer. Nonpalpable mammographic abnormalities are biopsied after a needle is placed using mammographic guidance (needle-guided breast biopsy) or, if the area is definable with ultrasound, with intraoperative ultrasonic guidance. Fortunately, less than 20% of breast biopsies are malignant.

The skin incisions used for excisional breast biopsy are determined by aesthetic and oncologic considerations. Aesthetically, the lines of tension of the skin of the breast run generally concentrically around the nipple. The least visible incision is along the areolar margin (i.e., a periareolar incision). Oncologically, the skin of the biopsy should be part of the excised tissue in the event a mastectomy later will be necessary, a consideration of diminishing importance with current breast cancer treatments. Most of the breast can be reached for biopsy via a periareolar incision of up to 50% of the circumference of the areola.

Deep breast lesions or those more than a centimeter or two from the areola will be exposed by a tunnel from the periareolar incision. After the specimen is removed, exposure of the biopsy bed may not be of the best quality and distortion of the breast by retractors can mask bleeding. This can be troublesome for the surgeon. Breast parenchyma is surprisingly vascular and there is no tamponade from adjacent structures, so any residual oozing can lead to a considerable hematoma. Closing the space left by the biopsy with sutures does lead to a small decrease in the incidence of breast hematoma but at the expense of significant distortion of the breast contour and increased asymmetry of the breasts. Use of local anesthesia containing epinephrine and of compression and drainage have no impact on the incidence or severity of postbiopsy breast hematoma. The old standbys for scrupulous hemostasis are electrocautery and suture ligature, as these are the only means of minimizing hematoma formation.

When they occur, breast hematomas present several problems. They can be exceedingly painful. They are slow to heal and lead to a broader scar. Managed without surgery, breast hematomas will slowly resorb over several months; however, a painful swollen breast from a hematoma is often best managed with reoperation. A short procedure under general anesthesia to evacuate the clot will rarely disclose any active bleeding, but will relieve the discomfort and lead to a better cosmetic result.

SUGGESTED READINGS

Bland KI, Copeland EM 3rd, eds. The Breast: Comprehensive Management of Benign and Malignant Diseases. 2nd Ed. Philadelphia: WB Saunders Company, 1998:802–816.

Strombeck JO, Rosato FE, eds. Surgery of the Breast: Diagnosis and Treatment of Breast Diseases. New York: Thieme, 1986:40–47.

71

PLACE THE MARKING STITCHES TO ORIENT THE SPECIMEN FOR PATHOLOGY *BEFORE* EXCISING A LESION THAT MAY BE MALIGNANT

MICHAEL J. MORITZ, MD

A biopsy is done to provide tissue for a histologic diagnosis and to guide further therapy. An open biopsy (excisional versus incisional) or needle biopsy (core for histology versus aspiration for cytology) is chosen based on factors related to patient, site, likely diagnosis, lesion size, and so on. For an open biopsy, there are additional considerations. These include the ability to excise the entire biopsy site and the provision of adequate tissue. If a biopsy has malignancy present at any margin, the malignancy has the capability to implant throughout the incision. Thus the incision chosen for open biopsy must be capable of being re-excised. In addition, an open biopsy specimen must be adequate for histology and for any additional studies. For example, estrogen and progesterone receptor analyses are most accurate on fresh tissue such as obtained at open breast biopsy. In contrast, the breast tissue in a mastectomy specimen will have additional ischemia while the axillary dissection is being performed, decreasing the accuracy of receptor analyses.

WATCH OUT FOR

For most malignancies, adequate local control requires a margin of normal tissue of 1 cm or greater thickness between the tumor and the edge of the specimen. More aggressive tumors require larger margins; for example, deep melanomas require a minimum margin of 2 cm. The orientation of the biopsy specimen is key if further surgery may be needed to provide the appropriate margins. If a biopsy has a positive margin, the next step in treatment (depending on the tumor type, location, curability, etc.) will often be a re-excision to remove residual cancer and obtain negative margins. While a positive margin "contaminates" the field and the entire biopsy site should be re-excised, extra tissue will be removed from the positive margin itself. Regarding the orientation of a pathologic specimen, *the onus is on the surgeon to provide the pathologist with the landmarks necessary to allow a meaningful interpretation of the biopsy.* Some biopsies will be partially oriented by the tissue; for example, skin orients superficial versus deep but not medial/lateral and superior/inferior. If no landmark is

included then the tissue's orientation will be impossible to discern unless the surgeon provides guidance by marking the specimen with clips or sutures.

An example of the importance of correctly marking specimens is a hypothetical 1.5 cm diameter subcutaneous tumor that extends near the muscle fascia. An excisional biopsy is done leaving tissue intact over the fascia. The biopsy is positive for cancer, and one margin is positive for tumor, but the specimen was not oriented. The patient needs a re-excision to negative margins in all directions. Had the deep margin been marked and negative, the fascia would not require excision, and the deeper tissue plane would not be violated at re-excision.

Orientation of a biopsy specimen must be clearly marked by the surgeon and the markers clearly described to the pathologist to facilitate proper pathologic interpretation. The proper handling and labeling of excised tissue is the surgeon's responsibility. To orient the specimen properly for the pathologist, the secure sutures or clips used as markers should be placed *before* the specimen is removed if possible; once removed, orientation can be lost. In complex specimens, the markers should be varied by type (sutures versus clips) or color (sutures come in many colors) to help the pathologist with the specimen. The surgeon should adopt a routine in orienting specimens (e.g., lateral margin marked with long suture, deep margin with double sutures). Care should be taken that the orientation markers are accurately listed on the pathology request that accompanies the specimen.

SUGGESTED READINGS

Luu HH, Otis CN, Reed WP Jr., Garb JL, Frank JL. The unsatisfactory margin in breast cancer surgery. Am J Surg 1999;178:362–366.

Neuschatz AC, DiPetrillo T, Safaii H, et al. Margin width as a determinant of local control with and without radiation therapy for ductal carcinoma in situ (DCIS) of the breast. Int J Cancer 2001;96:97–104.

72

DO NOT DO A SHAVE BIOPSY ON A LESION SUSPICIOUS FOR MELANOMA

X. D. DONG, MD

The incidence of melanoma and the mortality from this malignancy is rising. The lifetime risk of melanoma for individuals of white ethnicity is 1.74% for men and 1.28% for women. Over the past 30 years, the incidence of melanoma in the United States has been rising approximately 4% per year, from 5.7 cases per 100,000 population in 1973 to 13.3 cases per 100,000 in 1995. During the same time period, the mortality of melanoma has risen by 1.3% per year. The best strategy of dealing with melanoma is prevention through protection of the skin from sun exposure. As patients with localized, early stage disease have an excellent outcome, early detection is a critical determinant of the stage at diagnosis and, therefore, of prognosis. Melanoma detected at more advanced stages has a much greater lethality. Staging is a vital component of determining the extent of treatment needed to maximize the potential for cure. Proper staging of melanoma depends on the histologic determination of the depth and extent of invasion, which makes it imperative that a proper biopsy be performed for staging, prognosis, and treatment purposes.

Melanoma was first staged by Clark et al in 1967 based on invasion through the dermal layers, with progressively poorer prognoses correlated with invasion into deeper dermal layers. In 1970, Breslow et al described staging based on the depth of invasion measured in millimeters from the skin surface. In general, there is a good correlation between Clark level and Breslow depth, although Breslow's staging has mostly replaced Clark's in the current AJCC (American Joint Committee on Cancer) staging of melanoma due to its lower interobserver variability.

Prognosis for melanoma worsens with each advancing stage. Mortality rates associated with Breslow depth of invasion of 1 mm, 3 mm, and 6 mm are 10%, 45%, and 70%, respectively at 10 years. The new AJCC melanoma staging system is based on the thickness of the primary lesion, nodal status, and presence of metastatic disease. Changes compared with former AJCC systems include the addition of the following factors: ulceration in the primary, distinguishing microscopic from macroscopic lymph node metastases, and separating different sites of distant metastases.

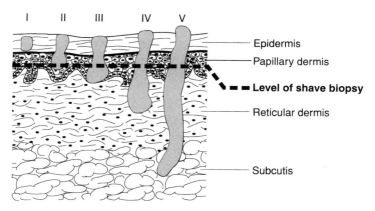

FIGURE 72.1. The Clark levels of invasion with typical depth of shave biopsy.

Given the implications from the proper staging of melanoma, it is important to perform the biopsy properly. However, biopsy techniques for skin lesions vary and can be an area of confusion. A brief description of standard skin biopsy techniques follows.

An **excisional biopsy** refers to complete removal of a suspicious lesion. This is performed with a narrow margin of clinically normal tissue, which in this context would be in the range of 2 mm (do not confuse with margins for wide local excision, which are measured in centimeters). An **incisional biopsy** is used to sample only a part of a suspicious lesion for histologic evaluation. Because it does not remove the entire lesion, incisional biopsies may limit the dermatopathologist's ability to detect a melanoma or to accurately determine depth of invasion, based on sampling error within a lesion. **Punch biopsy** refers to the use of a sharp circular instrument to remove a cylinder of tissue into the subcutaneous fat. Punches are available in diameters ranging from 1.5 mm to 1 cm. They are used for excisional or incisional biopsies. Punch biopsies can be closed with sutures or allowed to heal by secondary intention. **Shave biopsy** refers to a shallow removal of a lesion at a depth confined to the dermis. It can be performed by a scalpel, a Dermablade, a razor blade, or scissors. The biopsy site is not closed and is allowed to heal by secondary intention. The shave biopsy provides no information on the depth of a lesion; hence, any malignancy diagnosed via this technique will require re-excision. Specifically with melanoma, however, a prior shave biopsy will distort measures of the depth of invasion, making treatment decisions very difficult and making the prognosis uncertain(*Figure 72.1*).

Protruding raised skin lesions, such as low-grade basal cell carcinomas and squamous cell carcinomas, are often diagnosed based on shave biopsies. Shave biopsy is also appropriate for the management of benign lesions such as skin tags and seborrheic keratoses. However, any pigmented lesion that might be melanoma must *never* be subjected to a shave biopsy. Recognition that melanomas may be hypopigmented, variegated, or amelanotic (colorless, usually white) makes shave biopsy problematic for any lesion that might remotely be a melanoma.

Which lesions may possibly be melanomas? The **ABCDE** mnemonic can be helpful, remembering Asymmetry, Border irregularity, Color variation, Diameter (7 mm), and Elevation (although melanomas may also ulcerate) (*Figure 72.2*). Color variation includes both variation within a lesion and the spectrum from melanotic to amelanotic coloration amongst melanomas. In addition, MacKie described seven warning signs of melanoma. The three major signs are changes in the size, shape, or color of a mole. The four minor signs are the presence of inflammation as seen by a reddening of the mole; crusting or bleeding; a sensory change, sometimes felt as merely an increased awareness of the mole; and a diameter greater than 7 mm. In a study of 100 lesions, 94, 95, and 89 had changes in size, shape, and color, respectively, and all 100 had at least one of the minor signs. The current recommendation is that any one of the major signs is cause for referral, and the additional presence of a minor sign should provide added stimulus. The purpose of these criteria is not to diagnose melanoma, but to provide guidelines for the patient to decide whether to consult a physician and for the physician to decide if referral for biopsy and pathologic evaluation of the mole is warranted.

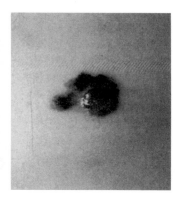

FIGURE 72.2. Irregular borders and satellite lesions in a melanoma.

Of course, the prudence of being examined regularly (at least once a year) by a dermatologist experienced in recognizing melanomas can not be argued against. However, of some consternation to surgeons is the frequency of referral from a dermatologist with a diagnosis of melanoma on a *shave biopsy*!

WHAT TO DO

Lesions that might be melanoma require a biopsy technique that includes the full thickness of the skin (to assess depth of invasion). For small lesions in little noticed areas, an excisional biopsy with a 2 mm margin, including subcutaneous fat, is ideal. Large lesions or those in cosmetically sensitive areas may be best approached with a partial, full-thickness biopsy (i.e., an incisional biopsy), again including subcutaneous tissue. A punch biopsy that is full thickness can also be acceptable. In any partial biopsy, inclusion of both uninvolved skin and the most suspicious portion of the lesion is necessary, but the potential for sampling errors is real. Overall, the prognosis is not greatly affected by the choice of technique between proper types of biopsy, specifically punch, incisional, excisional, and wide excisional biopsies; however, an excisional biopsy is slightly preferred as it provides the entire lesion without potential sampling error.

Biopsy-proven melanoma will generally be treated with a wide local excision including all of the biopsy site and a margin of uninvolved tissue (the size of the margin is determined by the location of the primary lesion and the depth of invasion), thus partial biopsies need to be planned with this in mind. Balch et al have examined the adequacy on a 2 cm margin for melanomas from 1 to 4 mm in depth and found it adequate to prevent local recurrence as compared to a 4 cm margin. Even with these recommendations, a 2 cm margin on all sides of a lesion would mean a skin defect more than 4 cm in diameter following excision of a 1 mm depth melanoma lesion. Hence, the biopsy must be planned with the possibility that the entire biopsy field will need to be excised in the future.

SUGGESTED READINGS

Balch CM, Soong S, Smith T, et al. Investigators from the Intergroup Surgical Melanoma Trial. Long-term results of a prospective surgical trial comparing 2 cm vs. 4 cm excision margins for 740 patients with 1-4 mm melanomas. Ann Surg Oncol 2001;8:101–108.

Helfand M, Mahon SM, Eden KB, Orleans CT. Screening for skin cancer. Am J Prev Med 2001;20:47–58.

Holmes EC, Moseley HS, Morton DL, et al. A rational approach to the surgical management of melanoma Ann Surg 1977;186:481–490.

Kim CJ, Reintgen DS, Balch, C.M. AJCC Melanoma Staging Committe. The new melanoma staging system. Cancer Control 2002;9:9–15.

MacKie RM. Clinical recognition of early invasive malignant melanoma. BMJ 1990; 301:1005.

Marinez JC, Otley CC. The management of melanoma and nonmelanoma skin cancer: a review for the primary care physician. Mayo Clinic Proc 2001;76:1253–1265.

Sabiston DC Jr, ed. Textbook of Surgery-The biological basis of modern surgical practice, 15th Ed. Philadelphia: W.B. Saunders, 1997:515–528.

73

HANDLE SUTURES WITH PROPER TECHNIQUE TO DECREASE FASCIAL DEHISCENCE.

RAMON RIVERA, MD

Healing of abdominal wounds requires adequate quality of the tissue edges and appropriate technical reapproximation. The two technical factors associated with fascial dehiscence are suture tearing through fascia in 70% to 90% of cases and suture failure in 10% to 30% of cases. The major technical factor causing suture tearing is excessively tight suturing with resultant fascial failure; this is independent of a running versus interrupted closure. The second technical factor, suture failure, occurs either from suture breakage or a knot becoming untied.

WHAT TO DO

Suture failure generally occurs only with monofilament suture. The type monofilament sutures (absorbable versus nonabsorbable) has not been shown to be a factor in fascial failure as long as the half-life of the suture is 6 weeks or greater. Monofilament sutures have a relatively high tensile strength and a relatively low shear strength. Monofilament failure usually occurs immediately adjacent to the knot, where tensile force is converted to shear stress and the shear is greatest. Monofilament is significantly weakened by physical damage, particularly crush, twist, and fray forces. Therefore, running monofilament closures must be carefully executed with correct handling of the suture material to avoid the above injuries and careful attention given to anchoring the knots. Before starting, the suture should be inspected to insure there is no preexisting damage from manufacturing. Every few bites the suture should be gently slid between the fingers toward the free needle to eliminate twists that increase shear stress. In addition, the suture should never be grasped with an instrument.

Suture slippage resulting in an "undone knot" results from improper knot-tying technique that allows the knot to slide and loosen. Proper knot tying is easiest with a two-handed technique, particularly for the crucial second throw to avoid the slip knots and jerking and straining associated with tying a one-handed knot under tension. Generally, sliding knots result from granny knots and from improperly tied square knots. Granny knots are formed from two suture throws in the same direction. Square knots result from two throws in opposite directions. It is important to note that when one of the strands of either one of these knots is held under tension and the other strand is tied around it (as with one-handed ties under tension), a slip knot results that can easily loosen. It is imperative that knots anchoring fascial closures are tied without excessive tension in a square and flat configuration.

To briefly review, the two monofilaments in common use for fascial closure are polypropylene (Prolene) and polydioxanone (PDS). Both are stiff and require multiple bulky knots for best knot security. Polypropylene is a permanent synthetic suture similar to nylon but with better handling properties. PDS is a slowly absorbed synthetic suture with handling slightly better than Prolene that retains approximately 50% of its strength 6 weeks after implantation. A third monofilament suture that may be encountered is Goretex (ePTFE). This is a permanent, synthetic, porous monofilament material with properties of both braided sutures (resistance to mechanical trauma, susceptibility to infection, ease of handling, inconspicuous knots, high tensile, and shear strength) and monofilament sutures (requires many throws to form a secure knot). The chief negative aspects of Gortex are that it is not as slippery as the other monofilaments and, if it becomes infected, it forms suture sinuses and must be removed.

One final note is that abdominal wound dehiscence is associated with several factors of patient origin including obesity, malnutrition, diabetes mellitus, corticosteroid use, chronic obstructive pulmonary disease, prior radiation therapy, and wound infection. Even a perfect technical closure has an increased risk of dehiscence in these patients.

SUGGESTED READINGS

Cameron JL, ed. Current Surgical Therapy. 7th ed. St. Louis: Mosby, 2001: 1196–2000.

Dinsmore RC. Understanding surgical knot security: a proposal to standardize the literature. J Am Coll Surg 1995;180:689–699.

Kon ND, Martin MB, Kawamoto E, et al. Abdominal wound closure: a comparison of polypropylene and Teflon-coated braided Dacron sutures. Am Surg 1984;50:549–551.

DO NOT REACH ONTO THE SCRUB NURSE'S TABLE WITHOUT PERMISSION

MICHAEL J. MORITZ, MD

Proper operating room (OR) etiquette holds that the Mayo stand is the province of the scrub assistant and no one else should reach onto the Mayo stand for anything. The Mayo stand, or its larger cousin the Gerhard, is the scrub assistant's primary repository for often used instruments during a procedure including clamps, sutures, ties, scalpels and so on. In an earlier time, etiquette in the OR was quite rigid and no one would dare to invade another individual's space or responsibility.

Today, the surgical team works in a more relaxed, less hierarchical atmosphere and etiquette matters less now than before. When the scrub is otherwise occupied, gowning and gloving other members of the team, receiving requested instruments, and so on, it is tempting to help oneself by taking what is needed from the carefully laid out instruments. However, this violates the rationale for leaving the Mayo stand exclusively for the scrub assistant—the scrub is responsible for passing instruments to the surgical team and cannot do so quickly if another person has altered the setup. If this happens, then the scrub must hunt among the rearranged instruments, frustrating the team and slowing the case. There are now additional important reasons to respect old customs, namely sharps (scalpels, suture needles, etc.) and the associated risk of accidental injury and bloodborne infections. When two individuals are competing for instruments on the Mayo, the possibility of accidental injury to the operator (whose hand is in an unexpected locale where it does not belong) is increased. The passage of sharps between the surgeon and the scrub has a defined technique. In some instances, the scrub will request or oblige a surgeon's request to create a landing area for sharps being returned to the scrub assistant. The landing area may be on the Mayo stand in certain circumstances but only with the expressed permission of the scrub. Trying to help by placing sharps in an unexpected locale does no one a favor. Helping oneself to instruments from the Mayo is an invitation to an accidental sharps injury and an undoubted irritated scrub.

SUGGESTED READINGS

Gruendemann BJ, Fernsebner B. Surgical instrumentation. In Comprehensive Perioperative Nursing, Vol. 2, Practice. Boston: Jones & Bartlett, 1995;13:15.

DO NOT CALL THE ANESTHESIOLOGISTS OR NURSE ANESTHETISTS "ANESTHESIA" OR "DR. ANESTHESIA"

CATHERINE MARCUCCI, MD

This is one of the simplest items pertaining to operating room (OR) etiquette, and it is astounding how often it is ignored. Nurse anesthetists are accustomed to being addressed by their first names, and anesthesiologists are generally split as to whether they prefer to be addressed by their first names or their professional titles. It is fine for the junior and senior members on a surgical team to discuss whether the OR has been called and "anesthesia" notified that a patient is coming up from the emergency room, and so on; but, once the surgeon enters a room with unfamiliar anesthesia personnel, an introduction should be proffered with care taken to learn the anesthesiologist's and nurse anesthetist's names. This is just common sense and common courtesy in addition to improving communication, outcomes, and preventing errors. These professionals are not ancillary members of the operating room team and should not be treated as such. To put this courtesy into perspective, if the interventional radiology attending physician or the gastroenterologist is called to do a procedure, would the surgeon and ask "Dr. Radiology" if the sheath had been withdrawn or "Dr. Endoscope" if the bleeding site in the colon had been identified?

EMERGENCY DEPARTMENT

OPERATING ROOM

MEDICATIONS

LINES, DRAINS, AND TUBES

BLEEDING

GASTROINTESTINAL TRACT

WARDS

INTENSIVE CARE UNIT

LABORATORY

76

Make sure that intravascular medications are not inadvertently placed in the extravascular space and extravascular medications are not placed intravascularly

Michael J. Moritz, MD

Although daunting to the novice, injections to the more experienced practitioner quickly become routine and mundane. Yet the complications of misplaced injections can be quite severe. Medications for intravenous injection are usually very different chemically from medications intended for extravascular (i.e., subcutaneous, intramuscular, intra-articular, etc.) routes of administration and contamination of all unintended sites can be quite problematic.

WHAT TO DO

Intravenous medications are often relatively concentrated, as they will be quickly diluted when given into the blood stream. Certain intravenous medications are very caustic when unintentionally administered extravascularly, with resultant local complications. For example, pressor agents (dopamine, epinephrine, and norepinephrine) are potent vasoconstrictors and are mixed in relatively concentrated solutions. When unintentionally given into soft tissues, usually as a result of an infiltrated intravenous catheter, the vasoconstriction will result in tissue necrosis if untreated. To prevent necrosis and tissue sloughing in the extravasated areas, the area should be infiltrated as soon as possible with 5 to 10 mg of phentolamine mesylate (Regitene) diluted in 10 to 15 ml of normal saline for injection. Phentolamine is a short-acting alpha-adrenergic blocking agent. A fine-gauge needle should be used to liberally infiltrate the area. The sympathetic blockade produced by phentolamine should cause rapid and conspicuous local hyperemic changes if the area is treated within 12 hours of the extravasation. The pediatric dosage of phentolamine is 0.1 to 0.2 mg/kg up to the adult dosage.

In addition, many of the intravenously administered chemotherapeutic agents are directly caustic to tissues when unintentionally administered extravascularly; again, necrosis of a significant amount of tissue should be expected. Classic examples of chemotherapeutic drugs with this potential are dactinomycin (actinomycin D, Cosmegen), daunorubicin (Daunomycin, others), doxorubicin (Adriamycin), mechlorethamine (Mustargen), mitomycin C (Mutamycin), paclitaxel (Taxol), plicamycin (Mithracin or mithramycin), vinblastine (Velban and others), vincristine (Oncovin), and vinorelbine (Navelbine). Extravasation necrosis is responsible for 2% to 5% of adverse reactions to chemotherapeutic regimens and has been noted in about 6% of peripheral intravenous infusions and in the same 6% of patients with access devices (ports, catheters, etc.). Lesser degrees of reaction (venous flare, phlebitis, cellulitis) must be distinguished from tissue necrosis. General treatment includes elevation of the extremity for 48 hours, cooling of the extremity (with the exception of mechlorethamine and mitomycin C; for vinca alkaloids, intermittent warming may be beneficial), and surgical consultation.

WHAT TO DO

In addition, several specific antidotes for extravascular administration of chemotherapeutic agents have been found useful. After mechlorethamine and mitomycin C injury, give 0.17 M sodium thiosulfate should be given intravenously through a new intravenous line and topical 50% to 90% DMSO (dimethyl sulfoxide) applied. After injury from doxorubicin and other anthracyclines, topical 50% to 90% DMSO should also be used. After vinca alkaloid injury, 150 units of hyaluronidase should be given intravenously. The administration of glucocorticoids has been promoted, particularly for doxorubicin, but lacks verification of efficacy.

WATCH OUT FOR

The reverse situation, intravascular infusion of an intended soft tissue injection creates different problems. Reactions can be systemic (from the systemic delivery of the drug) or locally related to vessel injury from the medication. A relatively common example is the intravascular injection of local anesthetics. With subcutaneous infiltration or field block, intravascular injection is unlikely to cause problems because the needle is steadily moving and only small vessels are in the subcutaneous space. Intravascular injection during a deep block (e.g., axillary, interscalene, stellate ganglion, deep cervical, etc.) is much more likely to cause a significant problem because of the larger vessels in proximity to the needle and the larger volume of anesthetic delivered. Systemic complications of local anesthetic infusion include central nervous reactions (typically seizures) and cardiac rhythm disturbance (e.g., bradydysrhythmias, cardiac arrest). Both neurologic and cardiac sequence can occur with intra-arterial or intravenous injection. If the local anesthetic contained a vasoconstrictor (usually epinephrine) when injected, systemic toxicity may also include hypertension, tachydysrhythmias, and myocardial ischemia. Local reactions to intra-arterial injection of epinephrine-containing solutions include arterial thrombosis.

Prevention of unintended intravascular injection requires an awareness of anatomy and the risks of the solution intended to be infiltrated into soft tissues. Aspirating through the needle *before* injecting is of some importance but does not insure that the needle tip is extravascular. Therefore, while aspirating first is useful, it does not replace thought and care. Reasons that aspiration may be unreliable in ascertaining an extravascular location of the needle tip include: (1) the tip is in a small vein, and aspiration collapses the vein around the needle; (2) the needle tip is plugged with a core of skin or subcutaneous fat; (3) small needles (e.g., 25 gauge or smaller) will frequently clot or be unable to reliably aspirate a viscous solution such as blood; and (4) the lumen of the needle may be partly intravascular and be unable to aspirate yet may still be capable of infusing intravascularly. Periodic aspiration while injecting will solve the second problem and may disclose the fourth problem; but, regardless, remember that aspiration that does not produce blood does not prove the needle lumen is extravascular.

One final note is that intramuscular injections of vaccinations or medications can produce nerve injury. In some instances, this may represent nerve trauma from the needle itself. Because these may present in a delayed manner, the medication injected may be responsible in some cases. The two classic examples are sciatic nerve injury from gluteal injection and axillary nerve injury from deltoid injection.

SUGGESTED READINGS

Abeloff JO, Armitage AS, Lichter AS, eds. Clinical Oncology. 2nd Ed. New York: Churchill Livingstone, 2000: 980–994.
Ben-David B. Complications of peripheral blockade. Anesthesiol Clin North Am 2002;20:695–707.
Dorr RT. Antidotes to vesicant chemotherapy extravasations. Blood Rev 1990;4:41–60.

77

DO NOT GIVE A VERBAL ORDER FOR A MEDICATION WITHOUT INQUIRING ABOUT THE PATIENT'S ALLERGIES

RACHAEL A. CALLCUT, MD

"Adverse drug reactions" include overlapping definitions, such as drug hypersensitivity (any immunologic type drug reaction) and drug allergy (classic IgE-mediated drug reactions). In addition, some drug reactions are nonimmunologic but mimic allergic reactions including: histamine release from opiates or from the solvent for some intravenous medications; "red man" syndrome from overly rapid administration of intravenous (IV) vancomycin (also a histamine release phenomenon); and some of the anaphylactoid vasodilator responses to iodinated radiocontrast media.

WATCH OUT FOR

Almost every medication can cause an allergic reaction. Antibiotics are the most common culprits in surgical practice. However, reaction to "safe" drugs such as acetaminophen and aspirin do occur and the cross-reactivity can be as high as 5% for these two compounds. The most common manifestation of an allergic reaction is a cutaneous drug reaction, which chronologically can occur any time from immediately after administration to up to 3 weeks after exposure. The spectrum of severity of cutaneous allergic reaction is wide, with the mildest form being a erythematous maculopapular rash that typically originates on the trunk and spreads centrifugally. Topical exposures can result in eczematous rashes from contact dermatitis. Urticaria are more serious and usually represent a true allergic (IgE-mediated) reaction. The most severe cutaneous reactions potentially involve skin loss and include the spectrum of erythema multiforme, which includes Stevens-Johnson syndrome/toxic epidermal necrolysis.

Other manifestations of drug allergy include fevers, arthralgias, wheezing, dyspnea, hemodynamic instability, laryngeal edema, angioedema, eosinophilia, hepatitis, and renal dysfunction. The most severe and immediate allergic reaction is life-threatening anaphylaxis. Onset usually occurs within seconds to minutes of exposure to the inciting drug. Patients generally develop an urticarial rash and respiratory distress followed by hemodynamic instability; however, vascular collapse can occur without respiratory distress.

Treatment of an adverse drug reaction consists of halting administration of the drug and antihistamines for mild reactions. Severe reactions may mandate use of intravenous steroids and epinephrine. Stevens-Johnson syndrome/toxic epidermal necrolysis should be treated as a severe burn and referred to a center with definitive burn care.

One final note is that many drugs have gastrointestinal adverse effects. While often unpleasant to the patient, these are best thought of as drug side effects (and may cause drug intolerance) and not allergic reactions.

SUGGESTED READINGS

deShazo RD, Kemp SF. Allergic reactions to drugs and biologic agents. JAMA 1997;278:1895–1906.

Fauci AS. Harrison's Principles of Internal Medicine. 14th Ed. New York: McGraw-Hill, 1998;304–310,1862–1868.

Reidl MA, Casillas AM. Adverse drug reactions: types and treatment options. Am Fam Physician 2003;68:1781–1790.

DO NOT PRESCRIBE A KAYEXALATE-SORBITOL ENEMA TO A KIDNEY TRANSPLANT PATIENT

DMITRIY A. NIKITIN, MD

Sodium polystyrene sulfonate (Kayexalate) is a sulfonated cation-exchange resin that is used to remove excess potassium. It is usually given orally with a suitable laxative, such as sorbitol, but can be given as an enema in the same sorbitol vehicle in ill patients or those with an ileus. Sorbitol is a hypertonic osmotic laxative.

SIGNS AND SYMPTOMS

Classically, Kayexalate-sorbitol–induced colonic necrosis occurs in the inpatient setting, where an early postoperative renal transplant patient with suboptimal graft function and an elevated serum potassium is administered a Kayexalate-sorbitol enema. In this complication, the clinical course is marked by administration of the enema, development or worsening of postoperative ileus, and then peritonitis and colonic necrosis, which may develop quite rapidly (within 36 hours of giving the enema). Signs and symptoms of colonic necrosis include abdominal pain, abdominal distention, ileus, fever, hypotension, and/or metabolic acidosis. Pathologic examination of involved intestinal specimens reveals extensive necrosis with areas of transmural infarction; amorphous or crystalline sodium polystyrene sulfonate has been found at necrotic mucosa sites.

The true incidence of colonic necrosis after Kayexalate-sorbitol enemas is unknown. A report by Gerstman et al noted a 0.27% overall incidence, with a higher (1.8%) incidence in the postoperative period. The exact pathophysiology of this colonic necrosis is unknown. Factors that may contribute include uremia, hypovolemia, peripheral vascular disease, and immunosuppression therapy. The hyperosmolarity of the enema in patients with sluggish colonic motility or impaired colonic wall perfusion may be the source of the damage. In view of this, some clinicians have suggested avoiding sodium polystyrene sulfonate in sorbitol enemas perioperatively, not only in patients undergoing renal transplantation but also in azotemic patients and the critically ill.

The manufacturer maintains the relative safety of giving Kayexalate-sorbitol enemas. They note that, in all cases of colonic necrosis reported to date, administration of a cleansing enema after the sodium polystyrene sulfonate retention enema was omitted. They maintain this should consist of up to 2 L of a non–sodium-containing solution to remove the resin after 30 to 60 minutes of retention. Although this may effect a thorough rinse of the colon, it is cumbersome for nursing personnel and inconvenient to the patient.

One final note is that, although Kayexalate-sorbitol enemas may seem an easier way to manage life-threatening hyperkalemia, dialysis to remove the excess potassium is what is truly needed; intravenous glucose/insulin/bicarbonate/calcium can be used to transiently manage the hyperkalemia until dialysis can be initiated.

SUGGESTED READINGS

Barbul A, Harrison MG, Dardik A, Moesinger RC, Efron G. Acute abdomen with colonic necrosis induced by Kayexalate-sorbitol. South Med J 2000;93:511–513.

Gerstman BB, Kirkman R, Platt R. Intestinal necrosis associated with postoperative orally administered sodium polystyrene sulfonate in sorbitol. Am J Kidney Dis 1992;20:159–161.

McEvoy GK, ed. Potassium-removing agents. In *AHFS Drug Information 2002*. Bethesda, MD: American Society of Health-System Pharmacists, 2002;40:18.

Rogers FB, Li SC. Acute colonic necrosis associated with sodium polystyrene sulfonate (Kayexalate) enemas in a critically ill patient: case report and review of the literature. J Trauma 2001;51:395–397.

79

REMEMBER TO CHANGE THE DOSAGE WHEN CONVERTING FROM THE INTRAVENOUS TO THE ORAL FORM OF IMMUNOSUPPRESSIVE AND OTHER DRUGS IN TRANSPLANT PATIENTS

DMITRIY A. NIKITIN, MD

Appropriate change of dosage when converting between the intravenous (IV) and oral (PO) forms of immunosuppressive drugs is important in managing transplant patients. Errors in drug dosages can result in danger to the graft or untoward side effects. Below are guidelines that can be used in patients taking little or nothing by mouth.

CYCLOSPORINE

Cyclosporine is available in three formulations: one intravenous and two oral forms. The two oral forms are the original cyclosporine (Sandimmune and generic) and the microemulsion form (Neoral, Gengraf, and other generics) that has higher and more reliable oral bioavailability. For cyclosporine, oral bioavailability is about one-third that of parenteral drug, therefore, the IV dose is one-third of the PO dose. It is important to monitor the trough level with both oral and intravenous forms. Oral drug is administered every 12 hours. The microemulsion form is well absorbed from the proximal gastrointestinal tract, so giving the usual every-12-hour dose orally or down a nasogastric tube (and clamping for 30 minutes) will often achieve adequate levels. Intravenous cyclosporine is typically given as a slow infusion to minimize the greater nephrotoxicity of the vehicle-related intravenous form. Early posttransplant, it is commonly given as a very slow infusion (e.g., over 20 hours or as 2 infusions every 12 hours over 8 to 10 hours), leaving a window for drawing a trough level. Late posttransplant, it can be infused over shorter time periods, such as every 12 hours over 4 to 6 hours.

TACROLIMUS

For tacrolimus (Prograf), oral bioavailability varies with indication—averaging 22% in liver recipients compared to 17% in kidney recipients. The intravenous form has greater neurotoxicity. Because it is well absorbed from the proximal gastrointestinal tract, it is usually possible to avoid the intravenous form by administration orally or down a nasogastric tube every 12 hours. If adequate levels cannot be obtained, the drug can be given intravenously beginning at one-fifth of the total daily dose as a slow infusion over 20 to 24 hours. Trough levels should be checked daily.

CORTICOSTEROIDS

For corticosteroids, the IV and PO dosages are the same. *Table 79-1* lists equivalence for glucocorticoid (not mineralocorticoid) properties. For example, for prednisone a switch to methylprednisolone at 80% of the dose is equivalent; for example, prednisone 10 mg PO daily is equal to methylprednisolone (Solu-Medrol) 8 mg IV daily. If a shorter-acting corticosteroid is desired, 4 times the daily oral prednisone dose as hydrocortisone (SoluCortef), given in divided doses every 6 or 8 hours, is sufficient (e.g., prednisone 10 mg PO daily is equivalent to hydrocortisone 10 mg IV every 6 hours).

SIROLIMUS

Sirolimus (Rapamune) is only available PO. Monitoring of blood sirolimus concentrations is recommended, given the drug interaction with cyclosporine (mutually increased levels) and the long half-life (.60 hours). Cyclosporine, tacrolimus, and sirolimus are all metabolized by cytochrome P450 3A4 (CYP3A4) and have drug interactions with inhibitors and inducers of CYP3A4.

TABLE 79-1 EQUIVALENCE VALUES FOR GLUCOCORTICOID PROPERTIES OF IMMUNOSUPPRESSIVE AND OTHER DRUGS

CORTICOSTEROID	RELATIVE POTENCY	EQUIVALENT DOSE	ROUTES
Cortisone	0.8	25 mg	PO, IM
Hydrocortisone	1	20 mg	PO, IV, IM
Prednisolone	4	5 mg	PO
Prednisone	4	5 mg	PO
Methylprednisolone	5	4 mg	PO, IV, IM
Dexamethasone	30	0.75 mg	PO, IV, IM

MYCOPHENOLATE MOFETIL AND AZATHIOPRINE

For both mycophenolate mofetil (CellCept) and azathioprine (Imuran), the PO dose is the same as IV dose with the same dosing interval. Serum levels are not tested.

OTHERS

Listed below are some guidelines that can be helpful with commonly used medications when transplant patients cannot take their PO medications:

- For **beta-blockers,** a switch to an IV form to avoid withdrawal effects (tachycardia, angina, etc.) is necessary. Every hospital has its own policies concerning which IV beta-blockers are permitted, and these policies differ among nursing units, depending on the availability of continuous ECG monitoring. Ask nursing or pharmacy before prescribing.
- For **calcium channel-blockers,** there is no risk of rebound withdrawal effects. The IV forms of calcium channel-blockers have short half-lives and are ill suited to the management of hypertension. The use of alternative parenteral antianginals or antihypertensives is recommended.
- **Digoxin** has a low therapeutic index; therefore, monitoring the serum trough level is essential. When changing from oral to intramuscular (IM) or IV, digoxin dosage should be reduced by 20% to 25%.
- For **phenobarbital,** the PO dose approximates the IV dose, and monitoring of serum trough levels is essential.
- For **phenytoin,** the PO dose approximates the IV dose, and monitoring the serum trough levels is essential. Phenytoin is a potent CYP3A4 inducer and is usually avoided in patients taking cyclosporine.

One final note is that serum levels are usually best drawn as trough levels (i.e., 30 to 60 minutes before the next dose).

SUGGESTED READINGS

D'Antiga L, Dhawan A, Portmann B, et al. Late cellular rejection in paediatric liver transplantation: aetiology and outcome. Transplantation 2002;73:80–84.

Higgins RM, Hart P, Lam FT, Kashi, H. Conversion from tacrolimus to cyclosporin in stable renal transplant patients: safety, metabolic changes, and pharmacokinetic comparison. Transplantation 2000;70:199–202.

Katzung, BG, ed. Basic and Clinical Pharmacology. 8th Ed. New York: McGraw-Hill, 2001;959–986.

McEvoy, GK, ed. AHFS Drug Information®. Bethesda, MD: American Society of Health-System Pharmacists, 2001.

80

DO NOT ALLOW ST. JOHN'S WORT TO BE COADMINISTERED WITH CYCLOSPORINE, TACROLIMUS, OR SIROLIMUS

NEIL SANDSON, MD

St. John's wort is a mild serotonin re-uptake inhibitor with additional mild monoamine oxidase inhibition, which appears to act as a reasonably effective antidepressant for many individuals with mild- to moderate-intensity depression. St. John's wort is available in the United States without a prescription and is one of the most common self-administered treatments for depression. Unfortunately, St. John's wort can produce tragic results in transplant recipients because it has significant drug interactions with immunosuppressive agents.

Specifically, St John's wort induces the liver to produce more of the cytochrome P450 3A4 enzyme. This is the primary enzyme responsible for metabolizing the immunosuppressive agents cyclosporine, tacrolimus, and sirolimus. In addition to this increased metabolism of immunosuppressive agents, St. John's wort induces the production of increased amounts of the P-glycoprotein transporter. This transporter is present in the enterocytes that line the gut lumen and acts to extrude substrates of the transporter from enterocytes back into the gut lumen, where they are then excreted. These immunosuppressive agents are also substrates of the P-glycoprotein transporter. Thus, St. John's wort decreases the absorption of cyclosporine, tacrolimus, and sirolimus from the gut, as well as increasing their rate of metabolism. These dual features of St. John's wort synergistically act to decrease the blood levels of these immunosuppressive agents, which can allow organ rejection. As a direct result of the St. John's wort–cyclosporine interaction, there have been two documented cases of heart transplant rejection and several cases involving rejection of other organs.

One final note is that depression is not uncommon in transplant recipients; however, and all transplant recipients must be *specifically* told to not medicate themselves with St. John's wort (or any other over-the-counter medications, herbal remedies, or dietary supplements) because of the increased risk of rejection.

SUGGESTED READINGS

Bolley R, Zulke C, Kammerl M, Fischereder M, Kramer B. Tacrolimus-induced nephrotoxicity unmasked by induction of the CYP3A4 system with St. John's wort. Transplantation 2002;73:1009.

Ruschitzka F, Meier PJ, Turina M, Luscher T, Noll G. Acute heart transplant rejection due to Saint John's wort. Lancet 2000;355:548–549.

Do not prescribe a nonsteroidal anti-inflammatory drug (NSAID) or an aminoglycoside to a patient with cirrhosis

Michael J. Moritz, MD

Standard, straightforward management of medical problems may not always be safely adopted in the cirrhotic patient. This principle of seemingly correct management that has a deleterious outcome is highlighted in the following clinical scenario:

WHAT NOT TO DO

An adult with Child's class C cirrhosis from primary sclerosing cholangitis (PSC) has significant ascites and is awaiting transplantation. His PSC is related to his Crohn's disease and an additional extra-intestinal manifestation is arthralgias. His physician prescribes naproxen for the arthralgias. He presents one week later with tense ascites and oliguric acute renal failure. He is admitted to the intensive care unit, requires dialysis, develops bacteremia, and expires.

This scenario highlights one of the common prescribing errors in cirrhotics that can have devastating results—NSAIDs should not be used in this patient population. Patients with cirrhosis and ascites have limited renal reserve and are at an increased risk of renal dysfunction.

Normal renal function and hemodynamics are a balance between renal vasodilatory and vasoconstrictive forces. Cirrhosis disrupts this relationship with marked vasoconstriction and an impaired ability to excrete sodium and water. The kidneys in patients with cirrhosis are more sensitive to nephrotoxins, with a greater degree and duration of injury occuring in response to an insult. A nephrotoxic insult in a patient with cirrhosis can cause acute renal failure, a complication with a high mortality in this setting.

NSAIDs alter intrarenal prostaglandin homeostatic mechanisms, even in noncirrhotics. NSAID-induced nephrotoxicity can have a range of manifestations but commonly presents as acute renal failure. Patients with volume contraction or preexisting renal compromise are at greater risk of NSAID nephrotoxicity. Additionally, cirrhotics are at high risk of gastrointestinal bleeding from a variety of etiologies. Given the gastrointestinal bleeding risk associated with NSAIDs and the potential nephrotoxicity, NSAIDs are contraindicated in cirrhotics. It is important for patients with cirrhosis to be advised to avoid NSAIDs, both prescription and over-the-counter forms.

Another classic prescribing error in cirrhotic patients is the use of aminoglycosides. These drugs are particularly tempting to use because they are familiar to most surgeons, widely available, active against Gram-negative infections, and cheap. Their well-recognized nephrotoxicity is particularly deleterious when coupled with the renal perturbations of cirrhosis as described earlier. Aminoglycoside use is both an independent and an additive risk factor for renal dysfunction in this population.

One final note is that patients with cirrhosis (or other disorders predisposing to NSAID-induced renal injury such as congestive heart failure, nephrotic syndrome, and other underlying renal diseases) need to be provided with written information listing generic names, trade names, and combination medications that contain NSAIDs so that they do not inadvertently ingest them.

SUGGESTED READINGS

Brenner BM. Brenner & Rector's The Kidney. 6th Ed. Philadelphia: W.B. Saunders, 2000:1581–1584.

Hampel H, Bynum GD, Zamora E, El-Sarag HB. Risk factors for the development of renal dysfunction in hospitalized patients with cirrhosis. Am J Gastroenterol 2001;96:2206–2210.

Laffi G, La Villa G, Pinzan M, Marra F, Gentilini P. Arachidonic acid derivatives and renal function in liver cirrhosis. Semin Nephrol 1997;17:530–548.

BE CAUTIOUS WHEN USING DEMEROL IN PATIENTS WITH RENAL INSUFFICIENCY

MICHAEL J. MORITZ, MD

Meperidine hydrochloride (Demerol) is a semisynthetic narcotic analgesic. It can be administered either orally or parenterally. It has approximately one-tenth of the potency of morphine (i.e., 1 mg of morphine is equivalent to 10 mg of meperidine). Meperidine is a short-acting narcotic with a half-life of about 3 hours. Meperidine is metabolized by the liver via several pathways, one of which generates the intermediate metabolite normeperidine, which has a half-life of 15 to 20 hours. Normeperidine has both renal and hepatic elimination pathways.

The use of meperidine can cause troublesome side effects, including tremor, muscle twitching, hyperactive reflexes, and seizures. These symptoms are due to accumulation of normeperidine. Seizures are most often seen in one of two settings. First, a patient taking relatively large doses of meperidine for chronic or recurring acute pain (e.g., chronic pancreatitis, sickle cell crises) develops progressive renal insufficiency, so a dose of meperidine previously used for analgesia now causes CNS excitation and seizures. With numerous other analgesics available, its use in patients with even a slight degree of renal insufficiency should be avoided. Second, a relatively healthy patient receives meperidine for acute pain (e.g., postoperatively) at a relatively high dose, often via a PCA (patient-controlled analgesia) pump and develops seizures. The maximum dose that even healthy patients receive should not exceed 10 mg/kg/day.

One final note is that hepatic insufficiency slows the metabolism of both meperidine and normeperidine but disproportionately so for meperidine; therefore, hepatic insufficiency more often leads to CNS depression from the narcotic's additive effect on encephalopathy.

SUGGESTED READINGS

Reisine T, Pasternak G. Opioid Analgesics and Antagonists. In Hardman J.G. and Limbird L.E., eds. Goodman & Gilman's The Pharmacological Basis of Therapeutics. 9th Ed. New York: McGraw-Hill, 1996;540–543.

Simopoulos TT, Smith HS, Peeters-Asdourian C, Stevens DS. Use of meperidine in patient-controlled analgesia and the development of a normeperidine toxic reaction. Arch Surg 2002;137:84–88.

Szeto HH, Inturrisi CE, Houde, R., et al. Accumulation of normeperidine, an active metabolite of meperidine, in patients with renal failure or cancer. Ann Intern Med 1977;86:738–741.

REMEMBER THAT ANTIBIOTICS CAN HAVE SEVERE AND IRREVERSIBLE SIDE EFFECTS WITH EVEN SHORT COURSES

MICHAEL J. MORITZ, MD

All medications have side effects and such side effects can be categorized in many ways; for example, by incidence, severity, or organ system affected. Many medications have rare, idiosyncratic side effects that can be life-threatening (e.g., Stevens-Johnson syndrome, pulmonary fibrosis, and hepatotoxicity). These side effects are not the subject of this topic. Rather, as antibiotics are widely and somewhat indiscriminately prescribed by physicians, it is important for physicians to be aware of uncommon but *severe and relatively irreversible side effects* that are specific to certain classes of antibiotics. Some examples are described below (see also *Table 83.1*).

WATCH OUT FOR

A classic example is chloramphenicol. Chloramphenicol has relatively common dose-dependent marrow toxicity, but the idiosyncratic development of irreversible, often lethal blood dyscrasias is rare. The spectrum of potentially fatal blood dyscrasias attributed to chloramphenicol includes aplastic anemia, thrombocytopenia, and granulocytopenia. The most common of these rare events is aplastic anemia, thought to occur in 1 in 20,000 to 1 in 40,000 exposures; the risk is higher with oral administration, followed by intravenous and perhaps even intraocular (eye drop) use. After years of relatively little use of this drug in the United States (in part because of the aplastic anemia risk), chloramphenicol use is again increasing because of its activity against some of the multiple antibiotic-resistant bacteria, for example, vancomycin-resistant enterococci. When used in this setting, its forgotten side effect of causing long-lasting, only partially reversible peripheral neuropathy is again becoming known. The neuropathy of chloramphenicol is relatively distal and is mixed between hypesthesia (numbness) and dysesthesia (pain).

Similarly, metronidazole (Flagyl) is a widely prescribed drug with the uncommon and little-known side effect of causing a long-lasting, partially irreversible peripheral neuropathy. The neuropathy tends to have a greater component of dysesthesia than hypesthesia. The risk of neuropathy is particularly related to the duration of the course and, to a lesser degree, to the dosage.

TABLE 83.1	SIDE EFFECTS OF ANTIBIOTICS				
	NEUROPATHY	CNS	OTOTOXICITY	TOOTH STAINING	APLASTIC ANEMIA
Quinolones		+			
Metronidazole	+				
Chloramphenicol	+		+		+
Aminoglycosides			+		
Tetracyclines			+	+	

Fluoroquinolones (quinolones) have an incidence of central nervous system reactions of approximately 0.5%. Most of these reactions are seizures, thought to be related to its property of displacing GABA (γ-aminobutyric acid) from its receptors, which is exacerbated by other drugs with similar properties (e.g., some nonsteroidal anti-inflammatories, caffeine, theophylline). However, some quinolones have been associated with rare, long-lived cases of depression, changes in personality, or difficulty with concentration. Ciprofloxacin (but not other quinolones) has been associated with Achilles tendon rupture.

The nephrotoxicity of aminoglycosides is well known. In contrast, one does not hear as much about their ototoxicity. Ototoxicity is less reversible than nephrotoxicity and, hence, physicians should be aware of this side effect. In patients receiving intravenous aminoglycoside and being prospectively studied with audiometry, the incidence of ototoxicity was almost 10%. The risk was highest in older patients and higher risk was also associated with higher trough levels.

Other drugs cause ototoxicity as well. In patients receiving oral neomycin, a small amount of drug will be absorbed. If given for a long course, the chronic exposure can cause ototoxicity. This has been seen in the treatment of hepatic encephalopathy. Ototoxicity also can occur with minocycline (a tetracycline) and intravenous erythromycin (a macrolide).

Tetracyclines are now well known to be incorporated into actively forming bones and teeth. When the drug was first released, it was prescribed to children and adolescents for various indications, including acne. When these children's permanent teeth appeared, they were often stained a mottled greyish color. As the discoloration is a result of the presence of the tetracycline in the tooth enamel, it cannot be removed but only covered by cosmetic dentistry. Tetracyclines are no longer prescribed to children in this country, but tetracycline (along with chloramphenicol) is widely available and inexpensive in most Third World countries.

Nitrofurantoin, when given in the presence of renal insufficiency and particularly with long courses, can cause peripheral neuropathy or pulmonary fibrosis.

One final note is that seizures are associated with a long list of antibiotics, all of which interfere with GABA and thus can cause central nervous excitation and seizures (penicillins, cephalosporins, quinolones, aztreonam, carbapenems, metronidazole, and isoniazid).

SUGGESTED READINGS

Christ W. Central nervous system toxicity of quinolones: Human and animal findings. J Antimicrob Chemother 1990;26(Suppl B):219–225.

Cunha BA. Antibiotic side effects. Med Clin North Am 2001;85:149–185.

Gatell JM, Ferran F, Araujo V, et al. Univariate and multivariate analyses of risk factors predisposing to auditory toxicity in patients receiving aminoglycosides. Antimicrob Agents Chemother 1987;31:1383–1387.

Pavithran K, Thomas M. Hematopoietic growth factors in drug-induced agranulocytosis. J Assoc Physicians India 2002;50:679–681.

84

CONSIDER PRESCRIBING *LACTOBACILLUS* (OR OTHER PROBIOTIC THERAPY) WHEN A PATIENT RECEIVES ANY DOSE OF ANTIBIOTICS

LISA MARCUCCI, MD

The overgrowth of *Clostridium difficile*, with its enterotoxin and the resulting colitis, that occurs in patients on antibiotics is one of the most troublesome (and potentially life-threatening) complications in patient care. It is also one of the most unnecessary. The incidence of this condition can be greatly reduced with a cheap and readily available regimen of Lactinex (a pharmaceutical grade probiotic), acidophilus (available "over the counter"), or yogurt (which contains the *Saccharomyces* yeast commensal). The concomitant use of one of these agents in patients on antibiotics has been reported to cut the incidence of antibiotic-related *C. difficile* colitis from 25 to 5%. Treatment protocols vary, but generally patients can be given two Lactinex (or acidophilus) capsules three times a day orally at the start of antibiotic treatment and for 14 days after completion of the antibiotic course. Lactinex capsules may be opened and slurry prepared for administration via a nasogastric or feeding tube if the patient cannot eat. Alternately, three standard-size containers of yogurt can be consumed daily. If *C. difficile* colitis does occur while the patient is on antibiotics and Lactinex, the Lactinex should be continued (or started if not already prescribed), with every attempt made to shorten or eliminate the course of the offending antibiotic. The appropriate treatment regimen *C. difficile* should then be started (see below).

When considering whether to use a probiotic, it should be noted that there are scattered reports of the development of polymicrobial invasive infections in immunocompromised patients and replacement valve patients where *Lactobacillus* has been isolated, although rarely with the common probiotic species of *Lactobacillus* acidophilus and with no established connection to an exogenously administered organism for *C. difficile* prophylaxis. The most worrisome of these infections is endocarditis, occurring in approximately 60% of the *Lactobacillus* infections. Due to the seriousness of vegetative valve lesions, some experienced infectious disease physicians believe that probiotics should not be used in transplant patients or patients with prosthetic valve.

C. difficile is an anaerobic, normally occurring gut organism that usually is not pathogenic. However if the gut flora is disturbed, overgrowth can occur with the development of friable, inflamed colon mucosa and the development of pseudomembranes. This is most often seen with administration of antibiotics that alter the number of the normally occurring flora. Classically, the antibiotic most associated with *C. difficile* was clindamycin, but essentially any antibiotic (even the antibiotics metronidazole and vancomycin that are used to treat this condition) can cause *C. difficile* colitis. It is important to note that it can occur after only a single dose of antibiotic (such as that given perioperatively), can present up to 4 weeks after antibiotics have been discontinued, and can relapse 3 to 14 days after apparent successful treatment. *C. difficile* colitis can also occur in the absence of antibiotics in severe, debilitating illness and some forms of malignancy.

SIGNS AND SYMPTOMS

Clinical presentation of *C. difficile* varies from constipation to a few mild episodes of diarrhea to fulminant pseudomembranous colitis. The most typical presentation is voluminous, foul-smelling, nonbloody diarrhea with abdominal cramps, abdominal tenderness, fever, and leukocytosis. Most experienced clinicians will treat based on clinical suspicion. Testing of a stool sample for *C. difficile* toxin A (using ELISA [enzyme-linked immunosorbent assay] technique) is the most readily available laboratory test with a sensitivity of 70% to 90% and a somewhat higher specificity. A tissue culture assay for the presence of *C. difficile* toxin B is the gold standard but is less readily available due to expense. Generally, repeat stool testing with the same assay does not increase accuracy of the *C. difficile* test.

To briefly review, the first-line drug treatment in a new onset case of *C. difficile* colitis is oral or intravenous metronidazole (effective in 85% of cases). The second-line drug is oral vancomycin (the intravenous form is poorly absorbed by the gut and is ineffective in treating *C. difficile* colitis). The third-line drug is oral rifampin (again, the intravenous form is not effective). In addition, cholestyramine can be used as adjunctive treatment because it will bind the *C. difficile* toxins; it should not be used with vancomycin because it also binds this drug. If patients become refractory to medical treatment and develop fulminant pseudomembranous colitis, subtotal colectomy is indicated. This is an ominous development for the patient, with 30% mortality even with prompt colectomy.

One final note is that patients with a known allergy to milk or Lactinex or who are lactose-intolerant should be not be given probiotics containing lactose (lactose-free products are available). The safety in nursing mothers and children under the age of 2 has not been ascertained, and thus these patients should not be offered this regimen.

SUGGESTED READINGS

Banerjee S, Lamont JT. Non-antibiotic therapy for *Clostridium difficile* infection. Curr Opin Infect Dis 2000;13:215–219.

Bergogne-Berezin E. Treatment and prevention of antibiotic associated diarrhea. Int J Antimicrob Agents 2000;16:521–526.

Braunwald E, Fauci AS, Kasper DL, eds. Harrison's Principles of Internal Medicine. 15th Ed. New York: McGraw-Hill, 2001:923–926.

Cremonini F, Di Caro S, Santarelli L, et al. Probiotics in antibiotic-associated diarrhoea. Dig Liver Dis 2002;34(Suppl 2):S78–S80.

Greenfield LJ, Mulholland MW, Oldham KT, eds. Surgery: Scientific Principles and Practice. 3rd Ed. Philadelphia: Lippincott Williams & Wilkins, 2001:196.

Marteau P, Seksik P, Jian R. Probiotics and intestinal health effects: a clinical perspective. Br J Nutr 2002;88(Suppl 1):S51–S57.

85

CHECK PEAK AND TROUGH LEVELS WHEN DOSING AMINOGLYCOSIDES (IF PHARMACOKINETIC OR ONCE-A-DAY DOSING IS NOT BEING USED) AND TROUGH LEVELS IN SELECT SITUATIONS WHEN DOSING VANCOMYCIN

HARSH JAIN, MD

For the aminoglycoside antibiotics (gentamicin, tobramycin, amikacin, kanamycin, and netilmicin), peak and trough levels and for the antibiotic vancomycin trough levels in select situations should be monitored to dose correctly. This will both ensure that appropriate efficacious levels are reached and that toxic side effects are avoided.

Vancomycin is a glycopeptide antibiotic derived from the fungus *Streptomyces orientalis*. It is a narrow-spectrum bactericidal antibiotic active against aerobic Gram-positive bacteria. Initial preparations of vancomycin contained as much as 30% of impurities that probably contributed to its toxicity ("Mississippi Mud"). With newer, purer vancomycin preparations, there is much less toxicity. Its mechanism of action is to inhibit bacterial cell wall synthesis by interfering with glycopeptide polymerization, thus it is active only against actively dividing bacteria. Vancomycin is the drug of choice for methicillin-resistant staphylococcal infections. In patients with penicillin and cephalosporin allergies, vancomycin is one of the alternative medications for methicillin-sensitive infections. Resistance to vancomycin has emerged in enterococci, more often in *Enterococcus faecium* (up to 50% of isolates) than in *E. faecalis* (less than 5% of isolates) and less common species. New antibiotics with activity against vancomycin-resistant enterococci (VRE) have been introduced, but the difficulty in treating VRE and the specter of vancomycin-resistant staphylococci should provide a major force to avoid the use of vancomycin when alternative antibiotics are available.

SIGNS AND SYMPTOMS

Vancomycin is cleared via glomerular filtration and has a half-life of 6 to 8 hours in patients with normal renal function. The most common side effects include chills, fever, and phlebitis at the site of administration. The so called "red man" syndrome (tingling, pruritis, erythema, flushing of the upper torso, angioedema, and hypotension) is not an allergic reaction but is related to overly fast intravenous administration of the drug. Ototoxicity, manifested by tinnitus and high-tone hearing loss that can progress to deafness, can occur, but is rare. Nephrotoxicity is rarely seen when vancomycin is used alone and serum concentrations and renal function are monitored. Aminoglycoside antibiotics used in conjunction with vancomycin may potentiate ototoxicity and nephrotoxicity. The use of peak and trough levels for vancomycin is rapidly decreasing; however, serum levels may be checked for hemodialysis patients as it is partially cleared during this modality. In non-dialysis patients, random serum levels may be checked to ensure that the drug level is greater than the MIC of the targeted microbe. Appropriate levels for redosing are 15 to 20 μg/mL. Some experienced hospital pharmacists maintain there is no indication ever to check peak levels for vancomycin.

SIGNS AND SYMPTOMS

Aminoglycoside antibiotics share many class properties. They are bactericidal and act by inhibiting bacterial protein synthesis. They are active against aerobic Gram-negative bacteria and, to a lesser degree, staphylococci and some streptococci. They are derived from soil fungi: gentamicin from *Micromonospora purpurea* and *M. echinospora*; tobramycin from *Streptomyces tenebrarius;* kanamycin from *S. kanamyceticus*; amikacin is a semisynthetic made by modifying kanamycin; and netilmicin is a semisynthetic derivative of sisomicin from *M. inyoensis*. All are cleared unchanged by the kidney and have half-lives of 1.5 to 3.5 hours in patients with normal renal function. Toxicity includes nephrotoxicity, ototoxicity, neuromuscular blockade, paresthesias, and peripheral neuropathy. The reported incidence of nephrotoxicity is between 5 and 25% and the risk of nephrotoxicity is increased with longer duration of therapy. Ototoxicity can damage the cochlear or vestibular systems, is usually irreversible, and has an incidence of 3 to 14%. Different aminoglycosides have different patterns of toxicity; for example, gentamicin more often causes vestibular toxicity, whereas amikacin more often causes hearing loss. In addition, neuromuscular blockade is a rare, dangerous effect of aminoglycoside administration that can occur with intraperitoneal irrigation. Risk of aminoglycoside toxicity is increased with concomitant vancomycin use.

Traditionally, aminoglycosides were administered every 8 hours in patients with normal renal function; however, once-a-day dosing appears to be as effective and less toxic, although not yet approved by the U.S. Food and Drug Administration (see *Table 85-1*). In addition,

TABLE 85.1	AMINOGLYCOSIDE ADMINISTRATION INCLUDING PEAK AND TROUGH LEVELS			
AMINO-GLYCO-SIDES	DOSING Q8H*	DOSING Q24H**	APPROPRIATE PEAK LEVEL	APPROPRIATE TROUGH LEVEL
Gentamicin, Tobramycin, Netilmicin	1–1.7mg/ kg q8h	5–7mg/ kg/d	5–10μg/mL	<2μg/mL
Amikacin, Kanamycin	7.5mg/ kg q12h	15mg/ kg/d	15–30μg/mL	<5μg/mL

* In adults with normal renal function only, not meningitis.
** In adults with normal renal function only, not meningitis.

some surgeons have switched to pharmacokinetic dosing with an initial dose of 4 mg/kg given with one and eight hour levels drawn to estimate drug clearance.

WHAT TO DO

If conventional aminoglycoside dosing is used, peak serum levels of aminoglycosides are drawn 30 minutes after completing an intravenous infusion. Peak levels are drawn to ensure that adequate concentrations for efficacy are achieved. Trough levels are drawn 30 minutes prior to a dose and excessively high trough levels are closely associated with toxicity. The two general means of adjusting dosing are to continue the same dose and extend (or shorten) the interval or to continue the same interval but increase (or decrease) the dose. Changing the dosing interval affects the trough value, whereas the peak value is more affected by the dose given. Given that vancomycin and aminoglycosides are cleared via the kidneys, dosing is dependent upon renal function.

In patients with impaired renal function, aminoglycoside dosing is more difficult because impaired clearance easily leads to high trough levels, with the consequent increased risk of nephrotoxicity further worsening renal function and predisposing to ototoxicity as well. The impairment in creatinine clearance must be estimated or measured before the aminoglycoside is measured. The basic methodology is to lower the daily dose in proportion to the impairment in creatinine clearance or to prolong the dosage interval without altering the daily dosage. See *Table 85.2* for the once-a-day dosing regimen of gentamicin in impaired renal function.

TABLE 85.2	ONCE-A-DAY DOSING OF GENTAMICIN IN PATIENTS WITH IMPAIRED RENAL FUNCTION.	
ESTIMATED CREATININE CLEARANCE (ML/MIN)		**ADMINISTER 7 MG/KG EVERY**
≥ 60		24 hours
40–60		36 hours
20–40		48 hours
<20		readminister dose when level <1μg/mL

SUGGESTED READINGS

Lundstrom TS, Sobel JD. Antibiotics for gram-positive bacterial infections. Infec Dis Clin North Am 2000;14:463–474.

Mandell GL, Bennett JE, Dolin R, eds. Principles and Practices in Infectious Diseases. 5th Ed. Philadelphia: Churchill Livingstone, 2000; pp.382–392,307–336.

Rybak MJ, Abate BJ, Kang SL, et al. Prospective evaluation of the effect of an aminoglycoside dosing regimen on rates of observed nephrotoxicity and ototoxicity. Antimicrob Agents Chemother 1999;43:1549–1555.

Avoid Long Courses of Antibiotics with Significant Antianaerobic Activity to Lessen the Risk of Vancomycin-Resistant Enterococcus

Michael J. Moritz, MD

Antibiotic-resistant bacteria are a growing threat. Increasingly liberal use of antibiotics in human health care and animal husbandry causes emergence of antibiotic-resistant bacteria. The increasing incidence of antibiotic resistance amongst pneumococci, the organism responsible for most community-acquired pneumonia, meningitis, and bacteremia, is well documented. Within U.S. hospitals, the three leading causes of nosocomial bloodstream infections are coagulase-negative staphylococci (80% of which are methicillin resistant), *Staphylococcus aureus* (30% of which are methicillin resistant), and enterococci (20% of which are vancomycin resistant). The mortality rates for these three infections are 20 to 30%.

Vancomycin-resistant enterococci (VRE) first appeared in 1986. Six types of vancomycin resistance have been described; VanA-E and VanG. VanA, VanB, VanD, VanE and VanG (but not VanC) are multigene traits acquired from other enterococci via transferable genetic elements. VanA is a cluster of seven genes on the transposable genetic element (transposon) *Tn1546*. This transposon is also transferable to other Gram-positive bacteria, and VanA-mediated vancomycin resistance has been transferred experimentally to *Staphylococcus aureus, Listeria monocytogenes*, and *Streptococcus pyogenes*. Fortunately, this transfer has not yet been observed outside of the laboratory, but the clinical ramifications are worrisome .

The epidemiology of VRE is quite different in the United States and Europe. In Europe there was widespread use of the glycopeptide antibiotic avoparcin in the poultry industry, with a large reservoir of VRE-colonized healthy people and farm animals. European outbreaks have been more sporadic and with fewer serious infections. Europe banned avoparcin in 1997, and there since has been a steady decrease in colonization rates. In the United States, vancomycin use is 5 to 10 times greater per capita than in Europe. In the United States, healthy individuals are only rarely colonized with VRE. However, VRE has become commonplace and difficult to eradicate in U.S. hospitals. The prevalence of VRE amongst nosocomial enterococci started near zero in 1990 and exceeded 25% by 1995, with VRE being more common in intensive care unit patients. *Enterococcus faecalis* comprises about 60% of enterococcal clinical isolates, *E. faecium* about 30%, and less common species the other 10%. However, VRE are predominately *E. faecium*, with approximately 50% of U.S. isolates having vancomycin resistance; less than 5% of *E. faecalis* isolates are vancomycin resistant.

<hr>
WHAT TO DO
<hr>

To control VRE, the most important concept is avoidance of antibiotic pressure that promotes the emergence of VRE. Enterococci are facultative anaerobes and normal inhabitants of the human intestinal tract. Obviously, vancomycin use, particularly long courses, promotes emergence of VRE. The use of oral vancomycin (for *Clostridium difficile* colitis) is particularly potent in promoting VRE, hence it should not be used except for metronidazole failures. The use of oral or intravenous antibiotics with significant antianaerobic activity has been shown to increase the density of colonization of VRE. Antianaerobic drugs/regimens include: piperacillin-tazobactam, ampicillin-sulbactam, ampicillin-clavulanate, imipenem-cilastatin, metronidazole, clindamycin, and cephalosporins such as cefoxitin and ceftriaxone. Antibiotics without antianaerobic potency do not promote VRE emergence and include the fluoroquinolones, methicillin, first-generation cephalosporins, cefepime, and trimethoprim-sulfamethoxazole. Further, when a course of antibiotic therapy with antianaerobic activity is needed, the course should be as narrow as practical and as short as possible.

In treating clinical VRE infections, identification of which enterococcal species is causative and delineation of the susceptibility/resistance pattern is critical. Although VRE infections from *E. faecalis* are uncommon as noted above, VRE *E. faecalis* often retains ampicillin or rifampin susceptibility. VRE *E. faecium* has variable sensitivity to chloramphenicol, tetracyclines, and a variety of combinations that include imipenem.

Three new antibiotics are active against VRE, and hopefully, will be reserved for treating antibiotic-resistant Gram-positive organisms. Quinupristin-dalfopristin (Synercid) is a combination of two streptogramin antibiotics (a new clinical antibiotic class) with activity against most isolates of VRE *E. faecium* (but *not E. faecalis*). This drug is only available intravenously; common side effects include thrombophlebitis, nausea, vomiting, arthralgias, and myalgias. It is eliminated via hepatic metabolism and interacts with other cytochrome

P450 3A4 drugs. Dosing is as high as 7.5 mg/kg/q8hours, reduced for side effects or decreased hepatic metabolism. Linezolid (Zyvox) is also a new class, an oxazalidinone, and is available both intravenously and orally at identical dosing, with near 100% oral bioavailability. A problem with its use is its monoamine oxidase (MAO) activity. Foods high in tyramine (aged cheeses, smoked meats, sauerkraut, red wine, beer, etc.) should be avoided. In addition, an exaggerated pressor response can occur in response to adrenergic drugs (e.g., pseude-phedrine), dopaminergic drugs (e.g., levodopa), and selective sero-tonin reuptake inhibitors (SSRIs); these must all be avoided when linezolid is being administered. Common side effects include nausea, vomiting, diarrhea, headache, and thrombocytopenia. Dosing is 600mg q12 hours or lower and its excretion is renally dependent. Daptomycin (Cubicin), also a new antibiotic class (cyclic lipopep-tide), is only available parenterally and is given as a single daily dose of 4mg/kg IV, reduced for creatinine clearance less than 30mL/min. Common side effects included myopathy and gastrointestinal distur-bances; neuropathy is uncommon.

Finally, the antibiotics most likely to have activity against VRE are chloramphenicol, quinupristin-dalfopristin, linezolid, and dapto-mycin. All four are bacteriostatic against most VRE. Accordingly, treatment of a VRE infection must include source control of the in-fection, a thorough search for drainable collections and spaces, and any reservoir of continuing infection must be drained and eliminated to promote clearance of VRE.

SUGGESTED READINGS

Bonten MJM, Willems R, Weinstein RA. Vancomycin-resistant enterococci: why they are here, and where do they come from? Lancet Infect Dis 2001;1:314–325.

Donskey CJ, Chowdhry TK, Hecker MT, et al. Effect of antibiotic therapy on the density of vancomycin-resistant enterococci in the stool of colonized patients. N Engl J Med 2000;343:1925–1932.

Murray, B.E. Vancomycin-resistant enterococcal infections. N Engl J Med 2000;342:710–721.

van den Bogaard AE, Jensen LB, Stobberingh EE. Vancomycin-resistant enterococci in turkeys and farmers (letter to the editor). N Engl J Med 1997;337:1558–1559.

Wenzel RP, Edmond MB. Managing antibiotic resistance (Editorial). N Engl J Med 2000;343:1961–1963.

DO NOT PRESCRIBE INTRAVENOUS VANCOMYCIN TO TREAT *CLOSTRIDIUM DIFFICILE*

MICHAEL J. MORITZ, MD

Antibiotic use leads to the development of antibiotic-associated diarrhea in up to 50% of patients. *Clostridium difficile* causes 20 to 30% of cases of antibiotic-associated diarrhea, 50 to 70% of cases of antibiotic-associated colitis, and greater than 90% of cases of pseudomembranous colitis. Pseudomembranous colitis is named for the endoscopic appearance of the colonic mucosa that exhibits 1 to 5 mm, raised, whitish-yellow plaques (pseudomembranes) that can progress to confluence and overlie colonic mucosa that is erythematous and minimally friable. A small fraction of cases may have other causes, such as staphylococci, but it is safe to assume that almost all cases of pseudomembranous colitis are related to *C. difficile*.

C. difficile colitis begins when an individual, susceptible because the normal colonic flora has been altered, ingests spores that then germinate and colonize the host colonic mucosa. *C. difficile* bacteria produce enterotoxins A and B which are responsible for the secretory diarrhea. The diagnosis is made by detecting the enterotoxins in the stool using a variety of assays. The most sensitive test is to assay for cytotoxicity resulting from the enterotoxins by adding filtered stool to plated tissue culture cells, but this assay is difficult to standardize and has a long turnaround time. Newer immunoassays for the enterotoxins are more specific but less sensitive, and most only assay for enterotoxin A. Only assaying for enterotoxin A will miss the uncommon *C. difficile* strains that only produce enterotoxin B.

SIGNS AND SYMPTOMS

Clinical colitis most typically begins 5 to 10 days after a course of antibiotics begins with fever, abdominal pain, and diarrhea. *C. difficile* colitis can begin up to several weeks after the discontinuation of antibiotic therapy. If the diagnosis is made early and the symptoms are mild and in a relatively normal host (immunocompetent, normal colon, not at extremes of age), discontinuation of antibiotics will aid in diminution of symptoms within one week. For most patients, even with improving symptoms it is appropriate to treat the *C. difficile* colitis with antibiotics.

C. difficile is sensitive to metronidazole, vancomycin and rifampin. First-line therapy is oral metronidazole (Flagyl) 250 mg four times daily for 10 days. This regimen is effective in 95% of cases with a relapse rate of about 10%. In patients unable to take oral medications, metronidazole may be given intravenously with the same efficacy. As metronidazole is well absorbed from the gut, its level in the stool is a function of transport into the colonic lumen and is related to the degree of colonic inflammation and secretory diarrhea. Metronidazole failures, defined as persistent or worsening symptoms, may be treated with *oral* vancomycin. When vancomycin is given orally, it is nonabsorbable and intraluminally reaches the colon mucosa. Intravenous vancomycin is *ineffective* in the treatment of *C. difficile* colitis. The usual dose of oral vancomycin for adults is 125 mg orally four times daily for ten days. A further concern about oral vancomycin is its proclivity to contribute to the development of vancomycin-resistant enterococci, hence it should be second-line therapy, and the length of the course not be overly long. Anecdotally, vancomycin given by enema has been used in patients who are refractory to other therapies.

Because *C. difficile* is a spore-forming bacteria, appropriate treatment can eliminate the bacteria but will not have any effect on spores that can persist on colonic mucosa. Days to weeks later, *C. difficile* colitis can recur. Recurrence is also possible if the patient is reinoculated from the same environmental reservoir. Generally, recurrence represents the reappearance of the same sensitive organism rather than antibiotic resistance, and the same treatment regimen that cleared the symptoms the first time should be repeated.

Please see Chapter 84 for information on the use of probiotics and *C. difficile* infection.

SUGGESTED READINGS

Guerrant RL, Lima AAM. Pseudomembranous enterocolitis *(Clostridium difficile colitis)*, in inflammatory enteritis. In Mandell, GL, Bennett, JE, Dolphin, R, eds. Mandell, Douglas, and Bennett's Principles and Practice of Infectious Disease. 5th Ed. Philadelphia: Churchill Livingstone, 2000, p.1131.

Stoddart B, Wilcox MH. Clostridium difficile. Curr Opin Infect Dis 2002;15: 513–518.

Thielman NM. Antibiotic-Associated Colitis. In Mandell, GL, Bennett, JE, Dolphin, R., eds. Mandell, Douglas, and Bennett's Principles and Practice of Infectious Disease. 5th Ed. Philadelphia: Churchill Livingstone, 2000, pp.1112–1126.

88

CONSIDER DOUBLE-COVERING
PSEUDOMONAS INFECTIONS

MICHAEL J. MORITZ, MD

Pseudomonas species produce an array of mostly nosocomial infections. *Pseudomonas aeruginosa* is the most common pathogen among the pseudomonads. The name *aeruginosa* comes from the fluorescent blue-green pigment pyocyanin that most strains produce. Pseudomonads grow well in moist environments and require limited nutrients. They are ubiquitous in nature and are normal commensal organisms in animals and humans. *P. aeruginosa* grows easily in water and colonizes faucets, tap aerators, sinks, ice machines, and kitchens. It can withstand many disinfectants; it has been reported to grow in Betadine when Betadine is kept in a warmer at 37°C. Pseudomonads are everywhere in hospitals. According to data from the Centers for Disease Control and Prevention (CDC), pseudomonads are the fifth most common nosocomial organisms, accounting for 9% of isolates. *P. aeruginosa* is the second most common cause of nosocomial pneumonia (17% of cases).

WATCH OUT FOR

P. aeruginosa does not cause infection in a normal human host, but a compromised individual is susceptible to invasive infection. Compromised conditions include immunosuppression and damaged skin or mucosal barriers. Common settings include neutropenia, chronic bladder catheters, cystic fibrosis, ventilator-dependent respiratory failure, invasive devices, and patients receiving broad-spectrum antibiotics. Transplant recipients receiving imipenem have a predisposition to acquiring multidrug-resistant *P. aeruginosa*.

The most common pseudomonad nosocomial infections are bacteremia, pneumonia, and urinary tract infections. Other infections include surgical infections (deep wound infections), external otitis, corneal keratitis, and hematogenously spread infections in a variety of sites, including endocarditis and osteomyelitis.

P. aeruginosa is known to have a relatively high rate of resistance to antibiotics. Since the late 1990s resistance of intensive care isolates has increased. Resistance to aminoglycosides is highly variable, ranging from 5 to 66%. Resistance to the antipseudomonal penicillins also varies, with piperacillin having 5 to 60% of strains resistant, ticarcillin 12 to 60% strains resistant, and mezlocillin still having general effectiveness. The variable coverage of antipseudomonal cephalo-sporins include ceftazidime (2 to 45% resistant), cefepime (10 to 50% resistant), and cefoperazone (5 to 35% resistant). Aztreonam (a monobactam) has resistance in 24 to 54% of strains. Ciprofloxacin is the fluoroquinolone with the best antipseudomonal activity, yet 8 to 75% of strains show resistance. The carbepenems (imipenem and meropenem) have similar resistance profiles (11 to 64% versus 5 to 48% respectively), with the newer drug meropenem retaining slightly higher effectiveness.

WHAT TO DO

In cases of suspected *P. aeruginosa* sepsis, and especially in septic shock, empiric therapy with a two-drug regimen is strongly advised. The decision for two-drug versus one-drug therapy is based on the severity of the patient's clinical infection and the magnitude of his or her underlying immunocompromised state. A two-antibiotic regimen has been reported to decrease the mortality of *P. aeruginosa* bacteremia by almost half (27% versus 47% mortality). Standard therapy is an antipseudomonal β-lactam (penicillin family or cephalosporin family) plus an aminoglycoside, but this is a generalization and each hospital's organisms will have a spectrum of resistance to guide empiric therapy. A monobactam, carbepenem, or antipseudomonal fluoroquinolone can be used in place of the β-lactam drug with an aminoglycoside. Non-aminoglycoside regimens will typically include two of the five groups mentioned above: penicillin, cephalosporin, carbepenem, monobactam, and quinolone. Resistance to nonaminoglycosides is more common and more quickly acquired than resistance to aminoglycosides; hence there is some risk to avoiding aminoglycosides. Antibiotic resistance is so common that any antibiotic regimen is empiric until sensitivities are determined.

One final note is that in addition to its intrinsic property of relatively high resistance, *P. aeruginosa* quickly acquires resistance via plasmid transfer when under antibiotic pressure. Interval cultures searching for emergence of resistance to the antibiotic regimen are needed. When considering empiric therapy, the intrinsic resistance pattern of pseudomonads in a given hospital and the degree of infirmity and compromised status of the patient must be considered.

SUGGESTED READINGS

Carmeli Y, Troillet N, Eliopoulos GM, Samore MH. Emergence of antibiotic-resistant *Pseudomonas aeruginosa:* comparison of risks associated with different antipseudomonal agents. Antimicrob Agents Chemother 1999;43:1379–1382.

Giamarellou H, Antoniadou A. Antipseudomonal antibiotics. Med Clin North Am 2001;85:19–42.

Goldman L, Bennett JC, eds. Cecil Textbook of Medicine, 21st Ed. Philadelphia: W.B. Saunders, 2000, pp.1709–1711.

Hilf M, Yu VL, Sharp J, et al. Antibiotic therapy for Pseudomonas aeruginosa bacteremia: outcome correlations in a prospective study of 200 patients. Am J Med 1989;87:540–546.

REMEMBER TO GIVE VACCINES FOR *HAEMOPHILUS INFLUENZAE*, MENINGOCOCCUS AND PNEUMOCOCCUS IN PATIENTS WHO UNDERGO A SPLENECTOMY, AND ALWAYS HAVE A HIGH INDEX OF SUSPICION FOR OVERWHELMING POSTSPLENECTOMY SEPSIS (OPSS) IN PATIENTS WITH SPLENECTOMY

HARSH JAIN, MD

Patients who undergo splenectomy must be vaccinated against *Haemophilus influenzae*, meningococcus, and pneumococcus. This is to reduce the risk of the potentially fatal syndrome known as overwhelming postsplenectomy sepsis (OPSS) or infection (OPSI).

SIGNS AND SYMPTOMS

OPSS is characterized by a brief period of low-grade fever and nonspecific symptoms such as chills, pharyngitis, headache, malaise, myalgias, abdominal pain, vomiting, or diarrhea that rapidly deteriorates into septic shock with concomitant seizures, coma, and disseminated intravascular coagulation that culminates in cardiovascular collapse. The time from initial prodromal symptoms to vascular collapse is very short, typically 1 to 2 days. Up to 50% of cases may be associated with pneumonia or meningitis, especially in children under 5 years of age. Previously it was reported that the mortality rate in full-blown OPSS, despite appropriate treatment and support, approached 70%. Newer reports suggest that with prompt medical attention the mortality is in the range of 10%. Greater awareness on the parts of patients and physicians is responsible for much of the improvement in outcome. Prompt recognition and treatment of OPSS is crucial.

The incidence of OPSS is controversial, with widely varying reports. The decrease in incidence in more recent reports presumably reflects the effectiveness of prophylactic antibiotics in children and the recommendation for and availability of vaccination for pneumococci and *H. influenzae*. The risk varies with age (exponentially higher with the very young) and diagnosis necessitating the splenectomy (higher with hematologic diagnoses than trauma and lower with longer distance of time from splenectomy). Children have a higher incidence of OPSS (lifetime risk approximately 5%, range 0.1 to 8.5%)

compared to adults (lifetime risk 0.9%, range 0.3 to 1.9%). Children less than 5 years of age may have a risk of OPSS approaching 10%. OPSS usually occurs in the first two years postsplenectomy. The risk, however, is a lifelong one, with approximately 40% of OPSS cases occurring more than 5 years postsplenectomy.

The most common causative organisms of OPSS are encapsulated bacteria. The single most important pathogen in OPSS is *Streptococcus pneumoniae*, which causes 50 to 90% of cases. Although it can be causative in all age groups, it is more common in older individuals. The second most common OPSS pathogen is *Haemophilus influenzae* type B, seen mostly in children less than 15 years of age. The third most common cause of OPSS is *Neisseria meningitidis*. Less common pathogens include group A streptococci and, rarely, *Capnocytophaga canimorsus* (from dog bites), group B streptococci, enterococci, and others including Gram-negative rods. The asplenic patient is also susceptible to serious parasitic erythrocyte infections (e.g., babesiosis and malaria).

WHAT TO DO

The diagnosis of OPSS relies upon a high index of suspicion. A history of splenectomy or functional asplenia in the presentation of fever should be considered a medical emergency and warrants the administration of appropriate parenteral antibiotics. A peripheral blood smear should be obtained and examined for the presence of bacteria. Blood cultures are generally positive within 24 hours. Supportive care should be undertaken for other symptoms; however, antimicrobial therapy should not be withheld during the diagnostic workup. Antibiotics should cover the three common causative agents, *S. pneumoniae*, *H. influenzae*, and *N. meningitidis*. Local resistance patterns should be used to establish treatment. If penicillin-resistant pneumococci are not prevalent, penicillin, ampicillin, or ceftriaxone can be given. If there is concern for resistance or in the presence of suspected meningitis, vancomycin *with or without* ceftriaxone should be given. Antibiotic therapy can be tailored once the causative agent is identified by culture. Intravascular volume depletion should be corrected aggressively and intense supportive care administered.

The incidence of OPSS can be minimized with vaccinations, antibiotic prophylaxis, patient education, and splenic salvage when possible. Vaccinations exist for the three common causative agents. In patients who are to undergo elective splenectomy, these vaccinations should be given at least 2 weeks preoperatively. In patients who undergo emergent splenectomy, it remains uncertain when vaccinations should be administered. Waiting until the acute postoperative catabolic state resolves may increase the vaccines' effectiveness but risks the patient becoming lost to follow-up and not being vaccinated. A reasonable compromise delays vaccination briefly until just before hospital discharge. Annual influenza vaccinations and booster pneumococcal vaccinations every 5 years are recommended. Vaccinations are not completely effective and failure (i.e., the development of OPSS) can occur in vaccinated patients.

Antibiotic prophylaxis was advised prior to the availability of vaccines, but its role is less clear at present. The effectiveness of antibiotics (penicillin or trimethoprim-sulfamethoxazole) has been compromised by community-acquired pneumococcal antibiotic resistance. Some still advise daily antibiotics for the first 2 years postsplenectomy in young children; others promote their use until a set age (e.g., 5 years or 18 years).

Patient education is also an important preventive measure. Asplenic patients should be advised:

1) The risk of infection is lifelong but is greatest in the first two years postsplenectomy.
2) Infections progress rapidly and are life-threatening.
3) The patient should seek immediate medical attention if febrile or feeling unwell.
4) If immediate medical attention is not available, begin self-administered antipneumococcal therapy. This requires having a supply while traveling or with limited access to healthcare.
5) All health care providers should be notified of the asplenic status, regardless of how long ago their splenectomy took place (Medic Alert bracelets are appropriate).

One final note is that patients who were splenectomized 10 to 15 years ago may not have had the full protocol of vaccinations and should be queried as to whether they have received all three current vaccinations. If they are lacking one or more, they should be administered.

SUGGESTED READINGS

Brigden ML, Pattulo AL. Prevention and management of overwhelming postsplenectomy infection–an update. Crit Care Med 1999;4:836–842.

Lynch AM, Kapila, R. Overwhelming postsplenectomy infection. Infec Dis Clin North Am 1996;10:693–707.

Styrt B. Infection associated with asplenia: risks, mechanisms and prevention. Am J Med 1990;88:33N–42N.

Williams DN, Kaur B. Postsplenectomy care: strategies to decrease the risk of infection. Postgraduate Med 1996;100:195–205.

CONSIDER THE USE OF FLUCONAZOLE PROPHYLAXIS IN INTENSIVE CARE PATIENTS WITH SEVERE PANCREATITIS, ABDOMINAL SEPSIS, OR NEED FOR MULTIPLE ABDOMINAL SURGERIES

LISA MARCUCCI, MD

There is growing awareness of the increasing role of fungal infections in morbidity and mortality of intensive care unit (ICU) patients. The use of the azoles in prophylaxis for fungal infection in immunocompromised patients is well described and has proven efficacy. In addition, there is an increasing body of work that azole prophylaxis may be of benefit in certain patient populations of immunocompetent patients as well. In both patient populations, infections caused by Candida species are thought to develop from endogenous colonization, yet the value of fungal surveillance cultures in critically ill patients is uncertain and lacks a high positive predictive value.

Fungal infections may develop in up to 30% to 35% of patients with necrotizing pancreatitis, with *Candida albicans* being the most frequently isolated fungal species by far. Two recent studies showed a significant decrease in fungal infections in a fluconazole prophylaxis group compared to a control group. In patients with septic shock from abdominal nonpancreatic sources, use of empiric fluconazole also showed a decreased incidence of candidemia and fungal-related deaths in three recent studies, although reduction in overall mortality was less certain. Some caution has been voiced concerning the prophylactic use of fluconazole in "moderately ill" immunocompetent patients because of the risk of developing drug-resistant (resistant to azole drugs) fungal strains, especially Candida glabrata, although Swoboda and colleagues have reported no shift to non-albicans pathogens with a decreased risk of mortality using prophylaxis.

Of recent interest to critical care physicians, is the emerging literature on the anti–inflammatory properties of fluconazole. It appears that, separate from its anti-fungal properties, use of fluconazole may improve outcomes in septic patients due to blunting of the systemic inflammatory response that typically occurs. In light of this effect and the high mortality of candidemia, it seems reasonable to institute a short (10 to 14 day) course of prophylactic oral azole therapy (initial bolus of 800 mg and then a minimum of 200 and preferably 400 mg/day of fluconazole) in patients with severe pancreatitis, abdominal perforation or anastomotic breakdown, and other abdominal catastrophes.

SUGGESTED READINGS

De Waele JJ, Vogelaers D, Blot S, Coladyn F. Fungal infections in patients with severe acute pancreatitis and the use of prophylactic therapy. Clin Infect Dis 2003;37:208–213.

He YM, Lu XS, Ai ZL, et al. Prevention and therapy of fungal infection in severe acute pancreatitis: a prospective clinical study. World J Gastroenterol 2003;9:2619–2621.

Swoboda SN, Merz WG, Lipsett PA. Candidemia: the impact of antifungal prophylaxis in a surgical intensive care unit. Surg Infect 2003;4:345–354

Sypula WT, Kale-Pradhan PB. Therapeutic dilemma of fluconazole prophylaxis in intensive care. Ann Pharmacother 2002;36:155–159.

91

DO NOT PRESCRIBE VIAGRA TO A PATIENT TAKING NITRATES AND VICE VERSA

ASHRAF I. OSMAN, MD

Sildenafil (Viagra) is a vasodilator and the first effective oral medication for erectile dysfunction. Erectile dysfunction can be categorized by mechanism: (1) vasculogenic as a result of occlusive atherosclerosis of the common and/or internal iliac arteries; (2) neurogenic, as in diabetic neuropathy, multiple sclerosis, and spinal cord injury; and (3) psychological. Sildenafil is effective in all three types of erectile dysfunction. Erectile dysfunction is common in men with cardiovascular disease; this combination provides the setting for a dangerous drug interaction.

Sildenafil produces vasodilatation by enhancing the effects of nitric oxide. During normal sexual stimulation, cells of the corpus cavernosum release nitric oxide, which activates the guanylate cyclase within smooth muscles and causes increased levels of cyclic guanine monophosphate (cGMP). Cyclic GMP causes smooth muscle relaxation in the corpus cavernosum, increased blood flow to the penis, increased intracavernosal pressure, and subsequent penile erection. Sildenafil enhances the effect of nitric oxide by selectively inhibiting phosphodiesterase type 5 (PDE-5), the enzyme responsible for degradation of cGMP in the corpus cavernosum.

WATCH OUT FOR

When sildenafil is taken without nitrates, it causes a small drop in blood pressure (approximately 8 to 10 mm Hg). When administered with topical, oral, or sublingual nitrates such as nitroglycerin or isorbide (mono- or dinitrate), which are ultimately converted to nitric oxide, there is a marked synergistic vasodilation that may cause a marked drop in blood pressure and malignant arrhythmias. In patients with coronary artery disease, any fall in blood pressure may result in angina, and the development of angina after taking sildenafil is a contraindication to taking nitrates. The risk of using sildenafil is high enough that the revised product insert for sildenafil (November 1998) identifies four groups of cardiac patients for whom sildenafil is contraindicated, even in the absence of nitrates: (1) patients who have suffered a myocardial infarction, stroke, or life-threatening arrhythmia in the past six months; (2) patients with resting hypotension (blood pressure less than 90/50) or hypertension (blood pressure greater than 170/100); (3) patients with cardiac failure or coronary artery disease causing angina; and (4) patients with retinitis pigmentosa (a minority of whom have genetic disorders of retinal phosphodiesterase). The two newer drugs vardenafil (Levitra) and tadalafil (Cialis) have similar pharmacology as sildenafil and the above cautions and warnings also apply.

WHAT TO DO   The half-life of sildenafil is 4 hours and five half-lives is generally used as the time needed to effectively clear a drug from the system. Thus 24 hours is a reasonable recommendation for the minimum time between administering sildenafil and nitrates. Sildenafil is 80% metabolized in the liver by the cytochrome P450 3A4 system and 20% metabolized in the kidney. Sildenafil metabolism is inhibited by tacrolimus, erythromycin, clarithromycin, ketoconazole, and other azole antifungals. Patients taking these drugs have an increased half-life of sildenafil and a 24-hour wait time is not sufficient for subsequent nitrate administration. Similar concerns apply to vardenafil (half-life of 5 hours) and tadalafil (half-life of 17 hours). Sufficient wait times for these drugs and the administration of nitrates are estimated to be 36 hours and 4 days, respectively, if no cytochrome P450 3A4 inhibitors are being taken.

Of recent concern to clinicians is that two over-the-counter dietary supplements for increasing sexual desire, confidence, and performance were recently and illegally found to contain sildenafil. These products were withdrawn from the market, but the potential for a dangerous drug interaction from a nonprescription compound in this consumer-driven market bears attention. It is best to query the patient or family as to use of any sexual enhancement products before prescribing nitrates.

One final note is that use of sildenafil, vardenafil, and tadalafil should be considered carefully when there is concomitant use of alpha-blockers that cause hypotension, such as terazosin (Hytrin), doxazosin (Cardura), and tamsulosin (Flomax).

SUGGESTED READINGS

Ament PW, Bertolino JG, Liszewski JL. Clinically significant drug interactions. Am Fam Phys 2000;61:1745–1754.

Cheitlin MD. The ten most commonly asked questions about sildenafil (Viagra). Cardiol Rev 1999;7:173–175.

FDA MedWatch website. 2003 Safety alerts for drugs, biologics, medical devices, and dietary supplements. Available at: http://www.fda.gov/medwatch/ SAFETY/2003/ safety03.htm. Accessed July 22, 2005.

How dangerous is Viagra? Harvard Heart Lett August 2000;10:5–6.

Muniz AE, Holstege CP. Acute myocardial infarction associated with sildenafil (Viagra) ingestion. Am J Emerg Med 2000;18:353–355.

DO NOT PRESCRIBE HYDROCODONE (VICODIN, LORTAB) OR TRAMADOL (ULTRAM) TO A PATIENT WHO IS TAKING FLUOXETINE (PROZAC), PAROXETINE (PAXIL), OR HIGH-DOSE SERTRALINE (ZOLOFT)

NEIL SANDSON, MD

Hydrocodone and tramadol are both prodrugs. They are relatively poor analgesics in their parent forms and require the intact functioning of the cytochrome P450 2D6 enzyme to be transformed into metabolites that are responsible for providing effective analgesia. Cytochrome P450 2D6 transforms hydrocodone (a component of Vicodin) into hydromorphone (Dilaudid). It also transforms Ultram into the active metabolite M1. Since fluoxetine, paroxetine, and sertraline (at doses of greater than or equal to 150 mg/d) significantly impair the functioning of cytochrome P450 2D6, their presence prevents both hydrocodone and tramadol from being converted to their metabolites and thus blocks them from acting as effective analgesic compounds. Other selective serotonin reuptake inhibitors (SSRIs), such as fluvoxamine (Luvox), citalopram (Celexa), and escitalopram (Lexapro), do not inhibit this cytochrome and do not prevent hydrocodone and tramadol from functioning in a normal manner and providing analgesia when coadministered.

A common clinical scenario in surgery where this P450 2D6 drug interaction is encountered is after breast biopsy. SSRI use is common in women, and hydrocodone is commonly prescribed for analgesia after breast biopsy. The patient should be specifically queried as to use of fluoxetine, paroxetine, and sertraline and an alternate analgesia strategy devised to avoid patient discomfort and inconvenience if one of these SSRIs is being taken.

One final note is that roughly 10% of individuals are born lacking P450 2D6, and in these individuals, hydrocodone and tramadol will generally be ineffective analgesics regardless of SSRI use.

SUGGESTED READINGS

Otton SV, Schadel M, Cheung SW, et al: CYP2D6 phenotype determines the metabolic conversion of hydrocodone to hydromorphone. *Clin Pharmacol Ther*, 1993;54:463–472.

Poulsen L, Arendt-Nielsen L, Brosen K, et al. The hypoanalgesic effect of tramadol in relation to CYP2D6. *Clin Pharmacol Ther*, 1996;60.

DO NOT PRESCRIBE MONOAMINE OXIDASE INHIBITORS (MAOIs) TO A PATIENT WHO IS TAKING A SELECTIVE SEROTONIN REUPTAKE INHIBITOR (SSRI)

NEIL SANDSON, MD

Monoamine oxidase inhibitors (MAOIs) work by inhibiting the breakdown and increasing body levels of monoamines. Common monoamines include serotonin and the catecholamines norepinephrine, epinephrine, and dopamine. Coadministration of an MAOI with a serotonergically active agent such as a selective serotonin reuptake inhibitor (SSRI) will cause two separate biochemical mechanisms that act to raise levels of serotonin and the catecholamines to act synergistically. This can cause dangerously high levels of serotonin that can lead to a central serotonin syndrome. This is characterized by fever (sometimes severe), confusion, diarrhea, flushing, myoclonus and, when severe, can lead to seizures, vital sign instability, and death.

MAOIs and compounds with significant MAOI-like activity currently available in the United States include the antidepressants phenelzine (Nardil) and tranylcypromine (Parnate), the antiParkinson agent selegiline (Deprenyl), and the antibiotic linezolid (Zyvox). The currently available SSRIs in the United States include fluoxetine (Prozac), sertraline (Zoloft), paroxetine (Paxil), fluvoxamine (Luvox), citalopram (Celexa), and escitalopram (Lexapro). Of particular note to surgeons is the MAOI effect of linezolid. Care should be taken to review the patient's medications for the commonly prescribed antidepressants or meperidine before starting this antibiotic.

One final note is that central serotonin syndromes also can occur when MAOIs are combined with other serotonergic agents such as venlafaxine (Effexor), nefazodone (Serzone), tricyclic antidepressants, dextromethorphan, and meperidine (Demerol).

SUGGESTED READINGS

Beasley CM Jr., Masica DN, Heiligenstein JH, Wheadon DE, Zerbe RL. Possible monoamine oxidase inhibitor-serotonin uptake inhibitor interaction: fluoxetine clinical data and preclinical findings. *J Clin Pharmacol*, 1993;13:312–320.

Bem JL, Peck R. Dextromethorphan: an overview of safety issues. *Drug Saf*, 1992;7:190–199.

Sporer KA. The serotonin syndrome: implicated drugs, pathophysiology, and management. *Drug Saf*, 1995;13:94–104.

GIVE PROPHYLACTIC PERIOPERATIVE BETA-BLOCKERS FOR PATIENTS AT RISK FOR CARDIAC ISCHEMIA.

MICHAEL J. MORITZ, MD

Assessment and management of perioperative risk of cardiac ischemia is a complex issue. Coronary artery disease (ischemic heart disease) may be clinically silent, present abruptly and atypically, and carry significant morbidity and mortality. Annually in the United States, there are about 50,000 perioperative myocardial infarctions (MI) with a mortality of 40%. The strongest risk factor for perioperative MI is a prior MI; the reinfarction rate is 25 to 35% for surgery within 3 months of an MI, 10 to 15% between 3 and 6 months postMI, and 5% thereafter.

WATCH OUT FOR

There have been numerous attempts to quantitate cardiac risk and devise algorithms for preoperative assessment and perioperative management. Even contemporaneous assessments of cardiac risk in noncardiac surgery patients such as the recommendations for a large number of the American College of Cardiology/American Heart Association (jointly, 1996) and the American College of Physicians (1997) differ substantially, offering divergent recommendations for a large number of patients. Patients at moderate or high cardiac risk are variably defined. Defining exact cardiac risk in terms of the benefit from perioperative beta-blockade is difficult. The list of cardiac risk factors includes the following: 1) History—a history of hypertension, MI, stroke, angina, congestive heart failure, valvular heart disease, or abnormal cardiac rhythm (excluding benign rhythms such as nonsinus atrial premature contractions or fewer than 5 premature ventricular contractions per minute); 2) a history of diabetes; 3) age over 70; 4) renal insufficiency (variably defined); 5) high risk surgical procedure, which includes all intraperitoneal, intrathoracic, aortic, and vascular procedures; and 6) emergency operations in susceptible patients.

Seperate from risk assessment is perioperative management. The use of beta-blockade has a low risk of adverse events and is low cost, and it seems reasonable to utilize them relatively liberally. Randomized trials of perioperative measures to reduce cardiac complications using beta-blockade do show a reduction in cardiac ischemic events.

The trials have used varying medications and regimens on populations undergoing varying surgeries, as described below.

According to Wallace and Colleagues (1988), atenolol (5 to 10mg given intravenously 30 minutes before the operating room and 50 to 100mg orally each day afterward for up to 7 days and adjusted to a target heart rate of 55 to 65) was effective in patients undergoing elective noncardiac surgery. It reduced postoperative cardiac ischemic events (24 versus 39%), cardiac deaths in the ensuing 2 years (4 versus 12%), and all causes of mortality over 2 years (9 versus 21%) as compared to controls with no difference in perioperative MI or death. Poldermans et al (1999) reported that bisoprolol (5–10mg given orally once daily started 7 days preoperatively and continued at least 30 days postoperatively in patients undergoing vascular surgery) reduced cardiac morbidity (nonfatal MI 0 versus 17%) and mortality (cardiac death 3.4 versus 17%) as compared to controls. In addition, intraoperative intravenous esmolol titrated to heart rate decreased the postoperative ischemia (Raby et al 1999, Urban et al 2000) in vascular surgery (postoperative cardiac ischemia 33 versus 73%) and knee replacement (who also received metoprolol postoperatively, postoperative cardiac ischemia 6 versus 15% and postoperative MI 2 versus 6%) as compared to controls.

WHAT TO DO

Regarding which beta-blocker to utilize and at which dose, the group of cardioselective (beta$_1$) blockers with low intrinsic sympathomimetic activity should physiologically provide the best risk-benefit trade-off. This group includes atenolol, esmolol, metoprolol, bevantolol, bisoprolol, and betaxolol. Choice of medication depends on drug availability, route of administration, need for continuous electrocardiographic (ECG) monitoring (depending on drug and route of administration), and timing of surgery. Consultation with the anesthesiologist is key. For patients on beta-blockade preoperatively for any indication, continuing beta-blockade is essential to avoid the known complications of abrupt withdrawal (tachyarrhythmias, MI, cardiac death).

One final note is that liberal use of perioperative beta-blockers is not a substitute for preoperative evaluation by a qualified physician, consultation with a cardiologist when indicated, and completion of the prescribed workup and therapy in advance. Emergent and emergency surgeries and other nonelective events preclude obtaining a complete cardiac assessment in advance and exemplify circumstances when such prophylaxis can be helpful.

SUGGESTED READINGS

Cohn SL, Goldman L. Preoperative risk evaluation and perioperative management of patients with coronary artery disease. Med Clin North America, 2003;87:111–136.

Gordon AJ, Macpherson DS. Guideline chaos: conflicting recommendations for preoperative cardiac assessment. Am J Cardiol, 2003;91: 1299–1303.

Poldermans D, Boersma E, Bax JJ, et al. Bisoprolol reduces cardiac death and myocardial infarction in high-risk patients as long as 2 years after successful major vascular surgery. Eur Heart J, 2001;22:1353–1358.

Raby KE, Brull SJ, Timimi F, et al. The effect of heart rate control on myocardial ischemia among high-risk patients after vascular surgery. Anesth Analg 1999;88:477–482.

Urban MK, Markowitz SM, Gordon MA, Urguhart BL, Kligfield P. Postoperative prophylactic administration of beta-adrenergic blockers in patients at risk for myocardial ischemia. Anesth Analg, 2000;90:1257–1261.

Wallace A, Layug B, Tateo I, et al. Prophylactic atenolol reduces postoperative myocardial ischemia. Anesthesiology 1998;88:7–17.

95

CONSIDER *N*-ACETYLCYSTEINE OR SODIUM BICARBONATE PROPHYLAXIS ALONG WITH ADEQUATE HYDRATION TO COMBAT CONTRAST-INDUCED NEPHROPATHY

MICHAEL J. MORITZ, MD

Contrast-induced nephropathy is the third most common cause of in-hospital acute renal failure and has been reported to occur in between 6% and 15% of patients receiving intravenous contrast dye. Iodinated contrast is used for arteriography (including cardiac catheterization) and venography, and is administered intravenously (IV) for contrast-enhanced computed tomography (CT) scans. All iodinated contrast agents used for intravascular radiography have potential nephrotoxicity. The mechanism of renal injury is unknown but may include oxidative injury, a prerenal component from the diuretic effect of the contrast agent, and other etiologies. Nephrotoxicity depends on patient factors and increases with the following: renal insufficiency; diabetes or myeloma as the etiology of chronic renal insufficiency; dehydration; and increasing age. Nephrotoxicity is also a function of the specific agent, with an increased incidence with the older, ionic, higher osmolarity agents, and a decreased incidence with newer, more expensive, nonionic, lower osmolarity agents.

WHAT TO DO

To reduce the risk of contrast-induced nephrotoxicity, patients should be adequately hydrated before exposure to contrast. Varying regimens have been used. One common regimen consists of 0.45% saline pre-exposure at 1 mL/kg/hr for 12 hours for inpatients or 2 mL/kg/hr for at least 4 hours for outpatients and postexposure at 75 mL/hr for 12 hours.

In addition to hydration, consideration should be given to administering *N*-acetylcysteine (NAC), especially in patients with renal insufficiency. One recent meta-analysis showed that NAC (which is relatively inexpensive and has few side effects if taken by mouth) reduced the risk of contrast-induced nephrotoxicity in patients with pre-existing chronic renal insufficiency. However, in this analysis, single doses varied widely, with oral doses of 400 to 1500 mg and IV doses of 50 to 150 mg/kg given at varying intervals and durations. Some clinicians recommend that if oral dosing is used, apparently more than one pre-exposure dose is needed. One common regimen consists of pre-exposure NAC 600 mg orally for two doses at least 4 hours apart and postexposure two doses 12 hours apart. For oral administration, NAC is best administered in a strongly flavored drink such as a carbonated cola or Fresca to partially mask the disagreeable odor and taste. In emergencies, IV administration of 150 mg/kg in 500 mL of 0.9% saline over 30 minutes pre-exposure and 50 mg/kg in 500 mL of 0.9% saline over 4 hours postexposure has been used, although IV use is more common for the treatment of acetaminophen overdose. Intravenous NAC has a higher risk of anaphylactoid reactions than does oral administration and the physician must consider the risk-benefit ratio of using IV NAC for renal prophylaxis.

Perhaps a better choice than using IV NAC for contrast prophylaxis is administering a sodium bicarbonate infusion of 3 amps of sodium mixed in one liter of D5W. A recent randomized controlled trial has shown the effectiveness of reducing contrast-induced nephropathy with the use of sodium bicarbonate in patients with both normal renal function and renal insufficiency pre-contrast administration. In this study patients received a bolus of 3 mg/kg/hr for 1 hour before iopamidol contrast followed by an infusion of 1 mL/kg/hr for 6 hours after the procedure. Contrast-induced nephropathy occurred in 1.7% of patients in the bicarbonate group, as compared to 13.6% in the control group of sodium chloride infusion. Use of sodium bicarbonate may have an advantage over NAC in the urgent setting because the pretreatment time is only one hour.

One final note is that NAC or sodium bicarbonate is not needed with magnetic resonance imaging contrast agents. These contrast agents are not iodine-based, but rather use a metal with magnetic properties (e.g., iron or the rare earth gadolinium) and have different toxicities.

SUGGESTED READINGS

Alonso A, Lau J, Jaber BL, Weintraub A, Sarnak MJ. Prevention of radiocontrast nephropathy with N-acetylcysteine in patients with chronic kidney disease: a meta-analysis of randomized, controlled trials. A J Kidney Dis 2004;43:1–9.

Fishbane S, Durham JH, Marzo K, Rudnick M. N-acetylcysteine in the prevention of radiocontrast-induced nephropathy. J Am Soc Nephrol, 2004;15:251–260.

MacNeill BC, Harding SA, Bazari H, et al. Prophylaxis of contrast-induced nephropathy in patients undergoing coronary angiography. Cath Cardiovasc Inter 2003;60:458–461.

Merten GJ, Burgess WP, Gray LV, et al. Prevention of contrast-induced nephropathy with sodium bicarbonate: a randomized controlled trial. JAMA 2004;291:2328–2334.

96

DO NOT USE "RENAL DOSE" DOPAMINE.

LISA MARCUCCI, MD

Although still commonly encountered in clinical practice (particularly in cardiac surgery) and widely used until the late 1990s, the use of renal dose dopamine as a renoprotective strategy in surgical patients must be discouraged. Its use in patients subject to renal stress was originally promulgated on the fact that, in studies in animals and healthy human volunteers, low dose dopamine (1–3 mcg/kg/min) increased renal blood flow and promoted natriuresis and diuresis. As renal ischemia is a common cause of renal failure, the extrapolation was made that it would protect renal cellular oxygenation and preserve glomerular filtration, even though there was a lack of studies to support this conclusion. A corollary argument often advanced was that, even if it did not provide much efficacy, the risks of using this drug at "less than pressor level" was minimal.

However, most of the recent work on the use of renal dose dopamine has made it abundantly clear that there is no clinically significant beneficial effect on kidney function. The Australia and New Zealand Intensive Care Society recently reported a large, controlled study of patients with early changes consistent with renal dysfunction that showed no difference in control versus renal dose dopamine treatment groups in multiple markers of renal failure including: peak serum creatinine; mean increase in baseline to the peak creatine concentration; number of patients whose serum creatinine rose to greater than 300 μmol/L; and the number of patients who required renal replacement therapy. In addition, there was no statistical difference between the control and treatment groups in duration of mechanical ventilation, survival to intensive care unit discharge, and duration of hospital stay. Additional studies arguing against the use of renal dose dopamine include the NORASEPT II study that looked at renal dose dopamine in the setting of acute renal failure and septic shock and a meta-analysis done by Kellum et al in 2001.

WATCH OUT FOR

In addition to exposing the lack of evidence-based medicine for the use of renal dose dopamine, investigators are better elucidating the risks of using this drug. These unwanted side effects include hypokalemia, hypophosphatemia, decreased respiratory drive, increased cardiac output and myocardial oxygen demand, onset of myocardial ischemia, onset of cardiac arrhythmias, and gut ischemia.

SUGGESTED READINGS

Bellomo R, Chapman M, Finfer S, Hickling K, Myburgh J. Low dose dopamine in patients with early renal dysfunction: a placebo-controlled randomised trial. Australia and New Zealand Intensive Care Society (ANZICS) clinical trial group. Lancet 2000;356: 2139–2143.

Kellum JA, Decker JM. Use of dopamine in acute renal failure: a meta-analysis. Crit Care Med 2001;29:1526–1531.

Marik PE, Iglesias J. Low-dose dopamine does not prevent acute renal failure in patients with septic shock and oliguria: The NORASEPT II study investigators. Am J Med 1999;107:387–390.

STOP METFORMIN (GLUCOPHAGE) BEFORE ANY ELECTIVE SURGERY (HOWEVER MINOR) OR INTRAVASCULAR CONTRAST STUDY TO AVOID LACTIC ACIDOSIS

MICHAEL J. MORITZ, MD

Metformin is an insulin-sensitizing agent in use for more than fifty years that increases peripheral glucose utilization and decreases hepatic glucose release. In overweight patients with type II diabetes, metformin has been shown to lower cardiovascular and diabetes-related deaths and has been considered the oral hypoglycemic agent of choice. It is also indicated to treat the insulin resistance of polycystic ovary syndrome. Metformin is renally excreted and has a half-life of 1.5 to 5 hours. Metformin is available as the branded drugs Glucophage and Glucophage XR (extended release) tablets and Riomet liquid. It is also a component of two combination drugs, Glucovance and Metaglip.

Lactic acidosis is a high anion gap metabolic acidosis. Lactate is produced by anaerobic glycolysis, and the development of lactic acidosis requires overproduction, slowed breakdown, or both. Chemically, metformin is a biguanide, a class of oral hypoglycemic agents. At high blood levels, metformin is capable of uncoupling oxidative glycolysis and producing severe, refractory lactic acidosis.

WATCH OUT FOR

Lactic acidosis associated with metformin appears to be rare (risk of 1 per 1,000 to 30,000 patient years) but has a mortality of 50%. Many cases are preventable. Situations that may lead to renal insufficiency and drug accumulation (e.g., surgery or exposure to iodinated radiologic contrast dye in such procedures as angiography and intravenous contrast for computed tomography scan) must prompt discontinuation of metformin. Other clinical situations that may precipitate this problem in patients taking metformin include shock with tissue hypoperfusion (septic, cardiogenic, etc.), hypoxia, liver disease, and alcohol abuse. According to the product insert, the use of metformin is contraindicated in patients with dehydration, renal disease, liver disease, congestive heart failure, binge drinking of alcohol, alcoholism, old age (unless renal function has been tested), and in individuals about to undergo surgery or be exposed to radiologic contrast.

For radiologic studies, metformin should be stopped 24 to 48 hours before the procedure, withheld for 48 hours, and restarted when renal function is known to be normal. For patients undergoing surgery, the preoperative fasting, postoperative reduced caloric intake, and the potential for perioperative hypoxia and tissue hypoperfusion lead to the same recommendations as for exposure to radiologic contrast; however, the drug should not be restarted until adequate oral caloric intake has resumed.

SUGGESTED READINGS

Bailey CJ, Turner RC. Metformin. N Engl J Med, 1996;334: 574–579.
Brown JB, Pedula MS, Barzilay J, et al. Lactic acidosis rates in type 2 diabetes. Diabetes Care 1998;21:1659–1663.
Nisbet JC, Sturtevant JM, Prins JB. Metformin and serious adverse events. MJA 2004;180:53–54.
Thomsen HS, Morcos SK. Contrast media and metformin: guidelines to diminish the risk of lactic acidosis in non–insulin-dependent diabetics after administration of contrast media. ESUR Contrast Media Safety Committee. Eur Radiol 1999;9:738–740.

MAKE SURE THE HEPARIN IS REMOVED FROM THE INTRAVENOUS FLUSHES AND HEPARIN-COATED LINES ARE REMOVED IF A PATIENT IS DIAGNOSED WITH HEPARIN-INDUCED THROMBOCYTOPENIA

HEATHER ABERNETHY, MD

One common cause of thrombocytopenia in the inpatient is due to the administration of heparin. Heparin-induced thrombocytopenia (HIT) is divided into types I and II and should be considered in all cases of low platelet count and heparin administration. Type I occurs in 10% to 20% of patients after receiving heparin. Mild decreases in platelet counts with an absolute count usually above $100,000/\mu L$ occur with type I HIT. This thrombocytopenia results from platelet aggregation and is usually temporary, resolving in a few days despite continued heparin administration. HIT type II is more clinically significant, with platelet counts usually less than $100,000/\mu L$. This is an immune-mediated response occurring in 1% to 5% of patients receiving heparin. The complex formed between heparin and the platelet-derived heparin neutralizing protein (platelet factor four [PF4]) is antigenic. The antibody then binds to and stimulates the Fc receptors on the surface of the platelet, which causes degranulation and platelet damage. Degranulation results in more PF4 release and a vicious cycle occurs that can result in thrombosis, the most severe complication of HIT. Promptly recognizing HIT and paradoxical thrombosis is vital since stopping heparin administration may reverse the syndrome. However, in HIT type II, it may take up to one month for the platelet count to normalize.

WHAT TO DO

Low–molecular-weight heparin is less immunogenic than unfractionated heparin and has a lower chance of causing thrombocytopenia. However, it is not a safe alternative in patients who have developed HIT. Many antibodies formed from exposure to heparin cross-react with low–molecular-weight heparin and may contribute to thrombocytopenia. If an anticoagulant is required, danaparoid (a heparinoid that prevents fibrin formation) or hirudin (a direct thrombin inhibitor) are safe alternatives. Any form of heparin administration, including routine intravenous heparin flushes, hemodialysis, subcutaneous ports, or heparin-coated catheters (including pulmonary artery catheters) can induce or promulgate HIT. Therefore, a specific order to avoid heparin flushes should be written if HIT is suspected and lines and catheters should be changed if heparin bearing. Although a laboratory test for the heparin antibody is available, it often takes several days to obtain test results. The best and easiest way to determine if a patient has HIT is to stop all heparin administration and monitor the platelet count to see if it increases.

SUGGESTED READINGS

Carey CF, Lee HH, Woeltje KF, eds. The Washington Manual of Medical Therapeutics. 29th Ed. Philadelphia: Lippincott-Raven, 1998:348–349.
Fauci AS, ed. Harrison's Principles of Internal Medicine. 14th Ed. New York: McGraw-Hill, 1998: 744:631–632.

HAVE A HIGH THRESHOLD FOR ADMINISTERING VITAMIN K INTRAVENOUSLY

MICHAEL J. MORITZ, MD

Anaphylactoid reactions in patients receiving intravenously (IV) administered vitamin K have been widely reported. A recent review of the literature along with the U.S. Food and Drug Administration (FDA) adverse drug reaction database uncovered a total of 155 cases, 27 of which were fatal and with the true number no doubt being much higher. The manufacturer has sufficient concern over the safety of IV administration of IV vitamin K that it was voluntarily removed from the Canadian market. Anaphylactic reactions and fatalities have occurred even when IV vitamin K was given at low doses and by slow dilute infusion. Of the reported 155 cases, 21 cases with four fatalities occurred in patients who received doses smaller than 5 mg of IV vitamin K. Reactions in patients receiving vitamin K by a nonIV route do occur but are much less common.

WATCH OUT FOR

The pathogenesis of this reaction is unknown and may be due to vasodilatation related to the solubilizing vehicle or immune-mediated (i.e., allergic) processes. The solubilizing agent is polyethoxylated castor oil (Cremophor EL). Despite rumors to the contrary, there has been no change in the formulation of the solubilizing agent in the last several years. Other drugs using this agent include paclitaxel, cyclosporine, and teniposide, and all three drugs, when administered by IV, have been associated with reactions including anaphylaxis. The incidence of anaphylaxis after IV vitamin K appears to be similar to that of other drugs known to cause anaphylaxis, such as penicillin or iron dextran. Routine pretreatment with antihistamines or corticosteroids before administration of vitamin K is not recommended.

Vitamin K is commonly used to treat overanticoagulation from warfarin, which can be life-threatening. The American College of Chest Physicians (ACCP) guidelines provide recommendations for vitamin K use in overanticoagulated patients but only for IV (despite the above described 155 cases) and oral administration. In addition to IV and oral administration, vitamin K can be given subcutaneously. However, subcutaneous vitamin K may have less reliable kinetics than the other routes. In addition, several reports have found that oral vitamin K has a more rapid effect on lowering the international normalized ratio (INR) than the subcutaneous route.

To reemphasize, the use of IV vitamin K should be avoided in almost all patients with overanticoagulation and should be reserved for those with serious hemorrhage, inability to take oral vitamin K, and inability to administer fresh frozen plasma. If IV vitamin K must be given, it should be administered mixed into a minibag of 100 mL of D5W or saline and given over a 30 minute period. Irrespective of the risk of an anaphylactoid reaction, there is no recommendation to pretreat patients with steroids or antihistamines before administering IV vitamin K.

SUGGESTED READINGS

Crowther MA, Douketis JD, Schnurr T, et al. Oral vitamin K lowers the international normalized ratio more rapidly than subcutaneous vitamin K in the treatment of warfarin-associated coagulopathy. a randomized, controlled trial. Ann Intern Med 2002;137:251–254

Fiore LD, Scola MA, Cantillon CE, Brophy MT. Anaphylactoid reactions to vitamin K. J Thromb Thrombolysis 2001;11:175–183.

Riegert-Johnson DL, Volcheck GW. The incidence of anaphylaxis following intravenous phytonadione (vitamin K1): a 5-year retrospective review. Ann Allergy Asthma Immunol 2002;89:400–406.

Wjasow C, McNamara R. Anaphylaxis after low dose intravenous vitamin K. J Emerg Med 2003;24:169–172.

100

DO NOT PUSH INTRAVENOUS VERAPAMIL WITHOUT THE PATIENT BEING MONITORED FOR CARDIAC RHYTHM AND BLOOD PRESSURE

RICHARD PUCCI, DO

Verapamil, one of the calcium channel blockers, inhibits the passage of calcium ions through the slow channels of conductive and contractile myocardial cells and vascular smooth muscle cells. In the sinoatrial (SA) and atrioventricular (AV) nodes, depolarization is largely dependent on the movement of calcium ions through these slow channels. Verapamil not only reduces the magnitude of the calcium ion current through the slow channel, but also decreases the rate of recovery of the channel. This "double-action" slow channel blockade accounts for verapamil's activity as an antiarrythmic agent.

WATCH OUT FOR

Verapamil has multiple other physiological and hemodynamic effects (depending on the route of administration) and should only be administered intravenously with continuous cardiac and frequent blood pressure monitoring. Verapamil decreases coronary vascular resistance, thereby increasing coronary blood flow. Intravenous (IV) verapamil causes a rapid decrease in arterial blood pressure because of a decrease in systemic vascular resistance (i.e., decreased afterload). However, the compensatory reflex tachycardia of this action is blunted by the direct negative chronotropic effect of the drug.

WHAT NOT TO DO

The intrinsic negative inotropic effect of verapamil described above, is partially offset by both a decrease in afterload and the reflex increase in adrenergic tone. Therefore, in patients without congestive heart failure, ventricular performance is not impaired and actually may improve. In contrast, in patients with congestive heart failure, IV verapamil can cause a marked decrease in contractility and left ventricular dysfunction. By slowing the AV node, verapamil may produce a second- or third-degree heart block, bradycardia, or (in extreme cases) asystole. This is more likely to occur in patients with sick sinus syndrome or AV nodal disease and is only partially reversible with atropine. In diseased ventricular tissues, particularly during acute ischemia, verapamil can diminish the conduction of recentrant impulses, but conduction within the normal ventricular conduction system is unaffected. After an IV dose, the electrocardiogram may show a slower heart rate and prolonged P-R interval. Because of its effects on conduction, IV verapamil should not be used in patients with second- or third-degree AV block and should be used with close monitoring in those with first-degree block. In addition, IV verapamil should be used with great caution after IV administration of any beta-blocker (aside from esmolol after an appropriate "washout" period).

Along with hypotension, bradycardia, and heart block, adverse reactions of verapamil include tachycardia, dizziness, headache, nausea, and abdominal discomfort. Compared with the other calcium channel blockers, use of verapamil results in greater impairment in contractility and cardiac conduction. In the calcium channel blocker class, verapamil has been linked with the most fatalities.

One final note is that calcium chloride, 500 to 1,000 mg (5 to 10 mL of a 10% solution), can limit or reverse some cases of verapamil-induced hypotension. Calcium salts attenuate the peripheral vasodilatory actions without altering the chronotropic (antidysrhythmic) effects of verapamil. If hypotension persists after calcium administration and IV fluids, a direct-acting vasopressor should be administered, with a search undertaken for an alternate explanation for hypotension (e.g., myocardial infarction, hypovolemia, or sepsis).

SUGGESTED READING

Marx JA, ed. Rosen's Emergency Medicine: Concepts and Clinical Practice. 5th Ed. Philadelphia: Mosby, 2002;1053–1098.

101

BE CAUTIOUS WHEN LOADING A PATIENT WITH INTRAVENOUS DILANTIN

AHMED MAMI, MD

Phenytoin sodium has a chemical structure related to the barbiturates. It is often referred to by its original brand name, Dilantin. Phenytoin inhibits the spread of seizure activity in the motor cortex by promoting sodium efflux and thereby causing stabilization of the neuron membrane. Since its anticonvulsant properties were discovered in 1938, phenytoin has been used to treat seizures and to prevent their recurrence. It is indicated for the control of status epilepticus of the grand mal type and the prevention and treatment of seizures.

Phenytoin has a plasma half-life ranging from 10 to 15 hours after intravenous (IV) administration. A serum level between 10 and 20 mcg/mL is recommended for optimum control without clinical signs of toxicity. The plasma level is affected by albumin level, hence free phenytoin is more accurate than total phenytoin level.

Phenytoin is a difficult pharmaceutical compound with which to work. The oral form became available in the 1930s, yet a parenteral form was not approved until 1956. Phenytoin is very soluble at a pH exceeding 10 and less soluble with lower pH. Further, at lower pH, phenytoin sodium hydrolyzes to free phenytoin, which is much less soluble. The IV form of phenytoin is a solution of phenytoin in 40% propylene glycol and 10% ethanol, with sodium hydroxide to adjust the pH to 12. Intravenous phenytoin should always be mixed with normal saline for adminisration because mixing phenytoin with dextrose-containing solutions will cause degradation or precipitation, possibly because of the lower pH of dextrose solutions. Intravenous use is associated with local and systemic complications, which are thought to be due more to the vehicle (especially propylene glycol) than the drug.

WATCH OUT FOR

Local problems include tissue destruction from extravasation and "purple glove" syndrome from local venous irritation without extravasation. Purple glove syndrome is poorly understood, occurs in up to 6% of patients, is characterized by progressive distal limb edema, discoloration, and pain, and is more common with infusion into small veins with cannulae smaller than 20 gauge. Systemic cardiovascular reactions include hypotension and bradycardia, and are more common in the young (less than 7 years), the old (greater than 60 years), and those with concurrent cardiovascular disease. The cardiovascular effects can be mitigated by slowing the infusion. The rate of IV administration should not exceed 25 to 50 mg/min in adults and 750 mcg/kg/min in children. Therefore, patients receiving intravenous phenytoin must be monitored for blood pressure, cardiac rhythm, and the status of the infusion site. The solution concentration should not exceed 5 mg/mL, and must be administrated using a filter.

Because of the difficulties of using phenytoin, consideration should be given to using fosphenytoin (Cerebyx), which has been approved by the U.S. Food and Drug Administration for status epilepticus. Fosphenytoin is only available parenterally. It is a phosphorylated phenytoin and is a prodrug, being rapidly hydrolyzed to phenytoin. However, it is water soluble, without the propylene glycol or ethanol solvents, and comes in a solution with a pH of 9.0. The bioequivalence is 1.5 mg of fosphenytoin to 1.0 mg of phenytoin. Unlike phenytoin, it can be given intramuscularly without major local reactions. Intravenously, it can be administered more rapidly, at up to 150 mg/min. The incidence of local reactions to intravenous infusion is much lower. Monitoring cardiac rhythm and blood pressure is still recommended during intravenous infusion. The cost of fosphenytoin is significantly higher (as much as 14 times higher), but the lower incidence of local and systemic reactions may make it more cost effective.

One final note is that the use of phenytoin is not first line treatment in transplant patients who are seizing and who are on cyclosporine or tacrolimus. Phenytoin induces cytochrome P450 3A4 and lowers drug levels. Also, these patients are likely to be total-body depleted of magnesium (regardless of serum magnesium levels) and should receive empiric IV magnesium (at least 4 mg) in the initial pharmacological treatment.

SUGGESTED READINGS

Carmichael RR, Mahoney CD, Jeffrey LP. Solubility and stability of phenytoin sodium when mixed with intravenous solutions. Am J Hosp Pharm 1980;37: 95–98.

Trissel LA, ed. Handbook on Injectable Drugs. 11th Ed. Bethesda, MD: American Society of Health-System Pharmacists, 2001;1051–1058.

Labiner DM. Data vs opinion, phenytoin vs fosphenytoin (Editorial). Arch Int Med 1999;159:2631–2632.

Meek PD, Davis SN, Collins DM., et al. Guidelines for nonemergency use of parenteral phenytoin products. Panel on Nonemergency Use of Parenteral Phenytoin Products. Arch Int Med 1999;159:2639–2644.

Pfeifle CE, Adler DS, Gannaway WL. Phenytoin sodium solubility in three intravenous solutions. Am J Hosp Pharm 1981;38:358–362.

102

MONITOR THE PATIENT WHEN USING PROTAMINE TO REVERSE HEPARIN

HEATHER ABERNETHY, MD

Systemic heparin use is widespread in health care (e.g., cardiac catheterization, cardiopulmonary bypass, vascular surgery, treatment of atrial fibrillation renal dialysis, and treatment of deep venous thrombosis and pulmonary embolism). When used as a continuous infusion, heparin may cause bleeding that is problematic or catastrophic (e.g., intracranial bleeding). In most circumstances, stopping the heparin infusion will control bleeding as heparin has a short half-life (30 to 60 minutes). In cases of significant bleeding heparin is reversible with protamine.

SIGNS AND SYMPTOMS

Mild hypotension with protamine administration is common because of vasodilatation and is related to rapidity of administration. There are three *serious* risks of protamine administration, in order of decreasing frequency: (1) severe systemic hypotension; (2) anaphylactoid reactions; and (3) pulmonary hypertension. Previous exposure to protamine, the use of NPH (Neutral Protamine Hagedorn) insulin, or a history of fish allergy (since protamine is commercially prepared from fish sperm) may increase the risk of adverse hemodynamic effects. In addition, men with a vasectomy are at a theoretically increased risk from protamine administration because approximately one-third of this patient group develops antiprotamine antibodies.

Protamine should be given only when really needed, slowly, and with appropriate monitoring. The dose of protamine can be estimated at 1 mg per 90 to 100 units of heparin administered in the preceding 60 minutes (if heparin was administered more than 60 minutes previously, the dose is lowered by 50%). The rate of administration should be less than 50 mg per 10 minutes, typically given as 10 mg over 1 to 3 minutes. To help guide therapy, an activated partial thromboplastin time (aPTT) or activated clotting time (ACT) should be obtained 5 to 10 minutes after protamine is given. During reversal with protamine, all patients should be monitored with telemetry, blood pressure, and pulse oximetry.

SUGGESTED READINGS

Hensley FA, Martin DE, eds. A Practical Approach to Cardiac Anesthesia. 2nd Ed. Boston: Little Brown, 1995;239:441–443.

Viaro F, Dalio MB, Evora PRB. Catastrophic cardiovascular adverse reactions to protamine are nitric oxide/cyclic guanosine monophosphate dependent and endothelium mediated: should methylene blue be the treatment of choice? Chest 2002;122:1061–1066.

CHECK FOR HISTORY OF MIGRAINE
BEFORE GIVING ZOFRAN

MICHAEL J. MORITZ, MD

Serotonin, or 5-hydroxytryptamine (5-HT), is a neurotransmitter derived from the amino acid tryptophan. Systemic 5-HT affects the cardiovascular, respiratory, and gastrointestinal systems, with vasoconstriction being the typical vascular response. Thus, 5-HT antagonists will cause vasodilation. In the gastrointestinal system, most serotonin receptors are of the $5-HT_3$ type. The strongest stimulus for emesis from both chemotherapy and postoperatively is serotonin release from the gut enterochromaffin cells. This release stimulates afferent vagal fibers via their $5-HT_3$ receptors that activate the vomiting center in the brain stem (chemoreceptor trigger zone). Thus, serotonin antagonists decrease nausea and cause vasodilation.

The three $5-HT_3$ antagonist drugs available in the United States are ondansetron (Zofran), granisetron (Kytril), and dolasetron (Anzemet). These $5-HT_3$ receptor antagonists are the most effective antiemetic drugs available. All three drugs are similar in effectiveness, cost, and side-effect profiles.

The $5-HT_3$ antagonists have relatively few side effects. The most common side effect is headache, occurring in 10% to 20% of patients receiving doses to prevent chemotherapy-induced emesis and in 10% of patients receiving the lower doses used for postoperative nausea and vomiting. In children particularly, a personal or family history of migraine headache leads to a much higher risk of ondansetron-related migraine at the antiemetic dosing for chemotherapy.

The interplay of the 5-HT receptor, vasodilation, and vasoconstriction can be seen in the management of migraine. The treatment of migraine blocks the vasodilation which causes the headache, typically with serotonin agonists. For example, sumatriptan succinate (Imitrex) is a $5-HT_1$ agonist that causes vasocontriction. Because the $5-HT_3$ antagonists cause vasodilation, their use should be avoided in patients susceptible to migraines.

SUGGESTED READINGS

American Society of Health System Pharmacists. Therapeutic guidelines on the pharmacologic management of nausea and vomiting in adult and pediatric patients receiving chemotherapy or radiation therapy or undergoing surgery. Am J Health Syst Pharm 1999;56:729–764.

Khan, RB. Migraine-type headaches in children receiving chemotherapy and ondansetron. J Child Neurol 2002;17:857–858.

Nissen D, ed. Ondansetron hydrochloride. In: Mosby's Drug Consult. 13th ed. St. Louis: Mosby, 2003.

104

BECOME FAMILIAR WITH THE ANTIDOTES TO COMMONLY PRESCRIBED DRUGS

MICHAEL J. MORITZ, MD

In the emergency medicine setting, an antidote is usually a counter-agent for a poison. However, elsewhere in the practice of medicine, an antidote is more commonly an agent to reverse or counteract a medicinal (rather than a poison). The need for reversal can be related to enhanced toxicity or intentional overdosage (suicidal attempt). In discussing antidotes, there are several vital factors to keep in mind. The inciting drug will have dose-dependent therapeutic effects and side effects. The reversal agent will also have different dose-dependent effects, side effects, and pharmacokinetics. Accordingly, reversal agents must be carefully titrated to the desired response and the patient carefully and intensively monitored until both drugs have been fully metabolized. The brief descriptions below and in *Table 104.1* are inadequate to fully describe dosing in adults and children, drug disposition and changes with organ dysfunction, side effects, adverse reactions, and so on. Rather, they are intended to provide familiarity with drug names and effects for reversal agents so that one can respond more quickly in an emergency while consulting the appropriate reference for details.

Atropine is an interesting drug. It is used both as an antidote and its use may require an antidote. It works by inhibiting the action of acetylcholine at postganglionic, parasympathetic sites including smooth muscle, secretory glands, and central nervous system (CNS) sites. These anticholinergic responses are dose related. Small doses of atropine inhibit salivary and bronchial secretions and sweating; moderate doses dilate the pupil, inhibit accommodation, and increase the heart rate (vagolytic effect); and large doses decrease motility of the gastrointestinal (GI) and urinary tracts. Atropine is used as a preanesthetic medication to reduce salivation and bronchial secretions. In poisoning by organophosphate cholinesterase inhibitors (found in certain insecticides) and by chemical warfare nerve gases, large doses of atropine relieve the anticholinergic symptoms and some of the (CNS) manifestations. It is also used as an antidote for mushroom poisoning due to species such as *Amanita muscaria*.

The usual adult dose of atropine is 0.4 to 1 mg when given intravenously (IV). When used as part of cardiac resuscitation, the usual

TABLE 104.1	DRUG NAMES AND EFFECTS FOR REVERSAL AGENTS		
DRUG	**CLASS**	**ANTIDOTE**	**CLASS**
Atropine	Anticholinergic	Physostigmine	Cholinergic
Organophosphate cholinesterase inhibitors found in certain insecticides and chemical warfare nerve gases	Cholinergic	Atropine	Anticholinergic
Heparin	Anticoagulant	Protamine sulfate	Reversal agent; directly binds and inactivates heparin
Narcotics	Analgesic; sedative anesthetic	Narcan (naloxone)	Reversal agent; receptor blocker
Benzodiazepines	Anxiolytic; anti-seizure	Romazicon (flumazenil)	Reversal agent; receptor blocker
Digoxin	Positive inotrope; cardiac rate control	Digifab (digoxin immune Fab [ovine])	Reversal agent; directly binds active drug
Vitamin K (phytonadione)	Procoagulant	Coumadin (warfarin)	Oral anticoagulant; vitamin K antagonist
Beta-blockers	Antihyper-tensive; negative chronotrope	Glucagon	Nonadrenergic positive inotrope and chronotrope

adult dose is 1 mg. As an antidote to poisoning, doses of 1 to 4 mg should be used and maybe repeated until the poison clears.

The action of acetylcholine is transient because of its hydrolysis by the enzyme acetylcholinesterase. **Physostigmine** is the antidote to atropine and reversibly inhibits acetylcholinesterase and prolongs and amplifies the effect of acetylcholine. Dramatic reversal of anticholinergic symptoms can be expected in minutes after IV administration of physostigmine if the diagnosis is correct.

The usual adult dose of physostigmine to reverse the anticholinergic effects of atropine is 0.5 to 3 mg IV given slowly (less than 1 mg/min). However, profound bradycardia, asystole, and seizures may occur (i.e., "cholinergic crisis"), for which the antidote is atropine!

The anticoagulant **heparin** is a heterogeneous group of straight-chain anionic mucopolysaccharides (glycosaminoglycans). Heparin is isolated from porcine intestinal mucosa or beef lung. Heparin dosing is most commonly expressed in units (some cardiovascular surgery sources still use milligrams [mg]). Both animal sources of heparin are around 150 units/mg.

Protamine is the antidote to heparin. Protamine is a combination of simple low–molecular-weight proteins rich in arginine (and thus strongly basic) isolated from the sperm of salmon and certain other fish. When administered alone, protamine is a weak anticoagulant. When given in the presence of (strongly acidic) heparin, a stable salt is formed, and the anticoagulant activity of both drugs is lost. Protamine has a rapid onset of action with neutralization of heparin within 5 minutes after IV administration. Too rapid administration of protamine can cause severe hypotension, bradycardia, dyspnea, and flushing. Overdose of protamine may cause bleeding as above (protamine is a weak anticoagulant), which must be distinguished from rebound anticoagulation that may occur 30 minutes to 18 hours following the reversal of heparin with protamine, so called reheparinization.

Each 1 mg of protamine neutralizes approximately 90 units of heparin from beef lung or about 115 units of heparin from porcine intestinal mucosa.

Naloxone (Narcan) is a pure narcotic antagonist (i.e., it does not possess any morphine agonist properties). In the absence of narcotics, it exhibits essentially no pharmacologic activity. The onset of action is rapid and apparent within 2 minutes when IV administered, and the onset is only slightly slower when given subcutaneously or intramuscularly. The duration of action is prolonged with intramuscular administration. The need for repeat doses of naloxone is also dependent on the amount, type, and route of administration of the narcotic being antagonized. The serum half-life is 30 to 60 minutes, hence redosing is usually necessary.

An initial dose of 0.4 to 2 mg of naloxone is given IV. If the desired degree of reversal and improvement in respiratory function does not occur, the dose may be repeated at 2- to 3-minute intervals. If there is no improvement after 10 mg of naloxone is given, the diagnosis of narcotic toxicity should be questioned. If no IV is available, the intramuscular or subcutaneous route can be used. In most adult hospital pharmacies, the usual vial size is 2 mg, although other sizes are available.

Flumazenil (Romazicon) is a benzodiazepine receptor antagonist. Flumazenil does not antagonize the effects of drugs that affect the CNS (e.g., ethanol, barbiturates, or general anesthetics) by means other than the benzodiazepine receptor and does not reverse the effects of narcotics.

In adults, doses of 0.1 to 0.2 mg partially antagonize and 0.4 to 1.0 mg completely antagonize therapeutic sedating doses of benzodiazepines. Reversal starts within 1 to 2 minutes after injection and peaks at 6 to 10 minutes. The duration and degree of reversal are related to the amount of benzodiazepine present as well as to the dose of flumazenil. The half-life of flumazenil is 40 to 80 minutes. If 3 to 5 mg have been given without clinical response, additional flumazenil is unlikely to have any effect. Resedation requiring redosing occurs in 10% to 15% of patients and is more common with larger doses of benzodiazepines (e.g., midazolam [Versed] greater than 20 mg) and longer procedures.

Digoxin is the prototype cardiac glycoside and acts by inhibiting cardiac sodium-potassium ATPase. The beneficial effects of digoxin result from direct actions on cardiac muscle and indirect actions on the autonomic nervous system. They result in: (1) an increase in the force and velocity of myocardial contraction (positive inotropy); (2) a decrease in the degree of activation of the sympathetic nervous system and renin-angiotensin system; and (3) slowed heart rate and decreased conduction velocity through the atrioventricular (AV) node, a vagomimetic effect. Toxicity may be manifest as rhythm disturbances (bradycardia, varying degrees of heart block, and less commonly, escape tachyarrhythmias), GI symptoms, and CNS symptoms. Particularly for rhythm disturbances, digoxin effects are amplified by hypokalemia, hypomagnesemia, hypoxia, and acid-base disturbances.

All patients with digoxin toxicity should be closely monitored, including continuous electrocardiogram (ECG) monitoring (telemetry), temperature, blood pressure, and potassium concentration. Factors that contribute to toxicity (especially hypokalemia) must be corrected. When the primary manifestation of digoxin toxicity is a serious cardiac arrhythmia, such as symptomatic bradyarrhythmia or heart block, consideration should be given to reversal of toxicity with **digoxin immune Fab (ovine) (Digifab)**, atropine, or the insertion of a temporary cardiac pacemaker. If the rhythm disturbance is a ventricular arrhythmia, electrolyte disorders must be corrected and reversal with Digifab considered. Other drugs used in treating digoxin toxicity include lidocaine, phenytoin, procainamide, and/or propranolol. Massive digoxin intoxication can cause hyperkalemia; potassium supplementation may be hazardous in this setting. After treatment with digoxin immune Fab (ovine), the serum potassium concentration will drop rapidly and must be monitored and addressed. The serum digoxin concentration must be obtained before administration of Digifab because results will be uninterpretable afterwards.

Digifab, digoxin immune Fab (ovine), is a preparation of antigen-binding fragments (Fab) from antidigoxin antibodies raised in sheep. Digifab also binds and inactivates digitoxin. Each vial contains 38 mg of antibody, which will bind approximately 0.5 mg of digoxin. Toxicity in a patient on chronic digoxin requires on average 6 vials, while acute overdosage requires an average of 20 vials. More specific dosing recommendations are given in the product insert.

Vitamin K (phytonadione) is used to correct overanticoagulation by the oral anticoagulants, the archetype being warfarin (Coumadin). Coumadin antagonizes vitamin K. Four clotting factors II, VII, IX, and X, are vitamin K dependent for their synthesis. Coumadin leads to depletion of these factors and the level of anticoagulation produced is proportional to the prolongation of the prothrombin time (PT), although the international normalized ratio (INR) is a more consistent measure of anticoagulation status. Moderate intensity anticoagulation is an INR of 2 to 3 and high intensity is an INR of 3 to 4. When Coumadin anticoagulation needs to be reversed, vitamin K can be used along with fresh frozen plasma. Dosing should be oral if at all possible. The IV route should be avoided because of a higher risk of anaphylaxis. The subcutaneous and oral routes work almost as quickly as parenteral and may have a decreased risk of anaphylaxis. The initial dose by any route is usually 2.5 to 10 mg. Frequency and size of subsequent doses is determined by the response of the INR or the clinical condition. If the INR has not fallen in 6 to 8 hours after parenteral administration (12 to 48 hours after oral dosing), the dose should be repeated. Parenthetically, the natural anticoagulant proteins C and S are also vitamin K dependent, which is likely the source of idiosyncratic hypercoagulation upon starting Coumadin (warfarin-induced skin necrosis) and the reason patients should be on heparin (or an equivalent) before starting Coumadin.

Overdose of a **beta-blocker** causes bradyarrhythmias and hypotension (cardiogenic shock) in addition to plus hypoglycemia and depressed respiration and mental status. Sustained release beta-blockers can result in delayed and/or prolonged toxicity. In beta-blocker toxicity, initial treatment starts with the proverbial ABCs of resuscitation ("airway, breathing, circulation"). Thereafter, treatment is difficult because catecholamines and atropine tend to be ineffective. **Glucagon** has positive chronotropic and inotropic effects that are not dependent on the beta-receptor and, in animal models and case reports, has been effective in treating beta-blocker toxicity. Doses of glucagon used to treat beta-blocker toxicily have varied, but one effective regimen is 5 to 10 mg IV over 1 to 2 minutes; and, if this initial treatment is effective, a drip of 2 to 5 mg/hr should be added. Side effects include nausea, vomiting, and hyperglycemia. Other treatments for beta-blocker overdose include high-dose catecholamines (dopamine, isoproterenol, norepinephrine, epinephrine), amrinone, calcium chloride, cardiac pacing, insulin plus glucose, aminophylline (also not dependent on the beta-receptor), and surgical interventions (intra-aortic balloon pump or cardiopulmonary bypass).

SUGGESTED READINGS

Bailey B. Glucagon in beta-blocker and calcium channel blocker overdoses: a systematic review. J Toxicol 2003;41:595–602.

Mosby's Drug Consult *2003*. Available at: http://www.mosbydrugconsult.com.

105

CONSIDER DRUGS AS A POSSIBLE
CAUSE OF LEUKOCYTOSIS

LISA MARCUCCI, MD

Causes of leukocytosis in the surgical patient are numerous, including infection, noninfectious inflammatory responses, trauma, malignancy, and physiologic stress. A surprising number of patients, however, will have an elevation of total white blood cell count or an elevation in a particular cell line due to pharmaceutical effect. One recent study of patients in a tertiary care setting found that 11% had drugs as the cause of their elevated white cell counts.

The classic drugs that cause leukocytosis are the glucocorticoids. The increase in total white blood cell count can be significant, with total white count in the range of 15,000 to 18,000 cells/mm^3. This mechanism involves an increased release from the bone marrow and a decreased egress from capillaries. The other classic drug associated with leukocytosis is lithium, with an increase to 12,000 to 14,000 cells/mm^3 being typical.

Other drugs that can cause an increased total white blood cell count are the nonsteroidal, anti-inflammatory drugs (NSAIDs). Included in this group are the commonly used ibuprofen (Advil), naproxen (Naprosyn), nabumetone (Relafen), dicloflenac sodium (Voltaren), and ketorolac (Toradol). Leukocytosis caused by NSAIDs is most typical in the setting of a relatively high-dose usage or in overdose. As some of these drugs are available on a nonprescription basis and are often overused to relieve pain in patients who are reluctant to present for care, the patient should be specifically queried about their use when a patient presents with pain and leukocytosis. Interestingly, these drugs in lower doses can also cause leukopenia.

In addition to NSAIDs, the beta-agonists are also well-known causes of increased white blood cell count. This group of drugs, which causes activation of the sympathetic nervous system, includes bronchodilators (terbutaline and albuterol) and cardiac pressors (dobutamine, isoproteronol, epinephrine and norepinephrine).

Drugs that are not commonly seen in the surgical setting that cause leuckocytosis include: efalizumab (Raptiva) for psoriasis; alpha$_1$-proteinase inhibitor (Prolastin) for alpha$_1$-antitrypsin deficiency; dexmedetodomidine (Precedex) for intensive care unit sedation;

fenoldopam (Corlopam) for severe hypertension and fluorouracil (leukopenia is more typical). Of course, granulocyte colony-stimulating factor (g-CSF; Neupogen) is given to raise the white cell count and often may cause a leuckocytosis.

In addition to an overall leukocytosis, some drugs cause an increase in specific types of white blood cells. A widely used drug that may produce this is ampicillin/sulbactam (Unasyn), which can cause an increase in lymphocytes, monocytes, basophils, eosinophils, and platelets (along with the well-described increase in transaminases and partial thromboplastin time [PTT]). Of note is that ampicillin/sulbactam use also may cause cytopenias.

SUGGESTED READINGS

Abramson N, Melton B. Leukocytosis: basis of clinical assessment. American Academy of Family Physicians Website. http//:www.aafp.org.

Goebel MU, Mills PJ, Irwin MR, Ziegler MG. Interleukin-6 and tumor necrosis factor-alpha after acute psychological stress, exercise, and infused isoproteronol; differential effects and pathways. Psychosom Med 2000;62:591–598.

Wanahita A, Goldsmith EA, Musher D. Conditions associated with leukocytosis in a tertiary care hospital, with particular attention to the role of Clostridium difficile. Clin Infect Dis 2002;34:1585–1592.

EMERGENCY DEPARTMENT

OPERATING ROOM

MEDICATIONS

LINES, DRAINS, AND TUBES

WOUNDS

BLEEDING

GASTROINTESTINAL TRACT

WARDS

INTENSIVE CARE UNIT

LABORATORY

DO NOT DRAW BLOOD PROXIMAL TO AN INTRAVENOUS LINE THAT IS INFUSING

GREGORY KENNEDY, MD, PHD

When blood samples are drawn proximal (or above) a running intravenous (IV) line, any laboratory values obtained from those samples may be inaccurate. An incorrectly drawn sample should be suspected and ruled out as a cause when laboratory results are unexplainable. Depending on which type of IV fluid or which antibiotic is infusing, the patient may appear to be hyperlipidemic, hyponatremic, hypernatremic, hyperkalemic, or hyperglycemic.

The most common clinical scenario of lab results happening is when there is an IV in the hand or forearm with an ongoing infusion and the blood sample is drawn from the ipsilateral antecubital vein by a medical student, who will invariably use the largest and "juiciest" vein regardless of site (professional phlebotomists are trained not to make this mistake). If the results of the blood draw are suspicious, the patient should be examined and the medical student or phlebotomist queried to determine from where the blood was drawn. If the site was close to an infusing IV, the blood should be redrawn at a site away from the infusion before correcting any laboratory abnormality (except profound hypoglycemia, which is too life-threatening to ever be ascribed to errors). If there are no other suitable sites for the blood draw other than immediately proximal to the IV site, the infusion should be stopped for 10 minutes before the blood samples are redrawn.

GO ABOVE THE RIB WHEN PLACING A CHEST TUBE OR NEEDLE INTO THE CHEST CAVITY

HEATHER ABERNETHY, MD

Introducing a chest tube (or needle or catheter) into the chest cavity is fraught with peril. Chest wall structures that can be injured include the intercostal nerve, artery, and vein that run along the inferior border of the ribs. These neurovascular structures are at risk both during introduction of the local anesthetic and during placement of a tube. An incorrect entry point of a chest tube, especially, can result in serious organ damage or even death. A chest tube should be placed with supervision until the surgeon is completely familiar and comfortable with a safe technique.

WHAT TO DO

One technique that can be used to minimize the risk of chest wall injury when a chest tube is being inserted is as follows (see *Figure 107.1*): The patient is placed in a supine position, then rolled slightly to the side with the ipsilateral arm positioned above his or her head. The skin is widely prepped with a sterile solution in the area the chest tube is to be placed, and the patient is draped. Lidocaine is used to anesthetize the skin, subcutaneous tissue, and the periosteum of the rib (the periosteum is well innervated and requires a generous amount of lidocaine to effect analgesia). A horizontal skin incision slightly larger than the diameter of the tube is made at the rib below the intercostal space that will be pierced. Using the closed tip of a clamp, a subcutaneous tunnel is made from the skin incision cephalad to the superior border of the rib (or the inferior border of the intercostal space). The clamp is then used to bluntly puncture the parietal pleura on the superior border of the rib in an "up and over the rib" direction.

When doing this procedure, if the neurovascular bundle is inadvertently pierced, a noticeable amount of blood may emanate from the skin incision. In this case, the chest tube (or catheter or clamp) should be left in place to partially tamponade the laceration and decrease the risk of massive hemorrhage or further nerve damage. A thoracic surgeon should be consulted immediately. Lack of immediate bleeding, however, does not rule out injury to the intercostals vessels. This may present with delayed bleeding, intrapleural bleeding, or a continuous

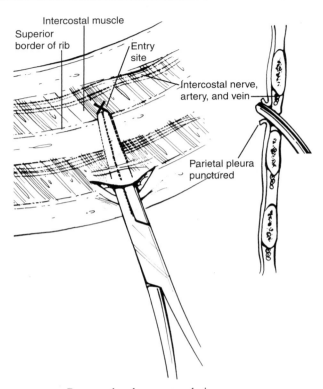

FIGURE 107.1. Proper tube placement technique.

bleed into the chest wall, where it escapes notice until hypovolemia and shock occur.

One further point bears highlighting. Similarly to inserting a chest tube, care must be taken when injecting lidocaine to stay immediately above the superior border of the rib and not stray toward the inferior border of the rib above. A large injection of lidocaine directly into the artery or vein can result in toxicity, including confusion, delirium, and seizures, especially if there is underlying liver dysfunction.

SUGGESTED READING

Elefteriades JA, Geha AS, Cohen LS, eds. House Officer Guide to ICU Care. 2nd Ed. Philadelphia: Lippincott-Raven, 1996:207–209.

108

DO NOT PUSH A MALPOSITIONED CHEST TUBE INTO THE THORACIC CAVITY

MICHAEL J. MORITZ, MD

Placing a chest tube is a not a trivial procedure. It is easiest on the surgeon and patient both when the tube is placed under anesthesia in the operating room, but the majority of chest tubes are placed at bedside, where, unfortunately, there is usually some attendant discomfort for the patient (and anxiety for the surgeon). Proper placement takes planning (gathering the sterile field, instruments, chest tubes, local anesthesia, Pleurevac), training, and experience. Properly introducing a chest tube includes inserting it the correct distance (far enough in that all the side holes are in the pleural space but not so far that the tip impinges on the mediastinum), correct orientation (anterior for air, posterior for fluid), and inserting it in the "free" pleural space (not into adhesions or into the fissure). Once completed, a chest radiograph is the next step so as to document proper position and improvement in the indication for insertion.

A chest radiograph showing a problem with chest tube position is disheartening, especially for the junior resident. Unless the tube is in too far, which can be corrected by cutting the anchoring sutures, withdrawing it a bit, and then resuturing it in place, the correct thing to do for an improperly positioned chest tube is to completely remove the tube and reattempt correct positioning with a new sterile tube. This means reconsenting the patient (and/or contacting the family), notifying senior house staff and the attending physicians, and repeating the whole involved process. It is therefore tempting to attempt to manipulate or push an improperly positioned chest tube further into the chest rather than redoing it.

This should not be done. Manipulating a chest tube is unlikely to succeed and very likely to breach the sterility of the pleural space. Never advance a chest tube farther into the chest once the sterile field has been broken. The position of the tube (anterior versus posterior) is mostly related to the influence of the layers of the chest wall on the course of the tube; if the course through the chest wall is tangentially posterior, for example, no amount of manipulation will convince that tube to go and stay anteriorly. Again, breaking the tube-to-Pleurevac-tubing connection to reposition a tube is likely to contaminate the tube and the pleural space. When a chest tube is inserted incorrectly, admit the error, and go about correcting it properly.

One tip to avoid not placing the tube into the chest tube far enough is to carefully examine the tube before inserting it. Look at the lines on the tube that are used to tell how far the tube is in the chest (they vary by manufacturer). In your mind, look at the patient's body size, recall the chest radiograph, and be aware of how far the tube should project into the pleural space. Add that distance to the length of the track through the chest wall which is measured with one's finger when insuring that your clamp is in the free pleural space. Orient the track in the direction you would like the tube to go, anteriorly or posteriorly, as it is uncommon to want the chest tube to lie straight laterally. Avoid the common and natural mistake of stopping insertion at the first rush of blood or air (this insures only that the holes closest to the tip are inside the chest cavity).

One final note is that the same admonition for chest tubes applies to all other sterile tubes entering sterile body cavities. Once the sterile field is broken, never advance the now nonsterile exterior tube into the body. The exterior part of a chest or catheter cannot be "sterilized" by using betadine, chlorhexidine, or other material.

109

Do not allow a patient to vomit around a nasogastric tube

Lisa Marcucci, MD

A fairly common occurrence after nasogastric (NG) tube placement is the ensuing call to the surgeon that the patient is vomiting around the NG tube, often accompanied by a request from the nurse for an antiemetic order. An antiemetic is inappropriate in this circumstance and a search for the underlying problem is needed because no patient should vomit around a properly positioned and functioning NG tube. Vomiting around an NG tube is not simply inconvenient or uncomfortable but is dangerous—the NG tube renders the lower esophageal sphincter incompetent, makes protection of the airway by the epiglottis difficult, and hence makes aspiration from vomiting more likely.

There are many reasons that an NG tube will not function appropriately to mechanically decompress the gastrointestinal tract. These include:

- Incorrect placement—usually the NG tube is not inserted far enough, but it also may be inserted too distally or be kinked or coiled. In intubated patients, it may have been inserted into the airway rather than the gastrointestinal (GI) tract.
- Mechanical obstruction of the tube from inspissated gastrointestinal contents, enteral feeds, medications, lubricant jelly, or blood clot.
- Obstruction of the sump port or having the sump port capped by the nursing staff to prevent linen soilage with GI contents.
- Malfunctioning wall suction or having a full canister.
- Cracks or breaks in the tubing or canister such that no suction is applied to the tube.

WHAT TO DO

The physician should use the following maneuvers to find and address the problem:

- First off it is important to remember to *never ever* adjust, move, replace, or reinsert an NG tube that is across, near, or adjacent to a fresh surgical anastomosis without notifying a very senior house officer or the attending surgeon—*there are no exceptions!*
- Inspect the tube. NG tubes are manufactured with four black lines toward the external end. In normal-sized adult patients, proper

placement of the NG tube in the stomach leaves two black lines in the patient and two black lines visible. Adjust the NG tube appropriately so there are two visible black lines unless the patient is extremely short or tall or the stomach lies in the chest (prior surgery, hiatal hernia, etc.). This adjustment fixes most malfunctioning NG tubes.

- Examine the tube to ensure that it is not clamped or mechanically blocked outside of the patient.
- Irrigate the tube to and fro with water or saline to ensure there is no blockage inside the patient.
- Make sure the suction is working and the canister is not full.
- If the sump port is capped, remove the cap. (The nurses will likely object but it should be removed nonetheless.) Make sure the suction is hooked up to the wall and is working and the sump lumen is functioning (one should hear a "whooshing" noise through the sump port). Irrigate the sump port with air, water, or saline as needed.
- Obtain a plain abdominal radiograph to check for positioning of the tip. (Auscultating with a catheter-tipped syringe over the epigastric area is a first step but is not entirely reliable for confirming correct position.)
- Replace the NG tube completely—remember to position with two black lines in and two black lines out of the patient and with radiographic confirmation if problems persist.

One final note is that, although a patient should always have sufficient mechanical decompression by an NG tube to prevent vomiting, he or she can have persistent complaints of nausea or retching without vomiting. Nausea has many causes other than gastric distention and some patients will retch from hypopharyngeal stimulation by the NG tube. If this occurs and the NG tube is functioning well, antiemetics may be appropriate and helpful.

SUGGESTED READINGS

Chen HE, Sonnenday C, Lillemoe K, eds. Manual of Common Bedside Procedures. Philadelphia: Lippincott Williams &Wilkins, 2000;43–50.
Joannabriggs.edu.au/protocols/protnasotube.php. September, 2004.

110

CONFIRM CORRECT PLACEMENT OF A FOLEY CATHETER BY RETURN OF URINE

LISA MARCUCCI, MD

WHAT TO DO

Placement of a Foley catheter drains the bladder when a patient is unable to void. It also allows accurate monitoring of a patient's urinary output, from which, one may partially judge volume status. Correct positioning of a Foley requires that the catheter tip with the drainage ports and the balloon lie within the bladder. To ensure successful placement, one commonly used insertion technique requires the catheter to be inserted all the way up to the side port, with the open end inspected for urine return. If the catheter was easily inserted without return of urine, manual pressure in the suprapubic area is applied to compress the bladder and force urine out into the Foley. When urine is seen, the balloon is then inflated with 10 mL of water and gently pulled back until resistance is felt. In this technique, the balloon should not be inflated until urine return proves the tip is in the bladder because balloon inflation in the urethra can damage or rupture this structure.

An enlarged prostate, urethral stricture, or previous urologic surgery may make insertion of a Foley difficult. When inserting the catheter, excessive force should not be used because a false tract can be created. Injecting a few milliliters of sterile lubricant jelly (sterilely packaged as Urojet) directly into the penile meatus can ease a tight passage. After generous use of lubricant, the jelly may clog the catheter to prevent the initial urine flow confirming placement. Irrigating the catheter with a bit of sterile fluid will clear the lumen, and urine flow will confirm bladder placement. A coudé catheter (similar to a Foley but with a curved, stiffer tip) can be used to overcome an enlarged prostate. If a bladder catheter cannot be inserted after two or three attempts, consultation with urology should be obtained for cystoscopy and placement of the catheter.

A careful history can identify a significant number of patients at risk for difficult catheter insertion, and urology should be alerted to be available. If insertion of a Foley was planned, it is generally not acceptable to proceed with an elective procedure with instructions to the anesthesiologist to "run the patient dry" to decrease urine output, because of the inability to place the catheter to be dealt with later. This underresuscitation may lead to needless hypotension, tachycardia, bladder distention (with its attendant autonomic problems), and bladder rupture.

An exception to inflating the Foley balloon without urine return is in patients receiving a kidney transplant. These patients should be queried preoperatively to ask if they are anuric. If so, their bladders are likely to be small and contracted from disuse. Therefore, insertion of the catheter should be done by an experienced member of the team.

Two final notes: (1) saline should not be used to blow up the catheter balloon because this may leach out of the balloon and cause the balloon to become deflated and the catheter to become dislodged; (2) urgent urology consult for urethral or bladder disruption should be obtained if a patient has a difficult catheter insertion and then develops increasing pain, scrotal edema, ecchymoses, or gross hematuria in the ensuing several hours.

SUGGESTED READING

Chen HE, Sonneday C, Lillemoe K, eds. Manual of Common Bedside Surgical Procedures. 3rd Ed. Philadelphia: Lippincott Williams & Wilkins, 2000;43–50.

111

BE RELUCTANT TO ALLOW MORE THAN 500 mL TO DRAIN OUT OF A NEWLY PLACED CATHETER OR DRAIN AT ONE TIME

LISA MARCUCCI, MD AND KEN MEREDITH, MD

Several potential morbid conditions are avoidable by proper management of tubes and drains. One often quoted "truism" concerns never draining more than 500 mL of fluid from a body cavity at one time (with some exceptions, notably large-volume paracentesis). Although recent evidence shows that complications from this are not common, cautious drainage of fluid collections should still be considered good care.

PLEURAL EFFUSIONS AND REEXPANSION PULMONARY EDEMA

Drainage of large pleural effusions mandates slow, incremental removal of fluid from the chest cavity to lessen the risk of reexpansion pulmonary edema, which carries a 20% mortality. A commonly used management plan is to limit fluid removal (to a maximum of 500 mL in the first 30 minutes over several increments) by intermittently clamping and unclamping the drainage tube or catheter. Full drainage of the effusion brings the visceral and parietal pleural linings into abrupt contact which can be very painful to the patient and can cause respiratory distress. Gradual removal of the pleural effusion is more comfortable for the patient. Development of respiratory difficulty or a "white out" on chest radiograph (pre- or postprocedure) mandates close observation of the patient.

BLADDER DISTENTION AND VASOVAGAL REACTIONS

Sudden decompression of an overly distended bladder can cause a vasovagal response with bradycardia and hypotension. Commonly used guidelines include clamping the bladder catheter for 5 to 10 minutes after each 500 mL of urine is drained to avoid this instability. Uncommonly, patients with long-standing bladder outlet obstruction may develop postobstructive diuresis after relief of the obstruction. Optimal management requires attention in this situation because the polyuric urine output may be quite high. Patients often have electrolyte derangements, and close monitoring of serum osmolarity, serum electrolytes, and cardiovascular status is mandatory. The elevated blood urea nitrogen (BUN) and creatinine usually return toward baseline within 24 to 48 hours.

STOMACH DISTENTION AND VASOVAGAL REACTIONS

Large return of gastric contents from a newly placed nasogastric tube is usually well tolerated, but anecdotal reports of transient vasovagal responses with bradycardia and hypotension do exist. Because even a transient episode of cardiovascular instability in precarious patients can be deleterious, a reasonable and common sense approach is to decompress a large reservoir of fluid in the stomach in increments of several hundred milliliters every 5 to 10 minutes.

SUGGESTED READINGS

Chen HE, Sonnenday C, Lillemoe K, eds. Manual of Common Bedside Surgical Procedures. 2nd Ed. Philadelphia: Lippincott Williams & Wilkins, 2000:43–50.
Heller BJ, Grathwohl MK. Contralateral reexpansion pulmonary edema. South Med J 2000;93:828–831.
Walsh PC, ed. Campbells Textbook of Urology. 8th Ed. Philadelphia: WB Saunders, 2002:454–456.

Obtain a Drain Study When the Output from a Drain in an Abscess Cavity Decreases Abruptly

Kenneth Meredith, MD and Lisa Marcucci, MD

Abscess cavities are usually drained via closed drainage tubes placed either intraoperatively by the surgeon or percutaneously by the radiologist. The surgeon caring for the patient after drain placement must know anatomically where the drain is positioned. Drain outputs must be recorded accurately by the hospital staff and the surgeon must be attentive to the quantity and nature of these outputs.

If the output from a drain that has had steady output stops acutely, mechanical malfunction or drain malposition must be assumed as drainage from slowly resolving abscess cavities typically falls gradually. The drain should not be pulled under the assumption that the abscess cavity has been obliterated. The two most common causes of mechanical malfunction are dislodgement of the drain from the abscess cavity and clogging of the drain with debris. Workup of a change in drainage can be via a fluoroscopic drain study or a computed tomography (CT) scan. A drain study may unclog the tube or allow the radiologist to exchange a clogged drain for a new one. A CT scan will allow the surgeon to assess if the abscess cavity has resolved or if the drain has become dislodged and a new drain needs to be placed.

Suggested Readings

Blackbourne LH, Fleischer KJ. Advanced Surgical Recall. Baltimore: Williams & Wilkins, 1997;25–29.

Chen H, Sonnenday C, Lillemoe K, eds. Manual of Common Bedside Surgical Procedures. 2nd Ed. Philadelphia: Lippincott Williams & Wilkins, 2000;43–50.

RELEASE THE SUCTION ON THE BULB BEFORE REMOVING A JACKSON-PRATT DRAIN

LISA MARCUCCI, MD AND KEN MEREDITH, MD

Jackson-Pratt (JP) drains are commonly used in surgery to remove fluid or blood from a closed body cavity or space. They are only effective when there is vacuum applied to the drain. The JP (see *Figure 113.1*) is placed on suction by squeezing the plastic bulb and then closing the air port by capping it with the attached plastic plug. Before removing a JP from a body cavity (e.g., the peritoneal cavity or subcutaneous tissue), these steps should be reversed; that is, the cap is taken off of the port, and the bulb is allowed to reexpand. If this is not done and the suction remains when the drain is pulled, tissue adjacent to the drain (such as omentum or even a surgical anastomosis) can be pulled into the drain tract causing pain and tissue disruption.

One additonal note is that JPs should not require much effort to remove. If left in place for more than one week, tissue will begin to grow into drain interstices and it will become slightly more difficult to extract. However, if the JP appears to be "stuck" despite steady, firm pressure, do not attempt to "yank it out". If a second inspection confirms that the anchoring suture for the drain has indeed been cut yet the drain can not be easily removed, a more senior member of the team should be contacted before additional attempts to remove the JP are undertaken. JP tubing easily can be unintentionally caught in the fascial closure and applying more force to such a drain will only lead to it breaking at the level where it is fixed.

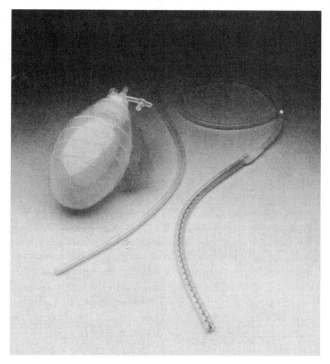

FIGURE 113.1. Jackson-Pratt drain.

SUGGESTED READING

Chen HC, Sonnenday C, Lillemoe K., eds. Manual of Common Bedside Procedures. 2nd Ed. Philadelphia: Lippincott Williams &Wilkins, 2000;43–50.

114

USE A DEDICATED, UPPER BODY, SINGLE LUMEN CENTRAL VENOUS CATHETER FOR ADMINISTRATION OF PARENTERAL NUTRITION

LISA MARCUCCI, MD

Although the use of parenteral nutrition was one of the milestone breakthroughs in the care of critically ill patients, serious morbidities are associated with its use. One troublesome complication is total parenteral nutrition (TPN) catheter–related sepsis, which is associated with poorer outcomes in patients, including longer intensive care unit stays, longer hospital stays, and higher mortality. To this end, some hospitals have developed entire care teams dedicated to the management of central venous lines used for TPN, including insertion procedure, skin site inspection, dressing changes, and evaluation of possible infection. Given the potential morbidities, numerous studies have been done to determine the best protocols for catheter care used for TPN.

From an accumulating body of research regarding how to reduce risks of infection, including TPN catheter tip infection, site infection, bacteremia, and catheter colonization, the following facts seems clear: (1) TPN should be initiated through a new catheter inserted via a clean stick, not a catheter changed over a wire; (2) TPN catheters should be inserted via subclavian (preferably) or internal jugular veins, not via femoral veins; (3) TPN should have its own dedicated lumen used for nothing else; and (4) a team dedicated to TPN central line care should be assembled to lower catheter infection rates. A 2003 study by Dimick and colleagues showed that single lumen subclavian catheters dedicated to TPN use and cared for by a dedicated team had a five-fold decrease in infection compared to other catheters that were used for multiple reasons.

One final note is that because the realities of care in seriously ill patients do not always allow for the placement of a dedicated TPN line, one port of a newly placed multiple lumen catheter can be designated for exclusive administration of TPN if no other options exist.

SUGGESTED READINGS

Clark-Christoff N, Watters VA, Sparks W, Snyder P, Grant JP. Use of triple-lumen subclavian catheters for administration of total parenteral nutrition. J Parenter Enteral Nutr 1992;16:403–407.

Dimick JB, Swoboda S, Talamini MA, et al. Risk of colonization of central venous catheters: catheters for total parenteral nutrition vs other catheters. Am J Crit Care 2003;12:328–335.

Kemp L, Burge J, Choban P, et al. The effect of catheter type and site on infection rates in total parenteral nutrition patients. J Parenter Enteral Nutr 1994;18:71–74.

BE METICULOUS IN TECHNIQUE WHEN INSERTING AND CARING FOR CENTRAL VENOUS ACCESS CATHETERS IN THE INTENSIVE CARE UNIT TO LOWER THE INCIDENCE OF INFECTION

LISA MARCUCCI, MD

Central venous catheters are associated with a significant rate of bloodstream infections, and an estimated 10% mortality in intensive care patients. Several strategies have been shown to be effective in reducing these infections and are summarized below.

USE FULL-BARRIER PROTECTION WHEN INSERTING CENTRAL VENOUS CATHETERS

This is the most bothersome protocol for most clinicians but should be employed except in the most emergent situations. Full-barrier protection consists of the surgeon and all assistants being fully gowned (with the ties fastened as in the operating room), masked, and gloved with sterile gloves and the patient fully draped with sterile drapes. If the procedure is a change of catheter over a wire, the surgeon should change gloves between removing the old catheter and inserting the new catheter.

USE CHLORHEXIDINE FOR SKIN PREP

Chlorhexidine has a decided advantage over aqueous iodine-based preps in reducing infection, and its use should be adopted routinely for subclavian catheters and should be strongly considered in internal jugular catheters, with extreme care to avoid contact with the eyes and the external ear canal. The prep should be applied via a concentrically larger circular motion for at least twenty seconds and should be allowed to dry without blotting or fanning. Alcohol-based iodine preps are effective but must be used on intact skin.

USE A STERILE DRESSING ON THE INSERTION SITE

Immediately after catheter insertion, the site should be protected with a transparent sterile dressing while the insertion site is still sterile. The sterile bandage should not be placed if the site is still oozing, and a sterile gauze should be used to remove blood (the ideal culture medium) before the sterile dressing is placed. Topical antibiotic ointment has not been shown to reduce infections and should not be used. Antiseptic impregnated dressings and disks are promising adjuncts to exit site care.

Use the catheter with the fewest number of lumens possible and consider treated catheters

The question of whether triple lumen catheters have higher infection rates compared to single lumen catheters is still somewhat uncertain, with the majority of studies showing higher infection rates for triple lumen catheters. Contradicting this are a few studies and one recent meta-analysis that found there is no strong evidence for an increase in infections in triple lumen catheters. This may be because the patient population studied in the literature is heterogeneous in the following variables—patient location (intensive care unit [ICU], inpatient, mixed), pulmonary artery catheters allowed, blood drawing allowed through catheters, types of catheters (antibiotic-impregnated, number of lumens), sites of catheters (peripherally inserted, centrally inserted), ports included or not, tunneled and/or cuffed catheters included or not, and so on.

In addition, catheters coated with a sterilant (e.g., silver) or an antibiotic (e.g., rifampin) are also effective at decreasing infections—cost-effectiveness will vary with an institution's infection rate.

Do not use stopcocks on the lumen ports

Use of stopcocks functionally increases the number of portals in a central venous catheter, with an attendant increase in contamination, and therefore should be avoided. Catheter hubs that incorporate an antiseptic barrier should be used whenever possible.

Suggested Readings

Chaiyakunapruk N, Veenstra DL, Lipsky BA, Sullivan SD, Saint S. Vascular site care: the clinical and economic benefits of chlorhexidine gluconate compared with povidone iodine. Clin Infect Dis 2003;37:764–771.

Dezfulian C, Lavelle J, Nallamothu BK, Kaufman SR, Saint S. Rates of infection for single-lumen versus multilumen central venous catheters: a meta-analysis. Crit Care Med 2003;31:2385–2390.

O'Grady NP, Alexander M, Dellinger EP, et al. Guidelines for the prevention of intravascular catheter-related infections. Pediatrics 2002; 110(5): e51.

Raad II, Hohn DC, Gilbreath BJ, et al. Prevention of central venous catheter-related infections by using maximal sterile barrier precautions during insertion. Infec Control Hosp Epidemiol 1994;231–238.

Sitges-Serra A, Hernandez R, Maestro S, et al. Prevention of catheter sepsis: the hub. Nutrition 1997;13:30S–35S.

Avoid the Subclavian Vein for Central Access of Any Type in a Dialysis Patient or Possible Dialysis Patient

Michael J. Moritz, MD

There are almost 300,000 hemodialysis patients in the United States today, and the number increases by about 4% to 5% annually. The median age of the dialysis patient in the United States has risen to 65 years. The aging population and the relative scarcity of renal transplants (about 10,000 done annually in the United States) means that dialysis will be required for longer periods of time and in many patients will be lifelong. In parallel, the critical nature of the vascular access in hemodialysis patients is amplified by longer dependence on this access for dialysis. Provision of vascular access is the greatest problem in dialysis today, with the solution involving the patient, nephrologist, surgeon, and interventional radiologist.

In the optimal situation, the patient presents early enough that the surgeon can place a permanent access in advance of dialysis. However, more commonly patients present with an acute need for dialysis that requires temporary dialysis access via percutaneous catheters. As the majority of these patients will go on to require chronic dialysis, it is vital that the temporary access catheter *not* compromise the anatomy required for permanent access procedures. The preferred sites for temporary access catheter placement are the internal jugular veins or the femoral veins—the subclavian veins should be avoided.

WHAT NOT TO DO

Temporary percutaneous dialysis access catheters are placed via central veins. They are very large in diameter compared to other venous catheters and are associated with significant damage to the cannulated vein and an increased risk of thrombosis or stenosis of the vein, which can occur acutely or can present much later. The venous damage can be at the site of entrance into the vein or more centrally. In studies examining damage from short term use (2 to 4 weeks), dialysis catheters placed by the subclavian route result in venous stenosis or thrombosis in 50% to 70% of veins, in contrast to a 0% to 10% incidence in catheters placed by the internal jugular route. Although the risk of injury to the vein is less than with dialysis catheters, in dialysis patients the subclavian vein should be avoided for placement of smaller bore central venous catheters such as triple lumen catheters, TPN (total parenteral nutrition) lines, or catheters that permit pulmonary artery catheters to be threaded through them.

Permanent accesses are arterial to venous connections, either as a fistula (direct artery to vein anastomosis) or via a bridge prosthetic graft between artery and vein. The best, longest-lasting permanent accesses are placed in the extremities, and upper extremities are preferred over lower extremities for reasons of infection, edema, and patient comfort. Permanent accesses create high flow through the vessels of the extremity, and the success of the access is highly dependent on adequate venous outflow from the access to the right atrium. Compromise of venous return results in access failure or edema of the access extremity to a degree that can be profound and limb-threatening. Thus subclavian vein stenosis or thrombosis (even if clinically silent) results in loss of all potential access sites in the ipsilateral upper extremity. Placement of a permanent access in such an extremity will result in immediate clinical symptoms of venous insufficiency (edema, cellulitis) and usually requires undoing the arteriovenous connection.

Patients who require a permanent dialysis access after prior subclavian venous puncture should be screened for patency of the central veins. Screening with Doppler ultrasound is noninvasive and is sensitive for veins that are easily visualized (e.g. jugular or axillary veins), but it is not sensitive for detection of venous stenosis or thrombosis of intrathoracic central veins such as subclavian and brachiocephalic (innominate) veins. If there is any reason to suspect problems with more central veins, a more sensitive study such as magnetic resonance imaging (MRI) or venography would be indicated.

Finally, patients with central venous occlusion may have spontaneous recanalization after 3 to 6 months, although the vein will never be completely normal. Patients with symptomatic stenosis of central veins can be treated with angioplasty and stent placement. The results overall are not as good as for arterial disease but can be helpful in patients with few or disappearing dialysis access alternatives.

SUGGESTED READINGS

Bander SJ, Schwab SJ. Central venous angioaccess for hemodialysis and its complications. Semin Dial 1992;5:121–128.

Cimochowski GE, Worley E, Rutherford WE, et al. Superiority of the internal jugular over the subclavian access for temporary hemodialysis. Nephron 1990;54:154–161.

Criado E, Marston WA, Jaques PF, et al. Primary venous outflow obstruction in patients with upper extremity arteriovenous dialysis access. Ann Vasc Surg 1994;8:530–535.

National Kidney Foundation. DOQI clinical practice guidelines for vascular access and anemia of chronic renal failure. Am J Kidney Disease 1997;30(suppl 3): 51:7–240.

Schillinger F, Schillinger D, Montagnac R, et al. Post catheterisation vein stenosis in haemodialysis: comparative angiographic study of 50 subclavian and 50 internal jugular accesses. Nephrol Dial Transplant 1991;6:722–724.

117

DO NOT ENTER THE FEMORAL ARTERY OR VEIN SUPERIOR TO THE INGUINAL LIGAMENT WHEN ATTEMPTING A NEEDLE CANNULATION

LISA MARCUCCI, MD AND KEN MEREDITH, MD

When attempting placement of a femoral arterial or venous catheter, correct technique is important to minimize complications and improve chances for cannulation on the first attempt, especially in obese patients. One of the keys to successful cannulation is to know the pertinent anatomy to correctly estimate the site of skin puncture to allow vascular access below the inguinal ligament. Needles inserted above the inguinal ligament risk puncture of the external iliac artery (instead of the desired common femoral artery), with the potential for retroperitoneal hemorrhage, hematoma, pseudoaneurysm, and (rarely) bowel perforation or bladder perforation. Puncture of the external iliac artery is harder to compress than the common femoral artery (the puncture above the inguinal ligament is often unrecognized) and any subsequent bleeding will be into the retroperitoneal space. Much greater blood loss can occur into the retroperitoneum than the thigh before it is discovered, with an increased risk of hypotension and cardiovascular collapse.

WHAT TO DO

A brief review of correct technique for accessing femoral vessels using the Seldinger protocol is as follows: After the patient is prepped and draped, palpate the femoral pulse at the midpoint along an imaginary line between the anterior superior iliac spine and the symphysis pubis. This line approximates the course of the inguinal ligament. Palpate the femoral pulse 1 to 3 cm distally from the inguinal ligament—this is the optimal level at which to enter the vessel. Administer anesthetic (1% lidocaine) with a 25-gauge needle into the skin and subcutaneous tissues along the course of the artery. Using the 18-gauge needle with a 5-mL syringe, puncture the skin 2 to 3 cm caudal to the point chosen to enter the vessel, about 3 to 5 cm below the inguinal ligament (farther in heavier patients, less in thinner ones), toward the pulsation when attempting arterial cannulation, and 1 cm medially from the pulsation when attempting venous cannulation. In obese patients, err in being too caudal instead of too cephalad on the initial skin puncture. Advance the needle cranially at a 45° angle to the long axis of the body while aspirating. If no arterial or venous blood is noted after 5 cm, withdraw the needle slowly and to the skin level, reassess your landmarks and repeat 1 cm more proximally. Once the artery or vein is cannulated, remove the syringe and thread the J-tipped guidewire (or straight guidewire if the patient has a previously placed vena cava filter). The wire should thread easily and should never be forced due to the risk of arterial or venous rupture. Continue the procedure as for other central venous access catheter placement.

When attempting femoral venous cannulation in coagulopathic patients, unintended arterial puncture can be catastrophic. The use of real-time bedside ultrasound to visualize the vascular structures and perform the vessel cannulation under ultrasonic visualization has been shown to improve safety and to lower incidence of unintended arterial puncture. In critical situations, use of ultrasound to decrease the risk of complications is appropriate in accessing the femoral vein or artery.

SUGGESTED READINGS

Chen HE, Sonnenday C, Lillemoe K. Manual of Common Bedside Surgical Procedures. 2nd Ed. Philadelphia: Lippincott Williams & Wilkins, 2000:43–50.
Hilty WM, Hudson PA, Levitt MA, Hall JB. Real-time ultrasound-guided femoral vein catheterization during cardiopulmonary resuscitation. Ann Emerg Med 1997;29:331–336.

118

IN A PATIENT WITH A PREVIOUSLY PLACED VENA CAVA FILTER, DO NOT USE THE J-TIP ON THE GUIDEWIRE WHEN USING THE SELDINGER TECHNIQUE TO PLACE A CENTRAL VENOUS CATHETER

LISA MARCUCCI, MD

Vena cava filters are placed for treatment of deep vein thrombosis and/or pulmonary embolism. Complications arising from the placement of these filters include migration, dislodgement, vena cava penetration, and vena cava thrombosis. One additional complication that has been increasing in frequency but is completely preventable is the ensnarement of the filter by guidewires being used to insert central venous catheters from the subclavian, jugular, and femoral approaches.

There are a variety of vena cava filters available in the United States. Some of the more commonly used filters include the Greenfield (both titanium and stainless steel models), Simon nitinol, Bird's Nest, Vena Tech LGM ,Vena Tech TrapEase and Gunther Tulip filters. Despite design differences, they are all similar in that they allow venous flow through the filter while capturing emboli via the radiating struts of the filter.

There are various guidewires that are used during the Seldinger technique, including straight guidewires and the more commonly encountered 1.5-, 3-, and 15-mm J-tip guidewires packaged in central venous catheter insertion kits (the number describes the radius of the curve of the J-tip). In vitro studies and case reports show that ensnarement of the guidewire in the filter struts is possible with all diameters of the J-tip guidewire used in placing central venous catheters and does not occur with straight guidewires. The filters with the highest likelihood of ensnaring the J-tip guidewires are the Greenfield and Vena Tech filters with only the Gunther Tulip reported as not entrapping the J-tip guidewire.

Ensnarement of an IVC filter occurs when the curved end of a J-tip guidewire (see *Figure 118-1*) is pushed through a strut opening with subsequent hooking of the wire onto the strut when the catheter is pulled back. This is noted clinically as the wire becoming "stuck" during wire withdrawal. If even slight resistance to removing the wire is noted further attempts to remove the wire must be halted immediately. Attempting to free the guidewire with force can cause shearing of the guidewire or dislodgement of the filter with potentially

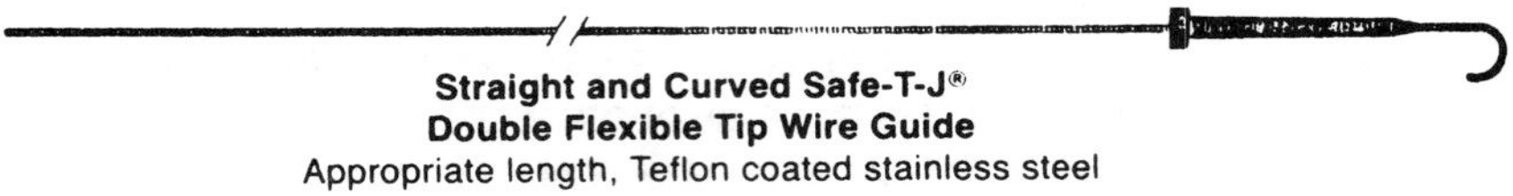

Straight and Curved Safe-T-J®
Double Flexible Tip Wire Guide
Appropriate length, Teflon coated stainless steel

FIGURE 118-1. Straight and curved J-tip double flexible tip wire guide.

catastrophic complications including filter caval disruption, perforation, arrhythmias, cardiac tamponade, and death. Although some clinicians advocate attempts to free the wire at bedside by pushing the wire caudally and applying torque to rotate the J-tip away from the strut, a more cautious approach demands urgent consultation with interventional radiology. Techniques used to remove ensnared guidewires include using fluoroscopic visualization and placement of a vascular sheath and snares to work the guidewire free.

WHAT TO DO

To help prevent ensnarement of a guidewire, all patients or patient families should be queried about the presence of a cava filter before elective insertion of a central venous catheter. With an increasing proportion of filters placed percutaneously, filter placement may not be elicited as part of a "past surgical history." In the event of an elective procedure in a patient where the history can not be obtained, a plain radiograph will show the presence of this device. Because patients usually do not know what model of vena cava filter they have received, they should be specifically asked about the placement of a "Greenfield, filter, or birdcage in the vena cava." If they answer in the affirmative, a straight guidewire (or the straight end of the J-tip guidewire) should be used to place the central venous catheter. Similarly, in emergent central venous catheter insertions a straight guidewire should be considered to prevent ensnarement.

SUGGESTED READINGS

Dardik A, Campbell KA, Yeo CJ, Lipsett PA. Vena cava filter ensnarement and delayed migration: an unusual series of cases. J Vasc Surg 1997;26:869–874.

Munir MA, Chien SQ. An *in situ* technique to retrieve an entrapped J-tip guidewire from an inferior vena cava filter. Anesth Analg 2002;95:308–309.

Stavropoulus SW, Itkin M, Trerotola SO. *In vitro* study of guide wire entrapment in currently available inferior vena cava filters. J Vasc Intervent Radiol 2003;14:905–910.

119

AIM FOR THE IPSILATERAL NIPPLE WHEN PLACING A CENTRAL VENOUS CATHETER IN THE INTERNAL JUGULAR VEIN

HEATHER ABERNETHY, MD

WATCH OUT FOR

There are not only a number of techniques by which a central venous catheter can be inserted, but also various sites available for cannulation. The right internal jugular is perhaps the most easily accessible, making its use convenient and relatively safe. Prior to inserting a catheter, the relative contraindications to internal jugular vein cannulation should be reviewed. These include prior neck surgery, thyromegaly, contralateral diaphragm dysfunction, carotid artery disease, and anticoagulation (due to the risk of carotid artery puncture). If the decision to proceed is made, one technique using the anterior approach to the right internal jugular vein using the Seldinger technique (which involves threading a catheter over a guidewire) is described below.

If available, telemetry pads should be placed on the patient and proper functioning of the electrocardiograph confirmed. The head is rotated to the left, and pillows under the head are removed. The patient is placed in Trendelenburg position, which distends the vein and decreases the risk of air embolism. The anatomic landmarks should be palpated; these are the clavicle and the two heads of the sternocleidomastoid muscle (which form three sides of a triangle). These landmarks may be verified, if the patient is awake and cooperative, by having them momentarily raise their head off the bed. If the bedside portable ultrasound machine is available and the surgeon is familiar with its use, this should be placed on the neck at this time (before prepping) to assess deep anatomy.

Complete aseptic technique in placing non-emergent internal jugular lines is mandatory including antiseptic skin preparation, sterile gloves, masks, and full-body drapes. A skin wheal with local anesthetic and deeper soft tissue penetration is done over the apex of the triangle and lateral to the pulsation of the carotid artery. A small gauge (21 or 23) "finder needle" is used to locate the internal jugular vein (with the help of bedside ultrasound, if available). This is done by slowly advancing the needle with constant negative pressure at a 45° angle to the skin surface in the direction of the ipsilateral nipple while manually "rolling" the carotid medially. Aspiration of dark, nonpulsatile blood indicates probable venous placement, but placement into the jugular vein and not the carotid must be confirmed by transducing the waveform or one of the other techniques available to insure venous blood (e.g., falling column of blood or rapid blood gas). An 18-gauge needle is then passed along the path of the finder needle until the vein is entered. A flexible wire is then passed through the hollow needle in standard fashion while monitoring the patient for arrhythmia (the wire should be immediately pulled back if an arrhythmia occurs). The J-tip of the wire should be used only after confirmation from the patient or reliable family that no previous caval filter has been placed (see Chapter 118 for further details). The balance of the procedure follows the standard protocol for the Seldinger technique. It is important to note that the jugular vein in thin patients is actually fairly superficial so the finder needle usually does not have to be inserted its entire length before puncturing the vein.

One final note is that if the carotid artery is somehow accessed, dilated, and is the receptacle of a central venous catheter, the catheter should be left in place and a consultation with a vascular surgeon should be obtained urgently. Inadvertent carotid catheters are most commonly removed in the operating room under direct visualization and with primary repair because many patients cannot tolerate the considerable degree of carotid pressure/occlusion that may be required to avoid formation of a life-threatening hematoma.

SUGGESTED READINGS

Duke J, ed. Anesthesia Secrets. 2nd Ed. Philadelphia: Hanley and Belfus, 2000:131–137.
Hensley FA, Martin DE, eds. A Practical Approach to Cardiac Anesthesia. 2nd Ed. Boston: Little Brown, 1995:111–115.

120

ADVANCE THE NEEDLE INTO THE VEIN WITH THE PLUNGER PULLED BACK GENTLY WHEN DOING CENTRAL VENOUS ACCESS

LISA MARCUCCI, MD

Careful attention to technique allows invasive procedures to be performed with the minimum number of complications. One simple maneuver to increase the success of placing a central line "on the first stick" is aspirating the needle as it is slowly being placed into the vein. The central venous system is usually under low pressure (5 to 15 mm Hg) even when the patient is in Trendelenberg position. This low pressure is usually insufficient to spontaneously fill a syringe and will not produce a "flash" of blood. Instead, if the syringe plunger is being pulled back while the needle is being advanced, the negative pressure generated will aspirate blood into the syringe when the needletip has entered the vein (and theoretically will lessen the chance of a back wall puncture). The negative pressure may also overcome the mechanical blockage in the needle lumen caused by a tissue plug that entered the needle as it was pushed through the subcutaneous tissue. The negative pressure on the plunger should not be overdone—gentle force on the syringe as it is slowly being advanced is best. Overuse of force causes two problems: (1) loss of touch and feel while manipulating the syringe (an experienced operator placing a line will feel the gentle pop of the anterior vessel wall and stop in the lumen, whereas the less-experienced will transpierce the vessel and find the lumen while withdrawing the needle); and (2) the increased chance of aspirating subcutaneous tissue into the needle as it is advanced with clogging of the needle and the inability to aspirate blood once inside the vessel.

A concern for every surgeon is if a rush of air occurs while the plunger is being aspirated and the needle is being advanced. In this case, the needle should be withdrawn immediately. The two most likely causes of this rush of air are: (1) loosening of the needle from the syringe; and (2) aspiration of intrathoracic air from the pulmonary parenchyma, raising the likelihood of a subsequent pneumothorax. Even if the needle is thought to have loosened from the syringe, an urgent portable upright chest radiograph should be obtained to evaluate for pneumothorax.

WHAT NOT TO DO

One final note is that if the first pass of the needle with the plunger being aspirated is not successful, the needle should be backed out completely before changing the angle and re-introducing it. Altering the angle of attack without complete withdrawal of the needle causes shear forces on the tissues impaled by the needle. If a vessel has been pierced through and through (i.e., out the back wall) and the needle is then moved sideways, the shear force on the vessel may lacerate it with resultant bleeding. Bleeding from punctures in a vessel wall are likely to stop, but vessel lacerations are more likely to cause significant bleeding.

SUGGESTED READING

Chen H, Sonnenday C, Lillemoe K. eds. Manual of Common Bedside Surgical Procedures. 2nd Ed. Philadelphia: Lippincott Williams & Wilkins, 2000:43–50.

121

MAINTAIN CONTROL OF THE WIRE WHEN PUTTING IN A CENTRAL LINE USING THE SELDINGER TECHNIQUE

LISA MARCUCCI, MD

There are many complications of central venous catheter insertion when using the Seldinger technique (pneumothorax, hemothorax, air embolism, cardiac tamponade, etc.) with an incidence of 1 to 2% even in experienced hands. One complication that should *never* occur is having a guidewire "lost" into the intravascular space. This most typically happens when the surgeon removes the hand holding the guidewire while reaching for an item on the central line tray or while threading the catheter over the wire just as the patient deeply inhales. The resultant fall in intrathoracic pressure is sufficient to suck the wire into the subclavian or jugular veins.

To lessen the chance of a surgeon letting go of the wire, the tray should be opened and organized before the venous puncture so that the needed equipment can be easily accessed. Before the central line procedure is started, an unopened spare kit should be nearby in the event something is dropped off the sterile field, and assistance should be within easy earshot in case a second pair of hands is needed. After the vein has been accessed with the needle and the wire inserted through the needle, the surgeon should have firm control of the distal wire while his or her second hand removes the needle from the skin and pulls it back up and over the wire. With this hand that is pulling out the wire he or she then grasps the wire proximal to the needle and removes the hand distal to the needle so the needle can be slid off completely. The surgeon (while still holding the wire) threads first the dilator and then the catheter onto the wire and slides it down the wire until wire is protruding from both ends of either the catheter or dilator. The wire is then grasped on the distal end, the hand closer to the skin is released, and the dilator or catheter is slid into the vein. All commercial kits have wires with sufficient length that the wire can always be seen and held without losing its position in the central vein. (See *Figure 121.1.*) *Never* lose sight of or let go of the wire!

If for some reason the wire or a piece of the wire or catheter is lost in the intravascular space, interventional radiology must be consulted emergently for retrieval. Catheter- and wire-tip embolism most typically occur when the guidewire or catheter is pulled back through the needle and the beveled needle edge shears the wire or catheter.

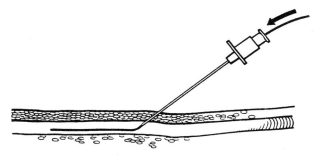

FIGURE 121.1. Guidewire protruding from both ends of needle.

Such separate motions should not be done. If the wire cannot be advanced or withdrawn easily, the needle and wire should be withdrawn together.

One final note is that the wires in the prepackaged kits for vascular access catheters and Cordis catheters are shorter than those in the triple lumen kits and cannot be used when a longer-to-shorter or shorter-to-longer catheter change is being contemplated. When a triple lumen catheter is being removed over a wire so that a Cordis or vascular access catheter can be placed, the wire from the Cordis or vascular access kit should be discarded and a wire long enough to "stick out both ends" of a triple lumen catheter should be used. This can be done by breaking into a triple lumen kit or obtaining a separately packaged "long wire."

SUGGESTED READINGS

Chen H, Sonneday C, Lillimoe K, eds. Manual of Common Bedside Surgical Procedures. 2nd Ed. Philadelphia: Lippincott Williams & Wilkins, 2000:43–50.

Doherty GM, ed, Washington Manual of Surgery. 3rd Ed. Philadelphia: Lippincott Williams & Wilkins, 2002:722.

http://www.fleshandbones.com/readingroom/pdf/947.pdf

122

CHECK FOR VENOUS BLOOD BEFORE DILATING THE TRACT WHEN INSERTING A CENTRAL VENOUS CATHETER

MICHAEL J. MORITZ, MD

Inadvertent carotid or subclavian artery puncture while attempting placement of a central venous catheter is not an insignificant problem; but, in patients with reasonably intact coagulation, it is usually manageable with withdrawal of the needle and direct digital pressure. However, not recognizing that the artery (rather than the vein) has been entered and proceeding with the remainder of the Seldinger technique for placement of a catheter can lead to serious complications. Dilatation of the carotid or subclavian artery can require formal surgical repair in the operating room.

WHAT TO DO

For successful placement of a central venous catheter, proper technique, including taking a history (prior unsuccessful attempts or known central venous thrombosis), performing a physical (dilated subcutaneous collaterals presaging central venous problems), and moderate Trendelenberg position, etc., is essential. For the internal jugular approach, use of portable ultrasound to visualize the neck structures has been shown to lower the incidence of unintended carotid artery puncture when placing an internal jugular venous catheter and should be used if possible. Two devices are currently available in the United States, SiteRite and SonoSite.

After placing the hollow needle intravascularly, discriminating between pulsatile, bright red, oxygenated arterial blood and nonpulsatile, dark, and relatively unoxygenated venous blood seems easy, but a variety of circumstances can make the distinction difficult. Venous blood can appear arterial in patients with very high partial pressure of arteral oxygen (PaO_2) from high concentrations of inspired oxygen, such as under general anesthesia, with mechanical ventilation, or from supplemental oxygen (nasal cannula, face mask, etc.). In these circumstances, venous blood will be almost fully oxygenated and will be bright red. Similarly, patients with right heart failure (e.g., severe pulmonary hypertension, tricuspid insufficiency) can have pulsatile central venous blood flow. It is harder to understand how bright red arterial blood can be misinterpreted as dark and venous except in the very hypoxic patient, but perhaps incomplete, partial, or tangential arterial puncture allows arterial blood to mix with venous blood and fool the operator into believing that arterial blood is venous.

There are at least five progressively more complex techniques (other than the estimating the color of the blood) that can be used to discriminate between arterial and venous puncture.

Option 1—connect sterile tubing to the hub of the hollow needle and watch blood fill the tubing. Then elevate the tubing and note if blood drains back ouf of the tubing. This is useful for inferring the pressure and pulsatility in the vessel (best with a cooperative patient or a patient under anesthesia). If the blood rises to a venous pressure in the tubing, the vein is most likely cannulated. Remember that each torr (1 torr = 1 mm Hg) is equal to 1.32 cm of water or blood and that venous pressure, even with the patient in Trendelenberg position, is unlikely to exceed 20 torr, or 28 cm of water. If the blood column rises above 30 cm or is pulsatile, the artery is most likely cannulated.

Option 2—connect the needle to sterile arterial line tubing, attach the tubing to a pressure transducer, and then inspect the waveform for venous versus arterial magnitude and morphology (venous waveform with both A and V waves compared to arterial waveform with the classic dicrotic notch present).

Option 3—withdraw blood and run a blood gas for the partial pressure of oxygen (PO_2) value. If it is arterial blood, PO_2 should be greater than 80 torr, but this number alone is not reliable if inspiring high concentrations of oxygen.

Option 4—place the wire through the needle (watching for cardiac dysrhythmias indicating that the wire is in the right atrium, confirming venous placement), withdraw the needle, and check with a radiograph. Venous placement will almost invariably show the wire in the right mediastinum, whereas arterial placement will usually show the wire in the left mediastinum.

Option 5—use contrast and fluoroscopy or radiography to demonstrate the needle's position. This is awkward outside the operating room where no C-arm fluoroscopy unit is available, but infusion of contrast while shooting a plain film will demonstrate the contrast flow toward or away from the heart.

If one of the these tests shows the carotid or subclavian artery has been punctured with the hollow needle but has not been dilated, it is usually safe to withdraw the needle at the bedside and hold point pressure over the puncture site for at least 5 minutes, and then watch for bleeding or hematoma. If problems occur after removal of the needle or if the artery has been dilated, consult vascular surgery emergently. Complications of arterial puncture include bleeding, pseudoaneurysm formation, and development of an arteriovenous fistula. In the neck (carotid), bleeding can compromise the airway; in the chest (subclavian), bleeding can be extensive and hidden until shock or cardiovascular collapse ensues.

SUGGESTED READINGS

Chen HE, Sonnenday C, Lillemoe K, eds. Manual of Common Bedside Surgical Procedures. 2nd Ed. Philadelphia: Lippincott Williams & Wilkins, 2000:43–50.

NICE technology appraisal guidance No. 49: guidance on the use of ultrasound locating devices for placing central venous catheters. National Institute for Clinical Excellence. London, U.K. Available at: http://www.nice.org.uk/pdf/ultrasound_49_GUIDANCE.pdf. Accessed July 24, 2005.

Randolph AG, Cook DJ, Gonzales CA, Pribble CG. Ultrasound guidance for placement of central venous catheters: a meta-analysis of the literature. Crit. Care Med 1996;24:2053–2058.

Do not push the dilator in the entire length when using the Seldinger technique to insert a central venous catheter

LISA MARCUCCI, MD AND KEN MEREDITH, MD

One of the steps in the Seldinger technique is the use of an 8 to 12 French (Fr) semirigid plastic dilator used to create a tissue tract between the skin and the central vein. After the dilator is threaded over the guidewire, firm twisting pressure is used to bluntly dilate the tissues to allow later insertion of the catheter. This is arguably the most dangerous step in the Seldinger technique. It is paramount that the dilator only be inserted until the tip of the dilator is in the vein lumen and no further. Fully inserting the dilator can cause rupture of the back side of the vein with hemorrhage (see *Figure 123.1*). It is important to note that bleeding is the most common cause of access-related deaths. Because of anatomic variation and differences in body habitus, placement of the dilator should be done under direct visualization if bedside ultrasound is available. If the dilator is being placed blindly, care should be taken to advance the dilator slowly until a subtle diminution in resistance is felt as the tip enters the vein lumen. The dilator should not be advanced past this point.

WATCH OUT FOR

Sudden decompensation of the patient during or soon after insertion is the cardinal sign of hemorrhage. If rupture of the back wall of the subclavian vein is suspected, a C-maneuver effected by placing the thumb and forefinger around the clavicle at the area of suspected perforation should be immediately performed with at least 15 minutes of firm pressure. Emergent chest radiograph and vascular consult should be obtained. If rupture of the jugular vein is suspected, point pressure should be placed at the site with care taken not to completely compress the carotid artery. Again, emergent vascular consultation is strongly recommended. If the dilator is inadvertently placed into the subclavian artery or carotid artery, it should be left in place and vascular surgery consultation obtained. The patient may need to be taken to the operating room for dilator removal and artery repair under direct visualization. If pericardial tamponade is suspected (hypotension, tachycardia, bulging neck veins, muffled heart sounds),

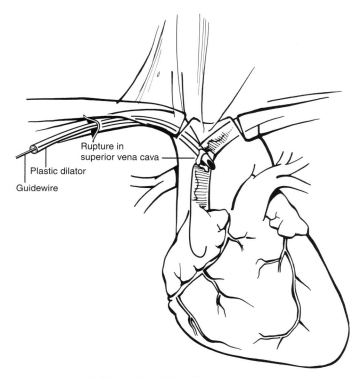

Figure 123.1. Full insertion of the dilator can cause rupture of the back side of the vein with hemorrhage.

needle pericardiocentesis can be performed while emergent cardio-thoracic surgery consultation is obtained.

SUGGESTED READINGS

Chen H, Sonnenday C, Lillemoe K, eds. Manual of Common Bedside Surgical
    Procedures. 2nd Ed. Philadephia: Lippincott Williams & Wilkins, 2000:43–50.
Doherty GM, ed. The Washington Manual of Surgery. 3rd Ed. Philadephia:
    Lippincott Williams & Wilkins, 2002:138.
http://www.fleshandbones.com/readingroom/pdf/947.pdf

124

SECURE A CENTRAL LINE WITH ANCHORING SUTURES AT FOUR SITES

LISA MARCUCCI, MD

Peripherally-inserted central catheters have, in some measure, replaced the need for placement of central venous catheters (CVCs). However, the use of CVCs is still quite common in intensive care units and in sicker patients. Even in experienced hands, the placement is uncomfortable for the patient, and the risk of serious complication such as pneumothorax and puncture of the artery is on the order of 1% to 2%. It is important that the patient not be exposed unnecessarily to repeat placement of a central line because the line was not secured properly and became dislodged. It should be the goal of every new surgical trainee to work their entire career without having a central line "fall out". If the plastic clasp included in some central line kits is used, a nylon stitch should be placed on both sides of it and the clasp should be secured to the line at the skin exit site. In addition, the flange on the catheter itself should be secured on both sides. If the plastic clasp is not used, the line should still be secured by four stitches as described below and in *Figure 124.1*.

1) A 2-0 or 3-0 suture (preferably nylon because it reacts less with the skin than silk) anchored to the skin should be placed at the exit point of the catheter from the skin and looped twice around the catheter to cinch (but not occlude) it circumferentially.
2) A 2-0 or 3-0 suture anchored to the skin should be placed at a gentle bend in the catheter 4 cm from the skin exit site; this serves to lessen tension on the exit site suture.
3) A 2-0 or 3-0 suture anchored to the skin should be placed on each plastic flange of the catheter; this will lessen the risk that a confused patient can get a sufficient grip of the catheter to pull it out.

Note that cuffed catheters should not have a suture placed at the skin exit site—it interferes with healing of the subcutaneous cuff.

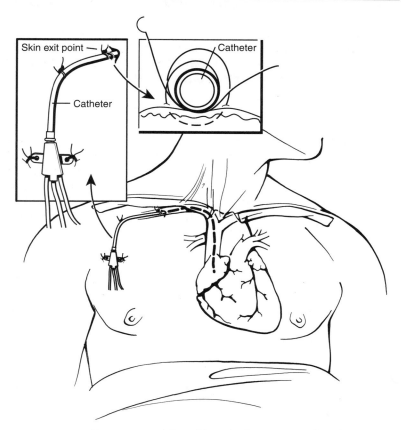

Figure 124.1. Secure a central line with anchoring sutures at four sites.

125

DO NOT INSERT, REMOVE, OR CHANGE A CENTRAL LINE IN THE UPPER TORSO UNLESS THE PATIENT IS LYING FLAT OR IS IN THE TRENDELENBERG POSITION

MICHAEL J. MORITZ, MD

Intrathoracic pleural pressure varies with respiration, typically in the range of 0 to -10 cm H_2O with quiet breathing. The maximal pressures that humans can generate are about -100 cm H_2O of inspiratory force and $+150$ cm H_2O of expiratory force. Intrathoracic venous pressure responds passively to changes in patient position, rising with lying flat or in Trendelenberg position and falling with the sitting or standing position. Intrathoracic venous pressure is the sum of the effect of patient position and the intrathoracic pleural pressure.

Any hollow needle or catheter in the central veins will allow air to enter the venous system when the intrathoracic pressure is below zero, as it is with every inspiration. Patient safety mandates that a needle or catheter in the central venous system must not have its lumen open to ambient air when the patient is inhaling (i.e., generating negative intrathoracic pressure). Retrospective analyses of episodes of air embolism from central venous catheters reveal that most air embolisms occur from three types of breaches in correct technique: errors during insertion, errors during removal, and unintentional disconnections in the system between the intravenous (IV) fluid bag or bottle and the patient.

Neither the rate that air can enter the venous system nor the volume of air capable of causing cardiac arrest has been rigorously studied, but available data indicates that greater than 100 mL of air per second are capable of entering an open catheter at relevant pressures, and that approximately 50 to 200 mL of air embolism is capable of causing cardiac arrest.

To help prevent this, when removing a central catheter, the patient should be placed flat or in Trendelenberg position. All lumens should be capped—or the catheter should not be disconnected from the IV line. When changing a catheter over a wire, the catheter will be open to air briefly while the wire is being introduced; the breach in the catheter should be timed to coincide with the expiratory phase or the patient should briefly hold their breath. The catheter should not be cut to thread the wire because even this small lumen is sufficient to allow a deadly air embolism. When a catheter is removed, the tract between skin and central vein does not remain open for more than a second or two; proper patient position, a finger exerting gentle pressure on the exit site, and a dressing are the sequence for keeping this simple procedure safe.

SIGNS AND SYMPTOMS

The astute clinician should be alert for the signs and symptoms of air embolism. Relatively minor degrees of air embolism result in dyspnea, tachypnea, and hypoxia. Larger degrees of air embolism collect in the right heart and cause hemodynamic instability and cardiac arrest, purportedly by filling the right ventricular outflow tract and pulmonary arteries. Significant air embolism is treated by: (1) eliminating the source; (2) 100% inspired oxygen; (3) if a central venous catheter is present, aspirating to attempt to remove air that is present; and (4) positioning the patient in Trendelenberg position with left side down to encourage air to accumulate in the right ventricle rather than the right ventricular outflow tract.

One final note is that thrombus that embolizes to the pulmonary circulation is filtered by the pulmonary vascular bed and cannot reach the systemic circulation in the absence of a macroscopic right-left cardiac connection (e.g., septal defect). Large air embolism *is* capable of reaching the systemic circulation through the pulmonary vascular bed and causing peripheral emboli.

SUGGESTED READINGS

Ely EW, Hite RD, Baker AM, et al. Venous air embolism from central venous catheterization: a need for increased physician awareness. Crit Care Med 1999;27:2113–2117.

Heckmann JG, Lang CJ, Kindler K, et al. Neurologic manifestations of cerebral air embolism as a complication of central venous catheterization. Crit Care Med 2000;28:1621–1625.

Toung TJ, Rossberg MI, Hutchins GM. Volume of air in a lethal venous air embolism. Anesthesiology 2001;94:360–361.

126

OBTAIN A CHEST RADIOGRAPH BEFORE SWITCHING SIDES WHEN ATTEMPTING ELECTIVE SUBCLAVIAN OR JUGULAR CENTRAL LINE PLACEMENT

LISA MARCUCCI, MD

Placing central venous catheters is an inherently dangerous procedure even in experienced hands using the latest visualization modalities (e.g., ultrasonic visualization). The combined complication rate for pneumothorax, hemithorax, and thoracic duct injury is on the order of 1% to 10% for a single attempt and is higher if the initial attempt is not successful and multiple passes are needed. Despite this risk of patient injury, there have been several recent reports from the gynecology literature suggesting that it is acceptable to omit the postinsertion chest radiograph based on the surgeon's estimation of the "danger" of the insertion. Concurrently, recent reports state that malpractice litigation for central vascular catheter insertion related injuries has resulted in escalating awards for high severity of injury and high mortality rate. This places some well-meaning surgeons in an awkward situation— whether to obtain a noninvasive, inexpensive, "defensive medicine" postinsertion radiograph that a minority of practitioners are postulating is not indicated.

Although the question of the usefulness of a chest radiograph when the surgeon has to switch to the other side has not been investigated in these recent studies, prudence dictates adhering to the previous standard of obtaining a chest radiograph for evaluation of possible complications (even if the surgeon has abandoned chest radiography after single-sided attempts). This common sense approach is based on the premise that complications may not cause immediate symptoms or signs; pneumothorax, hemothorax, cardiac tamponade, or carotid artery bleeding may not cause patient distress, discomfort, or changes in physical exam or vital signs until minutes to hours have passed. However, these complications can and do progress to life-threatening instability just before, during, or after the patient has an insertion attempt on the other side. In addition, if the patient should deteriorate *after* an insertion attempt is made on the contralateral side, the diagnosis of which side (or both sides?) is the source of the deterioration may be unclear based on physical exam and chest auscultation alone. This confusion then leads to a chaotic scene of emergent radiographs and empiric chest tube placements. It is far preferable to take the time

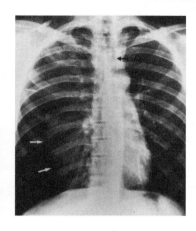

FIGURE 126.1.

to obtain the radiograph to find and treat any developing complication of a failed central venous access attempt before proceeding to the other side and to prevent the possibly graver clinical situation of a patient deteriorating while relatively inaccessible to exam and treatment due to positioning, drapes, and the like. (See *Figure 126.1.*)

SUGGESTED READINGS

Bailey SH, Shapiro SB, Mone MC, et al. Is immediate chest radiograph necessary after central venous catheter placement in a surgical intensive care unit? Am J Surg 2000;180(6):517–521.

Domino KB, Bowdle TA, Posner KL, Langan EM, Crane M. Injuries and liability related to central vascular catheters: a closed claims analysis. Anesthesiology 2004;100:1411–1418.

Puls LE, Twedt CA, Hunter JE. Confirmatory chest radiographs after central line placement: are they warranted? South Med J 2003;96:1138–1141.

Check for Left Bundle-Branch Block on an Electrocardiogram Before Placing a Pulmonary Artery Catheter

Michael J. Moritz, MD

The flow-directed pulmonary artery (PA) catheter, also called the Swan-Ganz catheter after its inventors, was introduced into patient care in 1970. Pulmonary artery catheters directly measure PA pressures, the pulmonary capillary wedge pressure, and the PA (mixed venous) oxygen saturation. Indirect measurements include cardiac output, parameters of left heart function, systemic vascular resistance, and peripheral oxygen consumption. Although in widespread use in the operating room and intensive care unit, the indications for its use remain controversial. Annually in the United States, 1.2 million PA catheters are used, costing more than $2 billion.

Regarding indications for use, prophylactic perioperative use of the PA catheter has not been shown to affect morbidity or mortality when studied in a variety of patient populations and surgical settings. The use of the catheter in the critically ill is more difficult to study prospectively but likely has greater utility in that the information provided by its insertion affects treatment in 30% to 62% of patients. Indications for use in the critically ill include hemodynamic monitoring for initial diagnostic and therapeutic purposes, as well as optimization of cardiac output and/or oxygen delivery when the diagnosis is known.

Insertion of a PA catheter is not without risk. Complications can be divided into those associated with obtaining access to the central veins, complications from catheter passage, and complications from catheter residence and use. Central venous access complications include the usual array of unintended punctures (e.g., artery, vein, lung, nerve, thoracic duct), hematoma, and air embolism. Complications associated with catheter use include thromboses, pulmonary artery damage, infections, and catheter knots. Complications of catheter passage are related to dysrhythmias. Premature ventricular or atrial contractions that resolve with passage or withdrawal of the catheter are common. Occasionally, a sustained run of ventricular tachycardia will require treatment. But the most dangerous cardiac disturbance associated with passage of the PA catheter is development of a right bundle-branch block (BBB).

The incidence of right BBB with catheter insertion has been reported to be in the range of 0.1% to 4.3%. Importantly, a new right BBB in a patient with preexisting left BBB can lead to complete heart block. The incidence of complete heart block in patients with left BBB who are undergoing PA catheter insertion has been reported to be 0% to 8.5%. Thus, patients in whom PA catheter insertion is contemplated need an electrocardiogram before insertion to look for a left BBB.

In a patient with left BBB, the indications for PA catheter insertion should be reconsidered in light of the risk of complete heart block. If the catheter is truly needed, then appropriate measures should be in place in the event heart block occurs, namely the availability of a temporary pacemaker. There are three basic types of temporary pacemakers. These are: an external transcutaneous pacemaker (also called a Zoll pacemaker after its inventor); a transvenous pacemaker; and a "pacing Swan" where the PA catheter itself is capable of functioning as an internal pacing wire. Care must be taken to assemble all components of the pacemaker chosen. For the Zoll pacemaker, the components are the pacemaker console (almost as big as a defibrillator but being rapidly downsized with new generations), wires to connect to the electrode pads, and the external pads that are applied to the skin. For a transvenous pacer, the pacer box (slightly larger in size than an MP3 player), the wires to connect to the internal component, and the sterile internal pacer are needed.

The efficacy and safety (it is noninvasive) of the Zoll pacemaker make it the first choice. However these units are not universally available, so locating a unit and ensuring that all the components are present is mandatory before insertion of the PA catheter. External transcutaneous pacing requires 65 to 100 milliampere (mA) of current (compared to 0.1 to 25 mA for transvenous pacers). This can produce significant pain from skeletal muscle contraction. However, virtually all patients can tolerate external pacing for at least 15 minutes. When using an older Zoll pacemaker, two pads are placed, one anteriorly just left of the sternum and one posteriorly inferior to the scapula so the heart is "in between" the pads. There are new combination units available that provide electrocardiogram, external pacing, and defibrillation capabilities. These units may require up to three different types of electrodes with differing pads. Familiarity with these systems by both physicians and nurses is critical *before* their use.

One final note is that if complete heart block occurs when placing a PA catheter, the catheter should be removed immediately and should not be reinserted without close consultation with a cardiologist.

SUGGESTED READINGS

American Society of Anesthesiologists Task Force on Pulmonary Artery Catheterization. Practice guidelines for pulmonary artery catheterization. Anesthesiology 2003;99:988–1014.

Bocka J. External pacemakers. eMedicine. Available at: http//www. Emedicine.com/emerg/topic699.htm. Accessed July 23, 2005.

Morris D, Mulvihill D, Lew W. Risk of developing complete heart block during bedside pulmonary artery catheterization in patients with left bundle-branch block. Arch Intern Med 1987;147:2005–2010.

Sprung CL, Elser B, Schein MH, Marcial EH, Schrager BR. Risk of right bundle-branch block and complete heart block during pulmonary artery catheterization. Crit Care Med 1989;17:1–3.

Thomson IR, Dalton BC, Lappas DG, Lowenstein E. Right bundle-branch block and complete heart block caused by the Swan-Ganz catheter. Anesthesiology 1979;51:359–362.

BE EXTREMELY CAUTIOUS WHEN MANIPULATING THE BALLOON USED IN PULMONARY ARTERY CATHETERS

LISA MARCUCCI, MD

The flow-directed, balloon-tipped pulmonary artery catheter introduced by Swan and Ganz in the 1970s is widely used in intensive care units and the operating room and in cardiac catheterization. It provides valuable information on the preload, contractility, and afterload of the heart through the measurement of filling pressures, stroke volume, cardiac output, and systemic vascular resistance. However, despite its utility, it is associated with infrequent but often catastrophic consequences if inserted and used improperly. A majority of these complications revolve around the manipulation of the latex balloon; therefore, careful attention to the correct techniques listed below can reduce these errors.

WHAT TO DO

1) Pulmonary artery catheters should not be used in a patient with a serious latex allergy. All commercially available catheters in the United States use latex in the balloon.

2) The integrity of the balloon should be tested *after* the balloon is slipped through the sterile extensor sleeve to insure that it was not damaged. If the balloon has been punctured as it was being passed through the sleeve, attempts to wedge it in the pulmonary artery will be futile (see *Figure 128.1*).

3) The balloon should be inflated with 1 to 2 ml of air only when the catheter is being advanced or the catheter is being wedged and then immediately deflated.

4) After wedging is confirmed, the balloon should always be left in an uninflated state, and this should be confirmed with the bedside nurse. Most commercial units have a lock mechanism that secures the balloon in either the uninflated or inflated state. Allowing an inflated balloon to remain in a pulmonary artery for more than 1 to 2 minutes can result in pulmonary infarct distal to the occlusion.

5) After the initial insertion of the inflated balloon and the subsequent deflation, remember that the tip will tend to migrate distally into increasingly smaller pulmonary arteries. Using the

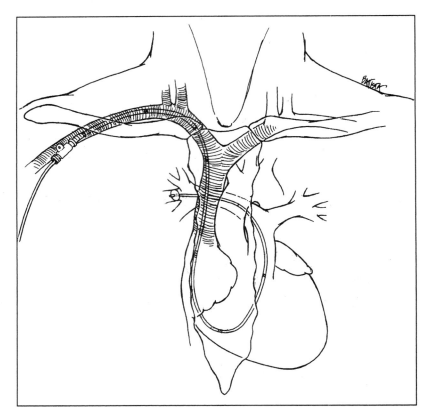

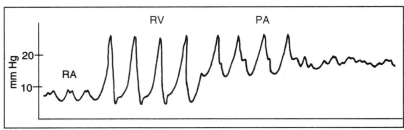

FIGURE 128.1. Wedged pulmonary catheter balloon and the characteristic waveforms. RA—right atrium; RV—right ventricle; PA—pulmonary artery.

same volume to inflate the balloon for the subsequent "wedges" risks pulmonary artery rupture. Thus, on every wedge attempt after the initial placement, the volume of balloon inflation should be as small as possible to wedge, or the catheter should be withdrawn several centimeters, inflated, and then allowed to float downstream to establish a new wedge position so as to avoid undue pressure on the wall of the pulmonary artery.

6) Patients with pulmonary hypertension, anticoagulation, and advanced age are at increased risk of pulmonary rupture during balloon manipulation, and extra care should be taken in these patient populations.

7) Pulmonary artery catheter bacterial colonization is uncommon for the first 4 or 5 days of insertion but rises dramatically for catheters in place longer.

8) Pulmonary artery catheter complications also include arrhythmias, catheter knotting, and catheter entanglement (with chordae tendineae, pacer wires, papillary muscle, etc.).

SIGNS AND SYMPTOMS

Pulmonary artery rupture is quite rare but has a high mortality. The presentation varies with the location of the rupture, the most common presentation being pulmonary interstitial hemorrhage with hemoptysis, which is life-threatening. If the visceral pleura ruptures, the patient presents with hemothorax with or without pneumothorax. Lesser injuries may cause the development of pulmonary artery pseudoaneurysms, which typically present with late rupture. Aggressive treatment is essential, starting with isolation of the lung with hemoptysis (right in more than 90% of cases) with a double lumen endotracheal tube. Reinflation of the catheter's balloon can provide temporary tamponade. The application of positive end-expiration pressure (PEEP) may help staunch the bleeding. The patient's underlying condition (e.g., pulmonary hypertension) and indication for catheter insertion may influence management, but thoracotomy to isolate, control, and repair or resect the damaged artery and pulmonary parenchyma may be necessary.

SUGGESTED READINGS

Bowdle, TA. Complications of invasive monitoring. Anesthesiol Clin North Am 2002;20:571–578.

Cissarek T, Saul FW, Hufnagel B, Mehlorn J, Losse B. Rupture of the pulmonary artery—fatal complication by pulmonary artery balloon-tipped catheter. Z Kardiol 2000:89:669–674.

Hannan AT, Brown M, Bigman O. Pulmonary artery catheter-induced hemorrhage. Chest 1984;85:128–131.

Ortmann C, Diallo R, Du Chesne A, Brinkmann B. Pulmonary artery catheters: are deadly complications avoidable? Anaesthesist 1996:45:755–759.

EMERGENCY DEPARTMENT

OPERATING ROOM

MEDICATIONS

LINES, DRAINS, AND TUBES

WOUNDS

BLEEDING

GASTROINTESTINAL TRACT

WARDS

INTENSIVE CARE UNIT

LABORATORY

129

REMEMBER THAT THE FIRST SYMPTOM OF A WOUND INFECTION IS PAIN, AND THE FIRST SIGN IS TENDERNESS (*NOT* ERYTHEMA)

HEATHER ABERNETHY, MD

In the United States, wound infections are the most common nosocomial infection in surgical patients. The risk of surgical site infection is dependent upon many factors, including the type of operation, length of operation, site of operation, elective versus emergent surgery, administration of appropriate prophylactic antibiotics, and multiple patient factors. These patient factors include coexisting infections (especially urinary tract infections), preoperative nutritional status, steroid use, diabetes, age, smoking history, and obesity. Overall the incidence of wound infection is estimated to be about 2% to 3%.

Simplistically, wound infections occur because the subcutaneous fat is more susceptible to infection than are the deeper fascial layers and the superficial (skin) layer, both of which heal quickly.

SIGNS AND SYMPTOMS

The astute clinician will recognize that the earliest sign of most wound infections is tenderness, and the earliest symptom is pain. Pain will be manifest as increasing discomfort, worse than the day before. Tenderness can be elicited by lightly but firmly tapping with one or two fingers along the entire length of the incision. Even relatively fresh postoperative wounds with staples in place will not be associated with much patient discomfort with light percussion. Later signs of wound infections include erythema, induration, discharge, fluctuance, cellulitis, leukocytosis, and systemic signs of infection, including fever. Delay in treatment can result in increased systemic signs of infection and can compromise the underlying fascia, increasing the risk of incisional hernia.

The treatment of a wound infection with a fluid collection involves opening of the wound to allow drainage. This decompresses the abscess and allows adequate inspection of deeper tissue. If necrotic tissue is present, debridement may be needed. Wounds should be left to heal by secondary intention and initially packed with wet to dry dressings to prevent closure of the skin and reformation of an infected space. For larger wounds, after an initial period of wet to dry dressing and elimination of purulent fluid, Vacuum Assisted Closure (VAC) dressings may be placed to speed formation of granulation tissue and secondary closure. Use of antibiotics is common even with open drainage of wound infections, with coverage narrowed as appropriate if wound cultures were obtained.

If the patient has pain and tenderness with skin cellulitis but no fluid collection, it is acceptable to start a short course of antibiotics (including coverage against staphylococci, streptococci, and Gram-negative coverage), with close follow-up without opening the wound.

SUGGESTED READINGS

Cameron JL, ed. Current Surgical Therapy. 7th Ed. St. Louis: Mosby, 2001;1277–1282.

Wilson MA. Skin and soft-tissue infections: impact of resistant gram-positive bacteria. Am J Surg 2003;186:35S–41S.

130

CONSIDER THE VAC DRESSING
FOR DIFFICULT WOUNDS

MICHAEL J. MORITZ, MD

Vacuum Assisted Closure (VAC) is a proprietary wound care system manufactured by KCI USA, Inc. The VAC system applies controlled negative pressure (vacuum) to suction away fluid that accumulates in a wound and to promote wound healing and it has been shown to accelerate wound healing in a variety of circumstances. It is not known whether the negative pressure or the removal of fluid or other factors are responsible for the positive impact of VAC.

WHAT TO DO

A VAC dressing starts with a sponge dressing (or if used on bowel an initial layer of film) that is cut to the shape of the wound and is directly applied to it. The sponge itself has a connector for the suction tubing that connects to the suction unit. A clear adhesive drape is applied that covers the wound and provides a seal. A suction canister collects the aspirated fluid. The negative pressure applied can be titrated, generally in the range of 50 to 125 torr, with 125 torr as the target but ratcheted down for pain or difficulty attaining a good seal (air leaks tend to dry out the wound). The VAC is intended to be attached to *continuous* suction; if off more than 2 hours a day, VAC dressing should be discontinued. The VAC dressing must be completely taken down and reapplied (new sponge cut to shape, new tubing, new adhesive drape) periodically, as often as every 12 hours for initially treated wounds or those with relatively active infection. Most wounds require dressing changes every 48 hours (except VAC over a new split-thickness skin graft may stay 4 to 5 days). The decreased frequency of dressing changes (compared to the standard twice a day wet-to-dry dressings) improves patient comfort.

The VAC may be *useful* for the following conditions:

- Chronic open wounds, including foot and ankle wounds (diabetic and peripheral vascular disease) and pressure sores
- Large, open, contaminated acute, and traumatic wounds
- Meshed split-thickness skin grafts
- Abdominal wounds, whether after dehiscence or difficult-to-close laparotomies
- High-output fistulas

The VAC is *contraindicated* in:

- Wounds with malignancy present in the base
- Exposed blood vessels or organs that must be covered with viable tissue (muscle, fascia, etc.)
- Bleeding wounds
- Necrotic or infected tissue with eschar present or needing surgical debridement

The VAC is not a panacea. The sponge is relatively stiff and can erode into adjacent or deeper tissues, particularly if the wound's base is damaged (e.g., by ischemia or prior irradiation). Wounds with inadequate perfusion will not heal, even with the VAC in place. Applying negative pressure to wounds that are bleeding, whether because of the nature of the wound or anticoagulation, can be dangerous because more bleeding can result.

The VAC is useful for wounds that produce a fair amount of exudative fluid because it will be suctioned away. The wound must be in a location such that the clear adhesive drape can be applied and a reasonably tight seal obtained (the seal does not need to be "hermetic"). Inspection of the wound at the time of dressing changes is important; healing wounds will need an incrementally smaller sponge shaped at each dressing change. It is not desirable to have granulation tissue or epithelium growing into the sponge.

SUGGESTED READINGS

Eginton MT, Brown KR, Seabrook GR, Towne JB, Cambria RA. A prospective randomized evaluation of negative-pressure wound dressings for diabetic foot wounds. Ann Vasc Surg 2003;17:645–649.

http://www.wounds1.com/care/kci/vac_therapy.cfm

Lionelli GT, Lawrence WT. Wound dressings. Surg Clin North Am 2003;83:617–638.

Morykwas MJ, Argenta LC, Shelton-Brown EI, McGuirt W. Vacuum-assisted closure: a new method for wound control and treatment: animal studies and basic foundation. Ann Plast Surg 1997;38:553–562.

EXAMINE THE WOUND WHEN A PATIENT HAS A HIGH FEVER, ESPECIALLY WITHIN 12 TO 24 HOURS OF SURGERY

RACHAEL A. CALLCUT, MD

High fever (greater than 102.5°F) in the early postoperative period can be the first sign of a necrotizing wound infection; "necrotizing soft tissue infection" (NSTI) is the preferred term over "necrotizing fasciitis" because the fascia is not invariably involved in these infections. A high fever requires a prompt and thorough inspection of the wound (including complete takedown of all bandages, dressings, and casts) in any postoperative patient because these infections are rapidly progressive, and delay in diagnosis can have fatal consequences. The overall mortality from NSTI approaches 30% to 40%. Palpation of the wound may reveal crepitus and patients may have significant pain despite a benign-appearing surgical site. Other signs include hypotension and skin bullae or necrosis, and laboratory findings include leukocytosis, hyponutrenia, and gas in soft tissues on X-ray or computed tomography (CT) scan. NSTI is usually polymicrobial, involving aerobic Gram-positive (β-hemolytic streptococci, group A streptococci, staphylococci, enterococci, etc.), Gram-negative (enteric facultative aerobes), and/or anaerobes (Gram-positive cocci, Gram-positive bacilli, Gram-negative bacilli). Less commonly, a single organism can be causative, including various streptococcal (e.g., *Streptococcus pyogenes*) or clostridial (e.g., *Clostridium perfringens*) species. Immediate and extensive surgical debridement is required in addition to high dose antibiotics. Other causes of early postoperative fever include atelectasis, thrombophlebitis, urinary tract infections, and line infections.

The treatment of an NSTI is immediate and extensive surgical debridement with a "second-look" operation usually within 24 hours. Early diagnosis and prompt surgical treatment is key. Important adjuncts to surgical treatment include high-dose antibiotics and, in some circumstances, hyperbaric oxygen.

SUGGESTED READINGS

Barie PS. The laboratory risk indicator for necrotizing fasciitis (LRINEC) score: useful tool or paralysis by analysis? (editorial) Crit Care Med 2004;32:1618–1619.
Cameron J, ed. Current Surgical Therapy. 7th Ed. St. Louis: Mosby, 2001;1277–1282.
Herndon D, ed. Total Burn Care. 2nd Ed. Philaelphia: WB Saunders, 2002;492–493.
Wall DB, DeVirgilio C, Black S, Klein SR. Objective criteria may assist in distinguishing necrotizing fasciitis from nonnecrotizing soft tissue infection. Am J Surg 2000;179:17–21.

Do not debride a dry/black eschar overlying a decubitus ulcer in a bedridden patient who has no evidence of underlying cellulitis

Nadine Semer, MD

The temptation for most general surgeons (and virtually all wound care nurses) is to debride dead tissue off wounds. In most circumstances, this is, in fact, the correct treatment. However, in the case wherein the patient is debilitated, demented, or has poor nutritional status and there is no evidence of purulence or surrounding cellulitis (erythema, warmth, induration, odor, leukocytosis, fever), this is the incorrect treatment. By debriding a noninfected eschar, or using creams that enzymatically degrade the eschar, you convert a dry, odorless, easy-to-treat wound to one that requires regular dressing changes. In a debilitated, bedridden patient, this can add to an already burdensome nursing regimen and adds to the cost of patient care.

A dry, uninfected eschar actually serves as a superb biological dressing and keeps the underlying wound in a moist environment that is conducive to healing. As the tissues underneath the eschar heal (through better nutrition, elimination of pressure at the site), the eschar will gradually separate and slough. If a previously uninfected eschar begins to show signs of infection, the eschar should be debrided and the open wound treated with appropriate dressing changes. In the case where the surgeon is uncertain if a decubitus ulcer eschar should be debrided, consideration should be given to consulting a plastic surgeon who is experienced in treating this condition.

STRONGLY CONSIDER THE DIAGNOSIS OF FASCIAL DEHISCENCE WHEN A WOUND DRAINS PINKISH OR SALMON-COLORED FLUID

MICHAEL J. MORITZ, MD

Dehiscence is defined as a splitting open or disruption. In medical terms, dehiscence generally means the disruption of something that has been surgically opened and then sutured closed. Skin closures can dehisce, uterine closures can dehisce, but the most common use of the word is to describe the disruption of the fascial layers of an abdominal wall closure. Synonyms include wound disruption, fascial disruption, and burst abdomen. Evisceration represents a subset of dehiscence when intra–abdominal contents are exposed.

The incidence of fascial dehiscence has been relatively constant during the successive decades of the 20th century despite the general improvements in patient care, antibiotics, and suture materials. The unchanging rate of dehiscence represents the competing forces of improved surgical practice (tending to lower the incidence) versus the increase in comorbid conditions of the patient (which increases the risk). The incidence of fascial dehiscence appears to be 1% to 4%, varying with the prevalence of comorbidities in the patient population.

The timing of dehiscence is only slightly earlier than that of wound infection, typically occurring 3 to 7 days postoperatively. This leads to some confusion in discriminating between the two entities and errors in management at the bedside.

There are a variety of presentations of dehiscence. The most important is disruption of the fascia with an apparently intact overlying skin closure. The cardinal event of a sudden gush of pink fluid through the wound is usually noted by the patient or patient's nurse, with a subsequent call to the surgeon. Upon examination, there may be no further drainage or only minimal drainage, and the skin closure appears intact. High on the differential diagnosis list for the inexperienced surgeon is a wound infection or wound hematoma (with opening the skin to drain the remaining fluid being desirable). However, usually in this situation if the physician opens a bit of the wound, more pink fluid will appear, followed by intra–abdominal contents.

WHAT NOT TO DO

A few common sense axioms should be considered when called to see these patients. Wound infections drain pus, not pink fluid. Wound hematomas, if sterile, do not benefit from bedside drainage. Dehiscences that may or may not be manageable conservatively get converted into eviscerations mandating emergency surgery with attendant increased risks if the staples are removed or the wound is probed by other manual palpation for nonapproximated fascial edges. The *history* of a sudden gush of pink fluid from an abdominal wound is almost pathognomonic of a dehiscence, thus no opening or probing of the wound is needed to make the diagnosis. The only decision making with this clinical finding involves the timing of reparative surgery; either urgent return to the operating room to reclose the fascia or an attempt to "conservatively" manage the wound with an abdominal binder, sterile dressings, and so on with the hope that the skin closure remains intact. If successful, this management will result in a large incisional hernia requiring late operative repair. If, at the time of dehiscence, the patient's general condition is so poor or if reversible or temporary factors are present that will impair healing of the reclosure, then an attempt at nonoperative management may be warranted.

Other presentations of dehiscence include simultaneous disruption of fascia and skin closures resulting in evisceration. Little decision making is needed in this situation because returning the abdominal contents to their domain is vital. Similarly, dehiscence of a wound where the skin has been left open to heal by secondary intention will manifest with drainage of pink fluid through the failing fascia. Examination will reveal the failing fascial closure and the need for urgent surgery to reclose the abdomen.

Fascial dehiscence can occur from failure of the suture or from the fascia tearing with intact sutures, this being the case in over 95% of dehiscences. There are numerous risk factors and associations with fascial dehiscence. Factors related to the wound itself (within the surgeon's purview) include superficial wound infection, wound hematoma, and a drain or an intestinal stoma brought out through the wound. The incidence of superficial wound infection can be lowered by avoidance of hypothermia, shorter duration operative procedures, and appropriate perioperative antibiotics. Most factors are patient related. General comorbidities include age greater than 65 years, obesity, chronic obstructive pulmonary disease (chronic cough, increased abdominal pressure, increased mechanical stress on the closure), pneumonia, sepsis, hypotension, hypoproteinemia (malnutrition), uremia, corticosteroids, and others. Specific abdominal factors include ascites, abdominal distention, abdominal malignancy, and the presence of an intra-abdominal infection. Half of patients with dehiscence have intra-abdominal infection; therefore at surgery, a thorough laparotomy is justified and nonoperatively managed patients must have intra-abdominal infection excluded.

Wound infections associated with fluid collections are diagnosed based on the inflammation surrounding the incision and the purulent fluid therein and should be promptly and widely opened so as to protect the underlying fascia from dissolution. Compared to failed skin closure, fascial dehiscence occurs much less often but is associated with a much higher rate of death. The mortality after dehiscence is reported to be 20% to 40%.

To reemphasize: the diagnosis of dehiscence is usually made on the basis of history, not by examination. Bedside or office opening or probing of wounds that may harbor a dehiscence is ill-advised. Believe the patient or nurse who tells of the brief flow of pink fluid onto bedding or clothing. Examine the patient with the diagnosis of dehiscence already in mind, evaluating for the timing of repair of the disrupted abdominal wall closure.

SUGGESTED READINGS

Carlson MA. Acute wound failure. Surg Clin North Am 1997;77:607–636.
Cliby WA. Abdominal incision wound breakdown. Clin Obstet Gynecol 2002;45:507–517.
Webster C, Neumayer L, Smout R, et al. Improvement Program. National Veterans Affairs Surgical Quality Prognostic models of abdominal wound dehiscence after laparotomy. J Surg Res 2003;109:130–137.

EMERGENCY DEPARTMENT

OPERATING ROOM

MEDICATIONS

LINES, DRAINS, AND TUBES

WOUNDS

BLEEDING

GASTROINTESTINAL TRACT

WARDS

INTENSIVE CARE UNIT

LABORATORY

LOOK FOR THE SOURCE OF A LOWER GASTROINTESTINAL BLEED IN THE UPPER GASTROINTESTINAL TRACT

RACHAEL A. CALLCUT, MD

Although upper gastrointestinal (GI) bleeding generally presents with melena and/or hematemesis, it can also present with hematochezia (bright red blood per rectum). In patients with a brisk upper GI bleed, approximately 10% will have hematochezia. When a workup for lower gastrointestinal bleeding is undertaken, a nasogastric (NG) tube should be placed and lavage performed to rule out an upper GI source. Correctly performed, NG lavage reliably excludes active bleeding proximal to the pylorus. Clear bile in the NG aspirate is strong evidence against a postpyloric upper GI source. If bleeding from a duodenal or proximal jejunal sources is brisk, it is more likely to reflux through the pylorus and be found in the NG aspirate, whereas slow bleeding from this area may only be detectable in the stool. Among the upper GI sources that may present as lower GI bleeding are gastric varices, esophageal varices, Dieulafoy's lesions, peptic ulcers, hemobilia, angiodysplasia, and aortoenteric fistulas.

Causes of lower GI bleeding include bleeding sites distal to the ligament of Treitz (although most originate in the colon). Lower GI sources are numerous and include neoplasms, inflammatory bowel disease, hemorrhoids, angiodysplasias, aortoenteric fistulas, vasculitis, mesenteric ischemia, diverticulosis, Meckel's diverticula, intussusceptions, arteriovenous malformations, and enteric infections.

SUGGESTED READINGS
Hamoui N, Docherty SD, Crookes PF. Gastrointestinal hemorrhage: is the surgeon obsolete? Emerg Med Clin North Am 2003;21:1017–1056.

Pianka JD, Affronti JS. Management principles of gastrointestinal bleeding. Prim Care 2001;28:557–575.

REMEMBER THAT BLEEDING IN THE RIGHT UPPER QUADRANT DIAGNOSED BY A BLEEDING SCAN CAN BE FROM THE HEPATIC FLEXURE OF THE COLON OR THE DUODENUM

MICHAEL J. MORITZ, MD

The bleeding scan is a nuclear medicine study where circulating blood is radiolabeled, serial images of the abdomen are obtained, and the bleeding site identified by the visualization of extravasated intraluminal tracer. The bleeding scan was developed to address the clinical problem of acute lower gastrointestinal (GI) bleeding. Acute GI bleeding is a common clinical problem. Most upper GI bleeding sources are readily seen endoscopically (e.g., ulcers, varices, tumors, and inflammation with the exception of Dieulafoy's ulcer). However, localization of lower GI bleeding is more difficult. The most common colonic bleeding sources (diverticulosis and angiodysplasia) bleed intermittently, can occur throughout the colon, and are difficult to diagnose endoscopically. The inability to identify which portion of the colon is bleeding is a major diagnostic problem, and continued or recurrent bleeding may lead to surgery and so-called "blind colectomy," which is resection without identification of the bleeding site. The morbidity of blind colectomy increases with resection of increasing colonic length, but shorter resections often fail to control the bleeding.

Current bleeding scan techniques use technetium-99m (^{99m}Tc) labeling of red blood cells. Current commercial kits for labeling autologous red cells are very efficient. Relatively crude (by today's standards) gamma cameras that could only image a portion of the abdomen at one time have been supplanted by extra-large–field-of-view detectors that image the entire abdomen simultaneously. These more sensitive cameras allow more rapid data acquisition to visualize extravasation more quickly. They also facilitate obtaining additional views (e.g., lateral and oblique) to distinguish between structures that overlap in the anterior-posterior view. Standardization of protocols for administration of tracer, rapid data acquisition, and (in select cases) delayed views all increase diagnostic yield.

WATCH OUT FOR

These newer techniques have eliminated many but not all of the sources of error. Common errors include confusion between overlapping

313

right upper quadrant structures, particularly the duodenum and the hepatic flexure, and accumulation of tracer distal to the bleeding site. Blood in the GI tract is an irritant and a purgative and is usually rapidly translocated in the anterograde direction. Occasionally, the blood will travel retrograde. In the past, intermittent or slow bleeding often was poorly visualized because it accumulated remote from the actual bleeding site. Thus, right lower quadrant tracer could be ascribed incorrectly to the cecum and proximal right colon or to a distal small bowel site when the bleeding was more proximal but pooled in the cecum. Jejunal bleeding sites were particularly difficult to diagnose. To add to the possibility of diagnostic error retrograde movement of tracer leads to further right upper quadrant accumulation, rapid anterograde movement may accumulate in the right lower quadrant, and accumulation in mid-abdomen can be confused with sites such as the transverse colon.

Adding to the uncertainty is that intermittent bleeding may not manifest during the initial imaging session. Plans for extending the imaging, or return for later delayed imaging should be made in conjunction with nursing staff and the surgical, GI, and other consultants. The half-life of ^{99m}Tc is 6 hours—images may be obtained for 18 to 24 hours after a single injection. The result of the scan must be fully discussed and reviewed with the radiologist. The surgeon must appreciate the subtleties of the nuclear medicine scan in deciding how much weight to give the result of the bleeding scan as part of the decision whether to operate and, if so, what operation to perform. To this end, many experienced surgeons will also attempt to localize a bleeding source using one of the several angiography modalities available.

One final note is that the first diagnostic maneuver for lower GI bleeding is placement of a nasogastric tube with lavage until bilious material is returned.

SUGGESTED READINGS

Gutierrez C, Mariano M, Vander Laan T, et al. The use of technetium-labeled erythrocyte scintigraphy in the evaluation and treatment of lower gastrointestinal hemorrhage. Am Surg 1998;64:989–992.

Holder LE. Radionuclide imaging in the evaluation of acute gastrointestinal bleeding. Radiographics 2000;20:1153–1159.

RECOGNIZE HERALD BLEEDING AND INSTITUTE THE APPROPRIATE DIAGNOSTIC AND THERAPEUTIC MANEUVERS

MICHAEL J. MORITZ, MD

Herald—one that precedes or foreshadows; one that gives a sign or indication of something to come; a harbinger.

Major arterial fistulae present with signs and symptoms of sepsis (often low grade) and bleeding. The most common situation is a small amount of bleeding that stops, the passage of a variable amount of time, and then massive hemorrhage. The first, small bleed is known as a "herald bleed" (or "sentinel bleed") as it presages the dramatic and ominous events to follow. If correctly diagnosed, the herald bleed allows time to initiate treatment before often life-threatening hemorrhage follows. Accordingly, in the appropriate setting, major arterial fistulae must be considered in the differential diagnosis of bleeding.

Two types of fistulae will be discussed: abdominal arterial, enteric fistulae, and thoracic tracheoinominate fistulae.

In the abdomen, primary fistulae are rare but can occur between arterial aneurysms and the bowel; for example, aortoduodenal or iliocolic (iliac artery to colon). More commonly, secondary fistulae occur between vascular grafts and the bowel. Most are aortoduodenal fistulae to the fourth portion of the duodenum, but fistulae can also occur to small bowel, colon, or esophagus (or to genitourinary structures such as ureter, bladder, etc.). Without repair the mortality is uniform; with repair the overall mortality rate is about 33%. Although the experience with endovascular stents for abdominal aortic aneurysm is still relatively small, aortoduodenal fistulae have been reported; no data exist on the relative risk of this complication for open versus endovascular repair.

SIGNS AND SYMPTOMS

Fistulae to the duodenum usually present with significant upper gastrointestinal (GI) bleeding but may less often present with lower GI or occult GI bleeding, as will fistulae to the small bowel or colon. The magnitude of the herald bleeding in the proper clinical setting prompts a workup. The diagnosis is usually made by upper GI endoscopy and/or computed tomography (CT) scan. Patients who are upper GI–endoscoped for GI bleeding and who have a history of aortic aneurysm or aortic surgery should be endoscoped down to the duodenojejunal junction (unless pathology is found more proximally) as the fistulae usually involve the fourth portion of the duodenum. In taking a history, remember that patients may have had aortic surgery using endovascular techniques so will not exhibit abdominal wall scars. Computed tomography scan typically shows fluid around the vascular graft. When obtaining this study, care should be taken to alert the radiologist that the intravenous dye should be given before the oral contrast to be sure that a small amount of dye leaking into the bowel is not obscured. While making the diagnosis should not be difficult, the magnitude of reparative surgery is so great that there is often reluctance to proceed without solid proof. Repair requires repair of the bowel defect, removal of the infected graft (when present) or infected vessel, and usually extraanatomic bypass, typically axillary artery to uninfected distal arteries at the femoral level or below.

Tracheoinnominate fistulae are almost always a consequence of a prior tracheostomy and are the result of erosion of the tube's cuff or tip inferiorly and anteriorly into the brachiocephalic artery. The incidence is less than 1% of tracheostomies. The classic time of presentation (75% of cases) is 3 to 4 weeks after the procedure. Factors that increase the risk of tracheobrachiocephalic fistula include high pressure in the tracheostomy cuff, excessive movement of the tube or the patient's head, and overly low placement of the stoma. Without repair, mortality is to be expected.

SIGNS AND SYMPTOMS

As with abdominal arterial fistulae, the initial presentation is bleeding, most commonly a short and brisk bleed into the airway (hemoptysis). This bleeding through a tracheostomy is often mistakenly attributed to trauma from suction catheters or other conditions (granulation tissue in the tracheostomy site, pneumonia, anticoagulation, etc.). Exsanguinating hemorrhage from the tracheostomy is less common as the presentation but is the inevitable outcome if not correctly addressed by investigating herald bleeding. Bronchoscopy and angiography may be negative, but the reemergence and volume of bleeding usually make the diagnosis. Tamponade of the bleeding brachiocephalic artery and control of the airway are critical; placement of an endotracheal tube distal to the fistula through the mouth or via the stoma controls the airway. Placing a finger into the stoma or overinflation of the tracheostomy balloon compresses the artery. Surgical repair via a sternotomy requires division of the inominate artery and separation of the artery from the trachea with healthy tissue.

To reemphasize: herald bleeding portends ominous events. Think of aortoenteric fistulae in the setting of aortic disease/aortic surgery and GI bleeding. Think of tracheobrachiocephalic fistulae when bright blood appears in or around a tracheostomy, particularly one placed relatively recently.

SUGGESTED READINGS

Cendan JC, Thomas JB, Seeger JM. Twenty-one cases of aortoenteric fistula: lessons for the general surgeon. Am Surg 2004;70:583–587.

Smith JW. Aortic graft–enteric fistula. In: Ernst CB, Stanley JC, eds. Current Therapy in Vascular Surgery. 3rd Ed. St Louis: Mosby-Year Book 1995;411–413.

Sue RD, Susanto I. Long-term complications of artificial airways. Clin Chest Med 2003;24:457–471.

137

DISCUSS WHEN AND HOW TO REANTICOAGULATE A PATIENT POSTOPERATIVELY WITH A SENIOR MEMBER OF THE SURGICAL TEAM

MICHAEL J. MORITZ, MD

Management of long-term anticoagulation perioperatively is difficult, with a paucity of clinical reports and widely varying recommendations. Given the absence of trials comparing perioperative anticoagulation regimens and the availability of newer agents, only broad recommendations can be made and a few caveats described. Generally, the risk and morbidity of perioperative thromboembolism must be balanced against the risk and morbidity of perioperative bleeding complications. For each patient, the individual's risks of thromboembolic complications must be assessed based on their disease process (the indication for anticoagulation), their medical histories, and individual risk factors as a function of the level of anticoagulation and the potential duration of subtherapeutic or discontinued anticoagulation. The individual's risk of bleeding perioperatively must be assessed based on the surgical procedure and the contemplated level and duration of subtherapeutic anticoagulation. From these assessments, an individualized plan should be discussed and developed with the most senior and/or experienced member of the surgical team.

WHAT TO DO

Conceptually, there are two options for managing perioperative anticoagulation for patients chronically maintained on warfarin for oral anticoagulation. The first option is to not interrupt anticoagulation and perform surgery during full or near full anticoagulation. This utilizes uninterrupted warfarin or bridging the patient with therapeutic doses of heparin or low–molecular-weight heparin (LMWH) to maintain a substantial level of anticoagulation at all times. Alternatively, warfarin dosing is halted and the patient is bridged through the preoperative period with heparin or LMWH, with therapeutic anticoagulation discontinued during the immediate perioperative period and reinstitution of heparin or LMWH postoperatively in either an incremental or full manner.

In assessing the perioperative bleeding risk of anticoagulation, the following factors increase the risk: concurrent use of antiplatelet drugs (e.g., aspirin, clopidogrel), advanced age, additional bleeding diatheses (e.g., renal or liver disease), and a history of bleeding complications. A hypercoagulable state as the indication for anticoagulation may lower the perioperative bleeding risk.

WATCH OUT FOR

In assessing the perioperative thromboembolic risk, data must be extrapolated from patients at risk of thromboembolism for whom anticoagulation must be stopped (e.g., for bleeding complications). Based on this information, patients at high risk for thromboembolic complications when anticoagulation is stopped include: mechanical prosthetic heart valves, atrial fibrillation, prior stroke or multiple risk factors for stroke, and deep vein thrombosis (DVT) or pulmonary embolism (PE) within 1 month. Unanticoagulated, the *daily* risk for a thromboembolic event is estimated to be in the range of 0.02% for mechanical valves, 0.003% to 0.05% for atrial fibrillation, and 0.2 to 1% for patients less than 3 months postDVT or PE. For mechanical valves, the risk is higher for tilting disk mitral valves and lower for bileaflet aortic valves.

SUGGESTED READINGS

Douketis JD. Perioperative anticoagulation management in patients who are receiving oral anticoagulant therapy: a practical guide for clinicians. Thromb Res 2002;108:3–13.

Kaboli P, Henderson MC, White RH. DVT prophylaxis and anticoagulation in the surgical patient. Med Clin North Am 2003;87:77–110.

138

CONSIDER A RETROPERITONEAL BLEED IF A PATIENT HAS NEW ONSET FLANK PAIN, ECCHYMOSIS, OR BACK PAIN

MICHAEL J. MORITZ, MD

SIGNS AND SYMPTOMS

Bleeding into the capacious retroperitoneal space can occur for a significant period of time before symptoms develop. The spectrum of presenting signs and symptoms of retroperitoneal hematoma vary widely including: cardiac arrest from hypovolemia; hypovolemic shock; unexplained drop in hemoglobin; pain in the back, flank, groin, or abdomen; femoral neuropathy (motor or sensory); abdominal mass; and ecchymosis of the flank, groin, or periumbilical area. The most common predisposing condition is therapeutic anticoagulation from an ever-enlarging spectrum of agents, including heparin, low–molecular-weight heparins, direct thrombin inhibitors, antiplatelet drugs, and oral vitamin K antagonists. The next most common etiology is iatrogenic, typically from high femoral artery or vein puncture, but numerous other diagnostic and therapeutic procedures have been reported to result in retroperitoneal bleeding. Finally and least common is truly "spontaneous" retroperitoneal bleeding in the absence of known risk factors for bleeding. A majority of these patients will have definable pathology, most commonly renal malignancies or vascular lesions (arterial aneurysms, venous varicosities), and a minority will have no identifiable cause.

Patients with retroperitoneal bleeding related to anticoagulation compared to those without are on average older, more commonly female, more likely to bleed within the psoas muscle, have more extensive bleeds, and are more likely to have femoral nerve involvement. On presentation, over half of patients with retroperitoneal bleeding on anticoagulation will be overanticoagulated (as measured by coagulation studies).

WHAT TO DO

The diagnosis is easily made by imaging, usually by computed tomography (CT) scan or by interventional radiologic dye study if arterial bleeding is suspected. When done with contrast, a small minority of patients have a localized blush of extravasated contrast indicating the site of bleeding. The treatment is appropriate fluid resuscitation, usually with transfusions of red blood cells for volume replacement, and fresh frozen plasma to reverse vitamin K antagonist (warfarin) anticoagulation. Short-acting antiplatelet agents will dissipate; aspirin can be partially reversed with desmopressin acetate (DDAVP) and platelet transfusions; however, clopidogrel (Plavix) is very difficult to reverse. If the bleeding is arterial, embolization should be entertained. Surgery for hemostasis or decompression is rarely indicated for several reasons: (1) the blood diffuses into numerous tissue planes, and there is not a single large hematoma present to evacuate; (2) the hematoma disrupts tissues, creating innumerable small sites of bleeding so surgical hemostasis is difficult and may traumatize tissue and result in more bleeding; (3) if the hematoma is decompressed, release of tamponade may stimulate more bleeding; and (4) surgery exposes the blood-suffused retroperitoneal tissues to the possibility of infection. For similar reasons, percutaneous decompression is equally futile and angiography to find the bleeding site for embolization is rarely successful.

The overall mortality of a retroperitoneal bleed approaches 20%. Prompt, appropriate fluid resuscitation and reversal of anticoagulation is key. After resolution of bleeding and stabilization, reinitiation of anticoagulation should be done with great trepidation. In patients without anticoagulation, the etiology of the retroperitoneal bleed is often obscured by the hematoma. Serial imaging over successive months will often show the pathology as the hematoma resorbs.

One final note is that, because these bleeds may be relatively asymptomatic, many surgeons will investigate the possibility of a retroperitoneal bleed with a screening CT scan in a patient on anticoagulation who has an unexplained loss of hemoglobin.

SUGGESTED READING

Gonzalez C, Penado S, Llata L, Valero C, Riancho JA. The clinical spectrum of retroperitoneal hematoma in anticoagulated patients. Medicine 2003;82:257–262.

139

DO NOT PRESUME THAT A GASTROINTESTINAL BLEED IN A PATIENT WITH KNOWN CIRRHOSIS IS FROM VARICES

MICHAEL J. MORITZ, MD

Upper gastrointestinal (UGI) bleeding is a serious problem. The overall mortality of a major UGI bleed is around 10% and this mortality has not substantially changed over the last several decades. The techniques of diagnosis have greatly improved with the widespread availability of endoscopy, but therapies have not greatly changed. UGI bleeding is most common in patients older than 60 years of age. The male–to–female ratio is 2:1.

Patients with cirrhosis and portal hypertension are prone to UGI bleeding. Over 50% of patients with cirrhosis and portal hypertension will have esophageal or gastric varices (24% to 80%, depending on diagnostic methods and criteria). The incidence of a first variceal bleed in patients with confirmed cirrhosis is approximately 35% over the first 2 years from diagnosis (range 15% to 68%). The mortality of a variceal bleed, defined as death within a 6–week period following the onset of bleeding, has fallen slightly over the past two decades but still exceeds 30%. The incidence of rebleeding from varices is 70% within the following year and rebleeding has the same risk of mortality as an initial bleed. While variceal bleeding in patients with cirrhosis is a major problem that requires vigilance, patients with portal hypertension are also at increased risk of UGI bleeding from other, nonvariceal sources, necessitating consideration because treatments for UGI bleeding vary with the etiology.

WHAT TO DO In UGI bleeding, while the history, physical examination, resuscitation, and stabilization are ongoing, plans for endoscopy for diagnosis and for potential treatment should be underway. Endoscopy is the test of first choice for both diagnostic and therapeutic purposes. It can help stop bleeding from esophageal varices, Mallory-Weiss tears, and peptic ulcers. Gastric lavage has not been shown to be effective in stopping bleeding but can still be useful by clearing the blood to increase the diagnostic accuracy of endoscopy. Lavage should not be done with iced solutions, which can cause hypothermia. Angiography and radionuclide imaging are rarely useful in UGI bleeding.

In cirrhosis, Mallory-Weiss tears account for 5% to 15% of nonvariceal cases of UGI bleeding. The tear is usually solitary, although up to 20% of patients may have more than one tear. The tear is usually in the stomach, but up to 20% of patients will have involvement of the esophagus. Usually the tear results from forceful vomiting or retching, and this history can be elicited in up to 90% of endoscopically-proven cases. A history of heavy alcohol use (very common in patients with cirrhosis) preceding the episode is reported in up to 60% of patients. Most Mallory-Weiss tears will stop bleeding spontaneously. Endoscopic treatments are effective at stopping bleeding, as is arteriographic embolization; accordingly, surgery is rarely necessary.

Peptic ulcer disease accounts for at least 50% of all UGI nonvariceal bleeding episodes in cirrhotics. Duodenal ulcers predominate, with a ratio of at least 2:1 over gastric ulcers. The three primary mechanisms for development of peptic ulcer disease are *Helicobacter pylori* infection, hypersecretion of acid, and nonsteroidal anti-inflammatory drug (NSAID) use, but only NSAIDs are associated with an increased risk of *bleeding* ulcers. Peptic ulcer disease is more common in both alcoholics and in patients with cirrhosis (alcoholic or nonalcoholic).

Gastritis or superficial gastric erosions account for up to 20% of all UGI bleeding episodes. Gastritis, hemorrhagic gastritis, erosive gastritis, and superficial gastric erosions are diagnoses with substantial overlap. Most cases of UGI bleeding from gastritis are relatively minor. The intensive care unit entity of "stress gastritis" can cause major hemorrhage but has fortunately become much less common in the last 20 years, presumably because of better prophylactic treatments (antacids, sucralfate, H_2-blockers, proton pump inhibitors, and others). The incidence of gastritis is high amongst heavy alcohol drinkers; at least 20% will have visible lesions on endoscopy.

Portal hypertension can cause UGI bleeding from esophageal varices, gastric varices, ectopic varices, and portal hypertensive gastropathy. Variceal bleeding is often more voluminous than nonportal hypertensive causes of UGI bleeding and can quickly devolve into shock. Rapid recognition, resuscitation, diagnostic endoscopy, and quick therapeutic endoscopy are key to minimizing the mortality of variceal bleeding, which exceeds 30%.

One final note is that to the degree that venous bleeding in a given nonvariceal lesion occurs, portal hypertension will greatly magnify the amount of venous bleeding from a given lesion. Thus, patients with cirrhosis and both gastritis and Mallory-Weiss tears will bleed more than patients without cirrhosis but with the same lesion. Coexistent coagulopathy will accentuate bleeding from all etiologies.

SUGGESTED READINGS

Cooper GS, Chak A, Way LE, et al. Early endoscopy in upper gastrointestinal hemorrhage: associations with recurrent bleeding, surgery, and length of stay. Gastrointest Endosc 1999;49:145–152.

Fallah MA, Prakash C, Edmundowicz S. Acute gastrointestinal bleeding. Med Clin North Am 2000;84:1183–1208.

Feldman M, Scharschmidt MF, Sleisenger MH. Sleisenger & Fordtran's Gastrointestinal and Liver Disease: Pathophysiology/Diagnosis/Management. 6th Ed. Philadelphia: WB Saunders, 1998:198–215.

140

HAVE A HIGH INDEX OF SUSPICION FOR LIVER INJURY IN CHILDREN WHO RECEIVE CHEST COMPRESSIONS

MARK SNEIDER, MD

Although distinctly uncommon, cardiac arrest does occur in children. As with adults, resuscitation protocols include chest compressions. One complication of chest compressions seen in children that is rare in adults is blunt liver injury and/or laceration (sometimes secondary to rib fractures). The overall mortality for children with isolated blunt liver injuries is 15%.

Children are more susceptible to abdominal injury caused by blunt forces than are adults. They have relatively compact torsos with smaller anterior-posterior diameters, which provide a smaller area over which the force of injury can be dissipated. They have softer, more compliant chest walls so that chest compressions cause more displacement of the anterior chest wall in the posterior direction. They have proportionally larger intra-abdominal solid organs, less overlying fat, and weaker abdominal musculature. In addition, compared to adults, a child's liver is relatively large and has decreased fibrous stroma. These differences make the child's liver more susceptible to laceration and bleeding in blunt abdominal trauma that occurs during cardiopulmonary resuscitation (CPR) than an adult's.

SIGNS AND SYMPTOMS

The signs and symptoms of liver lacerations are secondary to bleeding and include abdominal distention, pain, hypotension, and tachycardia. If clinically stable, children with suspected intra-abdominal injury after CPR should undergo emergent computed tomography (CT) scanning of the abdomen. Laboratory studies for these patients should include an immediate complete blood count, electrolyte panel, hepatic panel, amylase and lipase, coagulation profile, and a type and crossmatch for blood. Clinically silent liver injury may be identified by elevated serum transaminases. A CT scan of the abdomen should be done if aspartate aminotransferase (AST) levels are greater than 450 IU/L and alanine aminotransferase (ALT) levels are greater than 250 IU/L.

Nonsurgical observation of liver injuries in hemodynamically stable children after CPR is the mainstay of treatment and is generally safe. It is estimated that 90% of children with liver injuries can be managed nonoperatively. ICU monitoring, close monitoring of urine output, frequent serial CBCs, and follow-up CT scan is recommended. The decision to abandon conservative management and proceed to operation is based on hemodynamic instability or transfusion requirement of greater than 40 mL/kg of packed red blood cells.

Of note is that surgical treatment of liver injury in children and especially in young children is technically very difficult. If the decision for laparotomy is made, the most experienced pediatric liver surgeon available (even if this is an "adult" surgeon) should perform or supervise this high-risk procedure. Packing of a liver injury to control bleeding is part of the armamentarium of procedures, as is postoperative arteriography and embolization of bleeding branch arteries within the liver. Finally, adolescents and slender young adults are also susceptible to the same mechanism of injury secondary to chest compressions.

SUGGESTED READINGS

Gilles M, Hogarth I. Liver rupture after cardiopulmonary resuscitation during perioperative cardiac arrest. Anesthesia 2001;56(4):387–388.

Haller JA Jr, Papa P, Drugas G, Colombani P. Nonoperative management of solid organ injuries in children. Is it safe? Ann Surg 1994;219(6):625–631.

Holmes JF, Sokolove PE, Brant WE, et al. Identification of children with intra-abdominal injuries after blunt trauma. Ann Emerg Med 2002;39:500–509.

EMERGENCY DEPARTMENT

OPERATING ROOM

MEDICATIONS

LINES, DRAINS, AND TUBES

WOUNDS

BLEEDING

GASTROINTESTINAL TRACT

WARDS

INTENSIVE CARE UNIT

LABORATORY

141

TREAT MEDIASTINITIS FROM AN ESOPHAGEAL PERFORATION AS A TREATMENT EMERGENCY

MICHAEL J. MORITZ, MD

SIGNS AND SYMPTOMS

Infection of the mediastinum is serious and potentially fatal. Mediastinitis usually presents with fever, tachycardia, leukocytosis, and pain in the chest, back, epigastrium, or neck. When mediastinitis occurs postoperatively, wound infection and, if after a median sternotomy, instability of the sternum are often present. Contamination of the mediastinum with pathogens arises from a number of sites and etiologies. Perforation of the esophagus can be iatrogenic (from instrumentation) or from foreign bodies, penetrating or blunt trauma, leakage from an esophageal anastomosis, or from esophageal rupture (Boerhaave's syndrome, associated with forceful retching). Also, infections in the tracheobronchial tree and lungs and infections in the oral cavity, peritoneum, and parapharyngeal spaces can extend into the mediastinum.

WHAT TO DO

The cause of esophageal perforation leading to mediastinitis is most commonly iatrogenic (esophageal dilatation is riskier than other endoscopic interventions or endoscopy alone), followed by Boerhaave's syndrome, foreign bodies, and infections. Boerhaave's syndrome is "spontaneous" esophageal rupture following prolonged episodes of vomiting, with a transmural rupture in the distal left posterolateral intrathoracic esophagus. Boerhaave's syndrome is typically associated with heavy (binge) drinking, alcoholism, or peptic ulcer disease and presents with pain, vomiting, dyspnea (from mediastinitis and the left pleural effusion), and shock.

The diagnosis of esophageal rupture starts with plain radiography, which may demonstrate subcutaneous emphysema, pneumomediastinum, and pleural effusions. Contrast esophagography to pinpoint the site of perforation can be performed with water-soluble dye or barium, but is falsely negative in 10% of perforations. If the diagnosis remains unclear, a computed tomography (CT) scan should be performed. Analysis of pleural fluid (pH less than 6.0, high amylase, food particles) can be occasionally helpful. Endoscopy can be helpful with identifying the site of perforation but misses about 20% of perforations and can worsen a small perforation.

Nonoperative therapy of esophageal perforations has a place in the management of small contained leaks, particularly iatrogenic ones. Nonoperative management is predicated on defining the leak (there must be no extension to the pleural or peritoneal space), the absence of gastrointestinal obstruction distal to the leak, the absence of systemic signs of sepsis, and early prompt diagnosis and treatment. Nonoperative management has been reported to have an overall mortality of 5 to 26% in iatrogenic perforations; 0 to 14% in cervical esophageal perforations; and 13 to 59% in thoracic and abdominal perforations.

Surgery is indicated in virtually all cases of Boerhaave's syndrome and in patients who do not fit the criteria for nonoperative management and are reasonable candidates for surgery. Surgery consists of identifying and managing the perforation (primary closure, reinforced and patch closures, resection with anastomosis or exclusion, etc.) and widely and thoroughly draining the infected area. The reported mortality for surgical management is highly dependent on the time between perforation and surgery, ranging from 0 to 30% for less than 24 hours and rising to 26 to 64% after 24 hours.

The newest approach to managing esophageal perforation utilizes endoscopically placed expanding stents to cover the perforation plus drainage of the mediastinum in addition to supportive measures (e.g., nothing by mouth and antibiotics). A variety of different types of stents have been used in a variety of circumstances; the availability, the indications, and the outcomes are unclear at this time.

Regardless of the approach ultimately chosen to manage an esophageal perforation, the key variable in survival is the time between perforation and intervention, with mortality rising rapidly after 24 hours. Esophageal perforations are emergencies and prompt diagnosis and intervention is vital.

SUGGESTED READINGS

Duncan M, Wong RKH. Esophageal emergencies: things that will wake you from a sound sleep. Gastroenterol Clin 2003;32:1035–1052.

Gupta NM, Kaman L. Personal management of 57 consecutive patients with esophageal perforation. Am J Surg 2004;187:58–63.

Siersema PD, Homs MYV, Haringsma J, Tildnus HW, Kuipers EJ. Use of large-diameter metallic stents to seal traumatic nonmalignant perforations of the esophagus. Gastrointest Endosc 2003;58:356–361.

DURING RECTAL EXAMINATION, INITIALLY INSERT THE FINGERTIP JUST SLIGHTLY AND HOLD FOR SEVERAL SECONDS

RACHAEL A. CALLCUT, MD

Rectal exams are uncomfortable and embarrassing for the patient. An understanding of the involved anatomy and use of the proper technique in performing a rectal exam will decrease the pressure and fullness felt by the patient and will aid in performing a thorough exam. The astute clinician will recognize that the external sphincter is innervated by components of the somatic nervous system (inferior rectal branch of the internal pudendal nerve and perineal branch of the fourth sacral nerve) and is under voluntary control. The external sphincter is composed of striated muscle fibers and has three components: a deep external sphincter, the superficial external sphincter, and a subcutaneous external sphincter. In contrast, the internal sphincter is a 2.5 to 4 cm thickened portion of smooth muscle extending about 1.5 cm below the dentate line under the involuntary control of the autonomic nervous system.

WHAT TO DO

When performing a rectal exam the patient should be placed in a lateral decubitus position with knees drawn up. The fingertip should be inserted to the distal edge of the external sphincter and held for a few seconds to allow the external sphincter muscle to reflexively contract and subsequently relax. The clinician can then insert the finger fully to evaluate the sphincter muscles and anal canal. This includes palpating for any mucosal abnormalities, the prostate in men, the posterior vaginal wall in women, and obtaining a stool sample for a guaiac test for occult fecal blood.

SUGGESTED READINGS

Townsend C, ed. Sabiston Textbook of Surgery. 16th Ed. Philadelphia: WB Saunders, 2001:974–978.

Zuidema G, Yeo C, eds. Shackelford's Surgery of the Alimentary Tract. 5th Ed. Philadelphia: WB Saunders, 2001:332–354.

PERFORM ROUTINE RECTAL EXAMS

RACHAEL A. CALLCUT, MD

Colorectal cancer is the second leading cause of cancer death in the United States. As the stage of the cancer at the time of diagnosis and initial treatment is the most important determinant in survival, early detection is *key* to improving the outcome of this disease. Screening programs for colorectal cancer have suggested that tumors diagnosed in asymptomatic patients are less advanced, but the proof that early diagnosis in asymptomatic persons improves survival awaits the results of prospective controlled trials. Notwithstanding, the 5-year survival is greater than 90% if the disease is localized at diagnosis (Dukes' stage A, tumor limited to the mucosa). In contrast, the 5-year survival drops to less than 10% if the cancer is metastatic at diagnosis (Dukes' stage D).

Fewer than 10% of colorectal cancers have a familial link. Hereditary nonpolyposis colorectal cancer (HNPCC, or Lynch syndrome) accounts for 6% of colorectal cancers in the United States and is defined by the Amsterdam criteria: (1) at least three relatives with colorectal cancer, one of them a first-degree relative of the other two; (2) at least two successive generations with colorectal cancer; and (3) at least one individual with colorectal cancer before age 50 years. Two hereditary polyposis syndromes, familial adenomatous polyposis (FAP) and Gardner's syndrome, account for about 1% of cases. Thus, most (greater than 75%) cases are sporadic. Accordingly, for most cases of colorectal cancer, screening of asymptomatic individuals appears to be the only method to diagnose early stage cancers.

When asymptomatic adults over age 40 undergo colon cancer screening with guaiac-based fecal occult blood tests, about 1% to 3% have a positive test. Fewer than half will have a colorectal neoplasm with adenomas outnumbering carcinomas by 3:1. Thus, the proportion of positive guaiac tests attributable to colonic neoplasms (i.e., positive predictive value) is 30% to 35% for adenoma and 8% to 12% for cancer. As small (less than 1 cm) adenomas usually do not bleed, 75% of adenomas will be missed by guaiac testing. Accordingly, occult blood screening alone is not adequate to screen for colorectal cancer, and colonoscopy is complementary.

However, for any patient who presents to a surgical clinician for an abdominal complaint, rectal (or stomal) exam is warranted. Pathology detected on a rectal exam can include anorectal disorders, pelvic disorders, and (in men) prostatic disease. Along with digital exam, guaiac-based fecal occult blood tests also should be performed. For patients presenting to any clinician (surgical or not) for a periodic visit (including emergency department care), the examination is an opportunity for screening for colorectal cancer (however imperfect) with a digital rectal exam plus fecal occult blood testing.

SUGGESTED READINGS

Allison JE, Feldman RF, Tekawa IS. Hemoccult screening in detecting colorectal neoplasm: sensitivity, specificity and predictive value. Long-term follow-up in a large practice setting. Ann Intern Med 1990;112:328–333.

Cameron J, ed. Current Surgical Therapy. 7th Ed. St. Louis: Mosby, 2001;229–230.

Smith RA, Von Eschenbach AC, Wender R, et al. American Cancer Society Guidelines for early detection of cancer: update of early detection guidelines for prostate, colorectal and endometrial cancers. CA Cancer J Clin 2001;51:38–75.

Zuidema G, Yeo C, eds. Shackelford's Surgery of the Alimentary Tract. Philadelphia: WB Saunders, 2002:219–232.

144

Do not believe the old surgical dictum that it is not possible to reduce a hernia if it contains dead bowel

Michael J. Moritz, MD

Incarceration of a hernia is the entrapment of its contents within the sac and it can be either chronic or acute. Acute incarceration is a medical emergency because there is the likelihood of progression of incarceration to strangulation. The initiating event of incarceration is unclear. The entrapped tissue may become edematous or the venous return becomes compromised; but regardless, a vicious cycle develops in which edema compromises venous return and generates worsened edema. In a process that takes only a few hours from initiation, the bowel, omentum, or other tissue within the hernia sac is subject to venous infarction and gangrene. Local findings are extreme pain and tenderness, an enlarging hernia (from edema, increased intraluminal fluid, and incoming bowel contents in a closed loop obstruction), and lost ability to reduce the hernia. Erythema of the skin over the hernia is a late sign. Systemically, the patient will have a bowel obstruction, with the exceptions of a Richter's hernia (only a portion of the antimesenteric aspect of the bowel wall is entrapped, thus a portion of the bowel wall can progress to infarction without a bowel obstruction), a hernia with entrapped appendix, and non–bowel-containing hernias (e.g., ovary, bladder, omentum, etc.).

Every acutely incarcerated hernia requires urgent intervention. In the absence of contraindications (e.g., local inflammation about the hernia, peritonitis, and bowel obstruction with vomiting and abdominal distention), manual reduction may be attempted. If unsuccessful, surgery should follow.

The goal of manual reduction is to restore the hernia contents to their normal, unimpeded, intra-abdominal position. However, there are at least four major problems that can result from "successful" manual reduction.

1) **Successful reduction of the hernia's contents is accomplished, except the reduced bowel is necrotic.** Should this occur, peritonitis will develop relatively quickly. Fortunately, this is uncommon because bowel that has necrosed from venous infarction will usually (but not always) have too much edema for the

bowel to be reduced. Also, pain from the associated inflammation will usually preclude manual reduction unless the patient has received pain medication and sedation (as frequently occurs in the emergency room) before attempted reduction. A patient on corticosteroids might be more susceptible to reduction of necrotic bowel.

2) **Incomplete reduction can occur, in which most of the contents are reduced, except for residual and usually adherent bowel in the sac.** Another manner in which this can occur is with a complex multiloculated hernia (which are most often recurrent hernias), where most of the bowel is reduced but a loculation of the sac remains incarcerated. Again, in this situation, the potential exists for gangrene in the reduced or nonreduced bowel, and the patient should be promptly operated upon because of the nonreduced component. At surgery, a search for the previously incarcerated bowel to check its viability would be time well spent.

3) **It is possible to effect complete reduction of the hernia, hernia sac, and obstructing ring *en masse* by avulsion of the ring.** On examination, the hernia is absent, and the empty space may mimic the empty hernia sac that is appreciated after successful reduction. However, the incarcerated or strangulated hernia has simply been displaced and the strangulation/incarceration process will continue unabated. Bowel obstruction will continue or worsen and the likelihood of strangulation is increased. In a sense, the internal displacement of the bowel converts the hernia to an internal hernia, which has a higher incidence of strangulation than does an external hernia because the external physical signs are lacking.

4) **It is possible to effect displacement of the hernia sac inward or partial reduction of a complex hernia sac.** The hernia sac is less prominent, but the incarceration is not reduced. This rare event is limited to multiloculated hernia sacs or obese patients. Again, the incarcerated bowel has not been released and reduced, hence obstruction and progression to strangulation has not been interrupted.

Accordingly, a careful examination of the hernia site is needed after manual reduction. The sac should be empty, with the slippery feel of smooth peritoneal surfaces. Usually the narrow neck can now be easily appreciated. This examination should assure complete reduction of the sac's contents with the sac not having been displaced. The patient must be closely followed clinically until the question of whether the reduced bowel was gangrenous has been answered.

One final note is that, in children, most incarcerated inguinal hernias can be manually reduced. Some surgeons still admit such children to the hospital for elective hernia repair the following day. Others will discharge the child (after a suitable period of observation in the emergency room) with a plan for outpatient surgical repair within the following week. In girls, an incarcerated ovary can be difficult to manually reduce; however, if ultrasound shows it to be a normal ovary, the hernia and ovary can be dealt with electively. Suspected ovarian torsion is a surgical emergency.

SUGGESTED READINGS

Merriman TE, Auldist AW. Ovarian torsion in inguinal hernias. Ped Surg Int 2000;16:383–385.

Schumpelick V, Zinner, M. Atlas of Hernia Surgery. Philadelphia: B.C. Decker, 1990:23–4,199–208.

Schwartz SI, Ellis H. Maingot's Abdominal Operations. 9th Ed. Norwalk, CT: Appleton & Lange, 1989:252.

145

DO NOT USE HIGH-DENSITY BARIUM FOR AN INITIAL CONTRAST STUDY WHEN A GASTROINTESTINAL PERFORATION OR LEAK IS SUSPECTED

MICHAEL J. MORITZ, MD

There are several types of contrast agents of varying density used to study the gastrointestinal (GI) tract. Barium sulfate for upper GI or enema is a high-density suspension of water-insoluble particles. The barium solution used as an intraluminal contrast agent for computed tomography (CT) scanning is similar to that used in UGI except that it has a lower density. Water-soluble agents are lower density than any solution containing barium and are similar to angiographic contrast agents. Water-soluble agents utilize iodinated compounds. Correct use of these agents is critical in not adding to patient morbidity and mortality in suspected gastrointestinal perforation.

In the 1950s, reports in the medical literature noted a mortality of up to 50% in cases of GI perforation diagnosed by UGI or enema using barium. Intraperitoneal barium used in these studies was reported to coat the peritoneal surfaces and, when contaminated with feces, resulted in persistent infections, granuloma formation, and dense adhesions. During the 1980s and beyond, suspected GI perforations were often investigated with water-soluble (rather than barium) studies, with an improvement in mortality. In current practice, a CT scan using lower density barium has become common to aid in the diagnosis of perforated viscus, particularly colonic perforation. Although the final choice of contrast study is usually made by the radiologist, good practice requires that surgeons know what type of contrast is being used for tests ordered to evaluate for suspected GI perforation or leak. Usually, this does not include high-density barium.

SUGGESTED READINGS

Eklof O, Hald J, Thomasson B. Barium peritonitis: experience of five pediatric cases. Ped Radiol 1983;13:5–9.

Grobmyer AJ, Kerlan RA, Peterson CM, Dragstedt LR. Barium peritonitis. Am Surg 1984;50:116–120.

Rubesin SE, Levine MS. Radiologic diagnosis of gastrointestinal perforation. Radiologic Clin North Am 2003;41:1095–1115.

BE CAUTIOUS WHEN EVALUATING THE ABDOMEN OF A PATIENT TAKING CORTICOSTEROIDS

RAMON RIVERA, MD

Abdominal complaints and symptoms in a patient taking corticosteroids present a challenging diagnostic problem that requires more than a physical exam to rule out the need for exploration. The classical physical findings of an acute abdomen result from peritonitis: tenderness on palpation, rebound tenderness, rigidity, and guarding. All of these may be minimal or absent in a patient taking corticosteroids. Thus, a negative or unimpressive physical exam in a patient on corticosteroids complaining of any level of abdominal discomfort requires further diagnostic workup. This includes laboratory testing (complete blood count, lactic acid level, amylase and lipase, complete metabolic panel, liver panel) and an obstruction series. Patients taking corticosteroids may have baseline leukocytosis, adding to the diagnostic difficulty. Perforated bowel will be diagnosed as pneumoperitoneum by visualizing free air in the abdomen about 80% of the time. If the above workup is nondiagnostic, strong consideration should be given to obtaining a computed tomography (CT) scan with both oral and intravenous contrast as soon as possible after presentation and if no contraindications exist.

Corticosteroids are potent anti-inflammatory medications used in the treatment of numerous diseases, including allergic, autoimmune, and neoplastic disorders and also for posttransplant immunosuppression. Prior to the chemical synthesis of sterol hormones from soy bean derived precursors (androgens in 1939 and cortisone in 1949), corticosteroids were not available. Over the last 60+ years, it has been become well recognized that corticosteroid use increases the risk of gastrointestinal perforation, with the mortality reported in the range of 12% to 85%, depending on steroid dose. This causative association must heighten the suspicion that patients on corticosteroids (and in many surgeons' view other immunosuppressants like cyclosporine) who have abdominal pain may have an underlying gastrointestinal perforation.

SUGGESTED READINGS

Martin RF, Rossi RL. The acute abdomen: an overview and algorithms. Surg Clin North Am 1997;77:1227–1243.

ReMine SG, McIlrath DC. Bowel perforation in steroid-treated patients. Ann Surg 1980;192:581–586.

Rosen MP, Siewert B, Sands DZ, et al. Value of abdominal CT in the emergency department for patients with abdominal pain. Eur Radiol 2003;13:418–424.

Silen W, ed. In: Cope's Early Diagnosis of the Acute Abdomen. 21st Ed. New York: Oxford University Press, 2005:15–17.

DO NOT ALLOW A "NEGATIVE CT" (COMPUTED TOMOGRAPHY) TO PREVENT YOU FROM TAKING A CASE OF SUSPECTED APPENDICITIS TO THE OPERATING ROOM IF THE DIAGNOSIS IS SUPPORTED CLINICALLY

LISA MARCUCCI, MD

With the advent of 24-hour availability of computed tomography (CT) scan, emergency room (ER) physicians will often order this test to evaluate a suspected case of appendicitis before consulting a surgeon. A commonly repeated refrain by the ER physician then becomes, "I don't think it is anything right now. I thought it was a hot appendix; the story is right, and the patient has pain, but the CT is negative." This scenario, rather than encouraging the surgeon to acquiesce in a diagnosis on a patient he has not seen, should summon a prompt clinical history and exam by the surgeon. Although in many centers CT scan is a useful adjunct in evaluating appendicitis (see *Figure 147.1*) and other etiologies of abdominal pain, there are inherent limitations in its use. The decision to take the patient to the operating room must be made by the person who bears ultimate responsibility for diagnosing and treating surgical conditions. The importance of early diagnosis in appendicitis is not to be underestimated, as the morbidity of late appendicitis and rupture is considerably higher than diagnosis and treatment of an early appendicitis.

To be most helpful in diagnosing appendicitis, the CT scan should be performed with thin cuts (5 mm or smaller) taken through the area of the appendix and the pelvis and should be performed with triple contrast (intravenous, oral, and rectal to distend the cecum). Even with an optimal test, the sensitivity, specificity, and positive predictive value are in the 80–85% range. (For unknown reasons, these numbers are invariably higher in the emergency medicine literature, with some studies reporting values of 100%.) Recently, one major academic center reported 7 false negative CT scans in 104 patients who were evaluated for appendicitis. There are several possible reasons for these results. Gross pathological changes in early appendicitis can be relatively slight and beyond the resolution of the CT scan. Also, there is doubtless variability in the predictive value of a test that is a function of the skill, experience, and level of training of the person reading the test (this is particularly relevant if the person reading the "negative CT" is not a skilled radiologist).

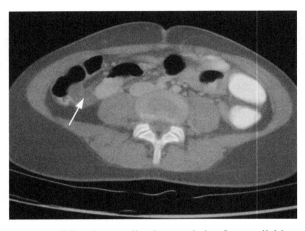

FIGURE 147.1. Dilated appendix characteristic of appendicitis on computed tomography (CT) scan.

SIGNS AND SYMPTOMS

To briefly review, the most common findings in appendicitis (except in the very young, the very old, and the neurologically or immunologically impaired) are pain in the abdomen (initially periumbilical and migrating to the right lower quadrant), anorexia, and tenderness to palpation (in the abdomen or in the rectum if the appendix is in the pelvis). Less common findings are nausea, vomiting, diarrhea, fever, urinary symptoms, and cervical motion tenderness. Common laboratory findings are leukocytosis (often mild) and microscopic hematuria.

SUGGESTED READINGS

Greenfield LJ, Mulholland MW, Oldham KT, Zelenock GB, Lillemore KD, eds. Surgery: Scientific Principles and Practice. 3rd Ed. Philadelphia: Lippincott Williams & Wilkins, 2001:1234.

Hale DM, Molloy M, Pearl RH, Schutt DC, Jaques DP. Appendectomy: a contemporary appraisal. Ann Surg 1997;225:252–261.

Maluccio MA, Covey AM, Weyant MJ, et al. A prospective evaluation of the use of emergency department computed tomography for suspected acute appendicitis. Surg Infect (Larchmt) 2001;2:205–214.

Perez J, Barone JE, Wilbank TO, et al. Liberal use of computer tomography scanning does not improve diagnostic accuracy in appendicitis. Am J Surg 2003;185:194–197.

HAVE A HIGH INDEX OF SUSPICION FOR ISCHEMIC COLITIS IF A PATIENT HAS A BOWEL MOVEMENT IN THE FIRST 24 HOURS POSTOPERATIVELY AFTER AN ABDOMINAL AORTIC REPAIR

MICHAEL J. MORITZ, MD

Colon ischemia after infrarenal aortic reconstruction can occur regardless of the indication for the procedure—aortoiliac occlusive disease or abdominal aortic aneurysm (AAA). Ligation of the proximal inferior mesenteric artery (IMA) obviously plays a role, but other local factors may include atheroembolism, interruption of internal iliac artery collaterals, and retractor placement; systemic factors include decreased cardiac output and blood pressure.

SIGNS AND SYMPTOMS

Prospective studies using colonoscopy have documented ischemic mucosal changes in 7% to 35% of elective infrarenal aortic reconstructions. Clinically manifest ischemic colitis occurs only in about 2% of elective infrarenal aortic reconstructions and up to 30% of ruptured AAA survivors. The classic presentation of ischemic colitis is bloody diarrhea early postoperatively, but this appears in less than 50% of patients. When it is present, it is highly suggestive of full-thickness colonic ischemia requiring surgical attention, thus this clinical event is not sensitive but is very specific. The other presenting signs are much less specific and include fever, renal insufficiency, hypotension, abdominal distention, leukocytosis, thrombocytopenia, higher than expected postoperative fluid or transfusion requirements, and lactic acidosis. The diagnosis of colonic ischemia is best made by *serial* colonoscopy—repeat studies at 1- to 2-day intervals will document resolution versus progression—and colonoscopy to 40 cm will diagnose over 95% of cases because more proximal ischemia without left colon involvement is rare.

Distinguishing full-thickness ischemia progressing to peritonitis and perforation from recoverable ischemic changes is dependent on serial abdominal examinations, serial colonoscopy, serial laboratory studies, and the clinical course (fluid requirements, renal function, etc.). Patients with recoverable ischemia are still at risk for late stricture formation as a consequence of mucosal loss and scarring.

Development of full-thickness colonic infarction has a very high-potential mortality when undertreated, but with prompt diagnosis and treatment, the reported mortality falls to under 50%.

Endovascular repair of AAAs is increasing in sophistication and use and has also been reported to result in colonic ischemia. Early reports place the incidence at or below the level seen in open AAA repairs (approximately 2%); but larger numbers of patients are having this procedure now and techniques are in rapid evolution, so definitive data are pending. Current endovascular techniques result in IMA occlusion at its origin and may occlude one or both internal iliac arteries, thereby putting the left colon at risk.

One difficulty in prompt clinical suspicion and diagnosis of colon ischemia is the length of postoperative paralytic ileus after open aorta infrarenal reconstruction. Ileus lasting 36 to 48 hours is common and all patients will have an ileus for at least 24 hours after an open infrarenal aortic reconstruction. Overly early return of bowel function after an open aortoiliac reconstruction should *not* prompt rapid advancement of diet, but rather consideration of ischemic colitis followed by watchful waiting, laboratory studies, serial examinations for a day or so, and possibly colonoscopy to ensure that the next bowel movement is not bloody and the patient is improving. Bowel movement within 24 hours of AAA repair is an ischemic colon until proven otherwise. Rigid or flexible sigmoidoscopy is diagnostic.

SUGGESTED READINGS

Bjorck M, Bergqvist D, Troeng T. Incidence and clinical presentation of bowel ischemia after aortoiliac surgery—2930 operations from a population-based registry in Sweden. Eur J Vasc Endovasc Surg 1996;12:139–144.

Champagne BJ, Darling RC, Daneshmand M, et al. Outcome of aggressive surveillance colonoscopy in ruptured abdominal aortic aneurysm. J Vasc Surg 2004;39:792–796.

Towne JB, Hollier LH, eds. Complications in Vascular Surgery. New York: Marcel Dekker, 2004:211–219.

149

DO NOT PERFORM ELECTIVE HERNIA REPAIRS OR HEMORRHOIDECTOMIES IN PATIENTS WHO HAVE CIRRHOSIS

MICHAEL J. MORITZ, MD

Overall, patients with cirrhosis have a higher mortality with abdominal surgery compared with patients without cirrhosis. Of note, patients with cirrhosis have only a slightly higher operative risk for cholecystectomy (as long as no other or more intrusive procedure is required), which is important because such patients have a higher incidence of gallstones and cholecystitis, may require cholecystectomy (if not end stage and/or awaiting transplantation), and have better outcomes with laparoscopic compared to open cholecystectomy. In addition to an increased incidence of gallstones, patients who have cirrhosis with ascites often develop hernias—umbilical, inguinal, and incisional. Except for incarcerated hernias, these hernias should not prompt surgery.

The perioperative mortality for nonliver abdominal surgery in patients with cirrhosis varies with severity of liver disease, as assessed by Child-Pugh or Child-Turcotte scores (based on bilirubin, international normalized ratio [INR], albumin, ascites, and encephalopathy), and is roughly 10% for class A, 30% for class B, and 60% for class C. Note that these survivals are quite similar to those experienced by Child with porta-caval shunts (published in 1954) and Pugh with esophageal stapling (published in 1973) in the treatment of bleeding esophageal varices. The operative mortality in these patients is about 50% for emergency procedures and about 25% for elective ones.

Why do cirrhotic patients have such a high mortality with abdominal surgery? One factor is the decline in liver function that often follows surgery, which may be related to the following: (1) the cirrhotic liver is much more dependent on hepatic arterial flow for oxygenation due to reduced portal perfusion of the parenchyma; (2) cirrhotic patients have a contracted intravascular volume with increased extravascular water and sodium; (3) hepatic arterial flow falls with general anesthesia and surgery; and/or (4) hepatic arterial flow falls with hypotension, decreased cardiac output, and the use of alpha-adrenergic vasopressors such as phenylephrine. Second, diminished liver function postoperatively plus the usual postoperative changes in the renin-angiotensin axis leads to fluid retention and manifests as ascites. Third, ascites often causes leakage through abdominal wall closures with resultant infection, dehiscence, and incisional hernia. Fourth, diminished liver function leads to coagulopathy. Fifth, cirrhotic patients are at increased risk of sepsis and renal failure.

Should people who have cirrhosis and hernias have elective repair to avoid the higher mortality with emergency procedures? The answer usually is no. Umbilical hernias can incarcerate, but the worse the preoperative ascites, the farther the bowel is from the abdominal wall and the less likely incarceration is to occur (a classic event is incarceration after large volume paracentesis). Inguinal hernias usually do not incarcerate; the internal ring tends to be dilated from the ascites. An additional reason to avoid hernia repairs in patients having cirrhosis is their protein catabolism, poor wound healing, and resultant much higher rate of recurrent hernia.

In addition to being predisposed to form hernias, patients with cirrhosis and portal hypertension are likely to develop hemorrhoids. One of the collateral venous routes in portal hypertension is the hemorrhoidal veins that collateralize with the perianal systemic veins. Plump hemorrhoids in such patients are under high (portal) pressure and may be associated with some bleeding; however, elective hemorrhoidectomy should not be done. The perioperative risks, particularly bleeding, are increased. Also, interruption of this collateral pathway may have untoward consequences because of the resulting higher portal pressure (e.g., precipitation of esophageal variceal bleeding). Treatment should be aggressive medical management as used in patients without cirrhosis, with surgery reserved only for severe and refractory cases.

SUGGESTED READINGS

Friedman LS. The risk of surgery in patients with liver disease. Hepatology 1999;29:1617–1623.

Mansour A, Watson W, Shayani V, Pickleman J. Abdominal operations in patients with cirrhosis: still a major surgical challenge. Surgery 1997;122:730–736.

Rizvon MK, Chou CL. Surgery in the patient with liver disease. Med Clin North Am 2003;87:211–227.

150

CONSIDER GASTRIC DILATATION WHEN A PATIENT IS HAVING RESPIRATORY DIFFICULTY

RACHAEL A. CALLCUT, MD

When patients experience respiratory difficulty, many different etiologies must be considered. In the surgical patient, gastric dilatation must be high on the list of possible causes. Gastric dilatation can be due to partial or complete small bowel obstruction, postoperative ileus, gastric outlet obstruction, and inhibition of the intrinsic pacemaker of the stomach (most commonly seen in diabetic neuropathy or after splenectomy and reflux operations including Nissen fundoplication). All of these conditions may cause an increase in intragastric pressure and, in the setting of a competent lower esophageal sphincter, a resulting enlargement of the stomach. As the stomach expands, it pushes against the inferior margin of the diaphragm (especially on the left side) and decreases its excursion. This in turn decreases lung expansion and may cause respiratory insufficiency or dyspnea in patients with borderline physiologic or anatomic pulmonary reserve.

WHAT TO DO

The best way to diagnose gastric dilatation on clinical exam is to check for a distended upper abdominal wall, sweating, hiccups, upper abdominal pain, and the presence of a succession splash. The best radiologic test is an abdominal radiograph, which will show a large gastric bubble (see *Figure 150.1*). The best treatment is urgent placement of a nasogastric (NG) tube with a sump port that is placed to wall suction. Placement of an NG tube should be undertaken without waiting for radiologic evaluation of a gastric air bubble if the patient is in extremis or one of the physical signs or symptoms is present. Confirmation of the correct placement of the NG tube must be obtained by aspirating gastric contents or radiologic confirmation of tube position. Auscultating air injected into the NG is less preferred as the sensitivity and specificity of this method for confirming intragastric placement is not ideal.

One final note is to have a high index of suspicion for gastric dilatation after reflux operations because relief of the bloat is much more difficult. Any patient with shortness of breath after this operation should get a radiograph, which usually establishes the diagnosis easily. Of course, one must always consider the diagnosis of pulmonary embolism also.

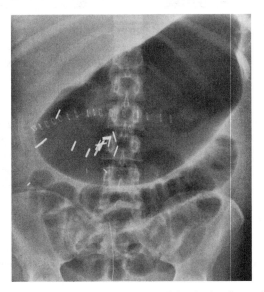

Figure 150.1. Acute gastric dilatation on abdominal radiograph.

Suggested Reading

Sabiston DL, Lyerly HK, eds. Surgery: The Biological Basis of Modern Surgical Practice. 15th Ed. Philadelphia: Saunders, 1997:355.

151

HAVE A HIGH INDEX OF SUSPICION FOR INCARCERATED OR STRANGULATED HERNIA IF A PATIENT HAS A BOWEL OBSTRUCTION AND NO PREVIOUS ABDOMINAL SURGERY

JAMES HERRINGTON, MD

In developed nations, the most common cause of bowel obstruction is postoperative adhesions from previous abdominal surgery. The second most common cause is an incarcerated or strangulated hernia, and a diligent search for a hernia is a mandatory component of the patient's workup in bowel obstruction. A missed or delayed diagnosis can increase the risk of bowel necrosis, sepsis, and death. Types of hernias that can cause bowel obstruction include inguinal (both direct and indirect), femoral, umbilical, and the rare obturator, spigelian, and lumbar hernias.

Inguinal hernias are the most common hernias in humans and a not infrequent cause of bowel obstruction, with about 10% of these hernias presenting with incarceration. A direct hernia is due to a weakness or defect in the floor of Hesselbach's triangle, with the hernia protruding medial to the inferior epigastric artery. Direct inguinal hernias typically have a broad neck, are not likely to incarcerate, and rarely cause bowel obstruction. The exception to this rule is a recurrent direct inguinal hernia. Most recurrences occur medial to the epigastric vessels, regardless of the original type of inguinal hernia, may have narrow necks, and are capable of incarceration and bowel obstruction. Indirect inguinal hernias course through the internal ring lateral to the inferior epigastric artery (i.e., they do not project through the floor of Hesselbach's triangle). Persistence of the normally obliterated processus vaginalis results in an indirect hernia in children and may contribute to indirect hernias in adults. Indirect hernias occur on the anteromedial aspect of the spermatic cord, usually have a narrow neck, and are prone to incarceration.

WHAT TO DO

Optimally, physical examination for nonincarcerated inguinal hernias should be performed with the patient standing and the clinician sitting. After visual inspection for a bulge or asymmetry, a finger is then inserted into the inguinal canal and the patient asked to cough. Although in many instances it is difficult to differentiate a direct from an indirect hernia with an experienced examiner, an indirect hernia may be appreciated as a mass or bulging felt with the fingertip moving from lateral to medial, whereas a direct hernia will be appreciated by the side of the finger and has a deep to superficial movement. The examination may be performed with the patient supine, but the hernia may not be as noticeable because the abdominal contents will not put as much pressure on the inguinal region as in the standing position. In this situation, the patient can be asked to perform a Valsalva maneuver to elicit the characteristic bulge in the inguinal canal.

Femoral hernias have a higher incidence in women than in men. Femoral hernias occur through the femoral canal, the space bounded medially by the lacunar ligament, posteriorly by Cooper's ligament (which runs along the anterior aspect of the pubic ramus), anteriorly by the inguinal ligament, and laterally by the femoral vein. This canal is rigidly bound on three sides and has a narrow neck, hence femoral hernias commonly present with incarceration. Physical examination reveals a mass inferior to the inguinal ligament. Uncommonly, the femoral hernia mass courses superiorly and is palpable at the level of or sometimes superior to the inguinal ligament. One-third of patients with an incarcerated femoral hernia will be unaware of its presence and will seek medical attention for symptoms of bowel obstruction.

Incarcerated umbilical hernias present with a tender, nonreducible mass at the umbilicus and are usually easily detected on physical exam. A patient with a bowel obstruction from other causes resulting in increased intra-abdominal pressure may present with a nonreducible umbilical hernia that is the result, rather than the cause of, the bowel obstruction.

SIGNS AND SYMPTOMS

Some of the rarer hernias may present with incarceration. They are more difficult to diagnose because their physical signs are more subtle and their rarity diminishes the physician's suspicion. Obturator hernias occur through the obturator foramen, inferior and medial to the femoral canal on the proximal inner thigh. The obturator nerve and vessels also pass through the foramen. An obturator hernia puts pressure on the obturator nerve, which is sensory to the medial aspect of the thigh, resulting in pain radiating down the medial thigh (Howship-Romberg sign). The mass presents in the very proximal medial thigh and may be palpable on vaginal or rectal examination.

Spigelian hernias occur through the junction of the semilunar line (longitudinally) and the semicircular line (transversely) where the internal oblique and transversus abdominus aponeuroses become part of the anterior rectus sheath. The surface landmarks for this point are the lateral border of the rectus sheath one-third of the distance between umbilicus and symphysis pubis. This rare hernia is difficult to diagnose because the external oblique aponeurosis remains intact, making the physical signs more subtle. Pain and a palpable abdominal mass in the correct location suggest the diagnosis and bowel obstruction is unusual.

Lumbar hernias are divided into superior and inferior hernias; both occur through a defect in the lumbodorsal fascia. Superior lumbar hernias occur through a triangle bounded by the paraspinal muscles medially, the internal oblique muscle laterally, and the 12th rib superiorly. Inferior lumbar hernia occurs through a triangle bounded by the external oblique muscle laterally, the iliac crest inferiorly, and the latissimus dorsi muscle medially. These hernias may present with pain and back or flank swelling. They can present with incarceration of large bowel with or without obstruction as a result of the posterior location of the hernia.

If the physical exam and history cannot elicit a hernia, an abdominal radiograph (see *Figure 151.1*) or, more optimally, a computed tomography (CT) scan is an important adjunct to physical examination in the diagnosis of hernia, particularly a recurrent or unusual hernia. Appropriate contrast either in the bowel or in the bladder can increase the accuracy of the CT scan tremendously. It is important to note that many hernias, particularly of the anterior abdominal wall, will spontaneously reduce in the supine position. Accordingly, the area of concern must be dependent for the CT scan to be helpful; for example, a spigelian hernia may only be seen on CT scan with the patient in the ipsilateral decubitus or prone position.

Manual reduction of incarcerated inguinal hernias is possible in about 25% of inguinal hernias and is much less likely for femoral hernias. If the patient appears toxic or there is significant concern that the bowel in the hernia is not viable (i.e., the patient needs surgery), no attempt should be made to reduce the hernia because the patient should be proceeding rapidly towards surgery. For manual reduction, the patient should be given sedation/analgesia with time allowed for the medication to work before proceeding, especially in younger patients. While waiting, the patient should be placed in gentle Trendelenberg position. For manual reduction, the patient is usually supine (for gravity to assist, the hernia should face the ceiling) and in a slight Trendelenberg position, with the abdominal wall maximally relaxed by flexing the knees and hips.

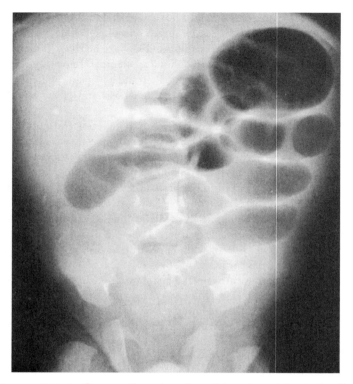

FIGURE 151.1. Gaseous distention of small bowel on abdominal radiograph secondary to an incarcerated inguinal hernia.

WHAT TO DO

To manually reduce a hernia, the nondominant hand grasps the hernia sac near the neck to form a funnel pointed at the neck. The dominant hand milks the hernia contents toward the abdominal cavity. Steady sustained pressure is more successful than abrupt movement. Success is presaged by the ability to return intraluminal gas or fluid first, and then the bowel as a second phase. If an incarcerated hernia cannot be reduced with 5 minutes of effort under the conditions described above, attempts at manual reduction should be abandoned with urgent surgery undertaken. Children with successful reduction may remain in the hospital for observation and subsequent hernia surgery. Adults may be discharged after observation with appropriate early follow-up for repair.

When reducing a hernia, one situation warrants consideration. Rarely, manual reduction can reduce the entire sac with the bowel still incarcerated within it. The patient will continue to have bowel obstruction, but the hernia will be empty. A high index of suspicion for this uncommon event is needed. (See Chapter 144 for more detail on these circumstances.)

SUGGESTED READINGS

Berry SM, ed. The Mont Reid Surgical Handbook. 4th Ed. Philadelphia: Mosby, 1997:519–525.

Cameron JL, ed. Current Surgical Therapy. 7th Ed. Philadelphia: Mosby, 2002:600–604,615,616–619.

Fitzgibbon RI, Greenburg AG, eds. Nyhus and Condon's Hernia. 5th Ed. Philadelphia: Lippincott Williams & Wilkins, 2002:71–79.

Schumpelick V, Truong S, eds. Atlas of Hernia Surgery. Philadelphia: BC Decker, 1990:41–50,51.

CONSIDER AN ANASTOMOTIC LEAK, INADVERTENT ENTEROTOMY, OR DEVITALIZED LOOP OF BOWEL IF TACHYCARDIA AND/OR TACHYPNEA THAT IS RESISTANT TO FLUIDS OCCURS AFTER ABDOMINAL SURGERY

MICHAEL J. MORITZ, MD

SIGNS AND SYMPTOMS

There are two early signs of intra-abdominal infection after abdominal surgery that usually precede the classic, later-occurring signs: tachycardia and tachypnea. Both are sensitive for intra-abdominal infection but are very nonspecific. Later signs of intra-abdominal infection include fever, increasing abdominal pain, signs of peritonitis (guarding, rigidity, rebound tenderness), development or worsening of paralytic ileus, altered mental status, and secondary organ dysfunction as a consequence of sepsis (e.g., renal insufficiency).

Persistent tachycardia with adequate hydration (neither hypo- nor hypervolemia) that occurs with no other cardiopulmonary explanation is often ascribed to postoperative pain and inadequate analgesia. While this may be true, pain is usually declining in the days postoperatively, whereas pain from intra-abdominal infection will be worsening. Also, if tachycardia is due to pain, then the tachycardia should fluctuate with the patient's analgesia. Persistent or worsening tachycardia must raise the suspicion of an intra-abdominal process. In this situation, tachycardia represents a systemic manifestation of a localized infectious process.

Postoperative tachypnea often accompanies tachycardia and is common after abdominal surgery. There are several likely culprits for which the patient should be evaluated. Atelectasis or its more severe cousin, lobar collapse, can cause tachypnea as compensation for a ventilation-perfusion abnormality. Pneumonia causes tachypnea for the same reason and additionally as a systemic response to the infection. The most common clinical presentation of pulmonary embolism is tachypnea with hypocarbia (not tachycardia or hypotension as often thought). Fluid, blood, or air in the pleural space (i.e., pleural effusion, hemo-, or pneumothorax) will cause tachypnea. Pericardial effusion may also cause tachypnea, particularly if tachycardia is blunted (e.g.. by beta-blockers). Fat embolism after trauma or orthopedic surgery and amniotic fluid embolism peripartum are less common causes of tachypnea. The evaluation for tachypnea will include pulse oximetry, chest radiograph, and when appropriate, arterial blood gases. Other diagnostic studies will be needed if specific diagnoses are entertained. Tachypnea with intra-abdominal infection represents a systemic response to infection and a local response to peritoneal irritation, with diaphragmatic splinting, use of accessory muscles, and shallow respirations.

The workup of isolated tachycardia overlaps the workup of tachypnea. Postoperative patients receiving narcotics will have some degree of respiratory depression that may mask tachypnea. Required studies include 12-lead electrocardiogram (ECG), pulse oximetry, and chest radiograph. In appropriate patients, other diagnoses (such as myocardial infarction or pericardial effusion/tamponade) may need to be excluded. In the days postoperatively, unexplained persistent tachycardia should not reflexively be thought of as pathologic and treated, for example, with beta-blockade, but as representing the patient's pathophysiologic response to an undiagnosed problem. In the patient with recent abdominal surgery, look there!

Postoperative abdominal infections can be loosely grouped into those that are relatively localized and those with diffuse peritonitis. Infections that have been walled off present more subtly, with tachycardia, paralytic ileus or poor gastric emptying, pleural effusion (if subdiaphragmatic), and localized pain. Patients with diffuse peritonitis present with more obvious sepsis, though may lack localizing signs. Computed tomography (CT) scan of the abdomen will often show small amounts of free air, but this is normal up to 7 days postoperatively. A pocket of air in an intraperitoneal fluid collection (not a loop of bowel) on CT scan is a common finding in making the diagnosis of a postoperative intra-abdominal abscess requiring intervention. Administering intraluminal contrast before the CT scan is valuable.

Patients with a single walled-off intra-abdominal collection (i.e., an abscess) can be managed operatively or by percutaneous drainage by interventional radiology. Patients with more complex problems such as multiple abscesses, collections not amenable to drainage via a percutaneous route, a question of compromised bowel viability, or a failing fascial closure may be best served by a prompt return to the operating room.

One final note is that experienced bariatric surgeons consider postoperative tachycardia very worrisome for anastomotic leak; therefore, development of this should be immediately reported to a senior member of the surgical team.

SUGGESTED READINGS

Holland AJ, Cass DT, Glasson MJ, Pitkin J. Small bowel injuries in children. J Paediatr Child Health 2000;36:265–269.

Hughes TMD, Elton C, Hitos K, et al. Intra-abdominal gastrointestinal tract injuries following blunt trauma: the experience of an Australian trauma centre. Injury, Int. J. Care Injured 2002;33:617–626.

Marvin RG, McKinley BA, McQuiggan M, Cocanour CS, Moore FA. Nonocclusive bowel necrosis occurring in critically ill trauma patients receiving enteral nutrition manifests no reliable clinical signs for early detection. Am J Surg 2000:179;7–12.

EMERGENCY DEPARTMENT

OPERATING ROOM

MEDICATIONS

LINES, DRAINS, AND TUBES

WOUNDS

BLEEDING

GASTROINTESTINAL TRACT

WARDS

INTENSIVE CARE UNIT

LABORATORY

153

CONSIDER CONSULTING PSYCHIATRY ON ADMISSION OF THE PATIENT TO EVALUATE FOR COMPETENCY

NEIL SANDSON, MD

In this litigious age, malpractice attorneys search the informed consent process for mistakes by the treating surgeon as evidence of liability or negligence. One common problem for surgeons is the confusion concerning competency and mental status.

A patient is considered competent to consent to a procedure based on two essential criteria. First, the patient must be able to comprehend the risks and benefits of both undergoing and not undergoing the procedure. Thus, an acutely delirious patient may not be able to properly consent to a procedure as a result of his or her state of cognitive compromise. Conversely, an initially competent patient who grants consent for a procedure and, who then becomes delirious before the procedure, can nonetheless appropriately be brought to the operating room. Second, the patient must be in a state that allows him or her to make meaningful choices. Using these criterion, a patient may be cogent and oriented to time and place but may still not be considered competent. Examples include serious psychiatric conditions such as major depression, bipolar disease, and schizophrenia. In these patients, their expressed wishes may be compelled by their active illness and therefore are not a true choice that accurately reflects their beliefs and desires if they were not in a suicidal or manic state.

One strategy for surgeons to avoid cancelled cases and successful litigation by malpractice attorneys over competency issues is to carefully review medications and ask about a psychiatric history before the perioperative period. If the patient reports a significant number or dose of psychiatric medications, previous psychiatric history, or dementia or brain injury, consideration should be given to having a trained professional interview the patient for competency. When a patient's confusion, dementia, depression, or other condition that might render the patient unable to grant consent (e.g., multiple sclerosis, HIV/AIDS, brain tumor) is discerned, the surgeon must seek appropriate consultation and simultaneously seek out next-of-kin, guardians, or powers-of-attorney.

One final note is that, in a true emergency situation where competency issues are ambiguous, a physician's good intentions are usually honored and generally not subject to successful litigation. However, a psychiatric consult should be obtained in any nonemergent case in which competency issues are not straightforward.

SUGGESTED READINGS

Grisso T, Appelbaum PS, Hill-Fotouhi C. The MacCAT-T: a clinical tool to assess patients' capabilities to make treatment decisions. Psychiatr Serv 1997;48:1415–1419.

Reid-Proctor GM, Galin K, Cummings MA. Evaluation of legal competency in patients with frontal lobe injury. Brain Injury 2001;15:377–386.

154

DO NOT DISCHARGE A PATIENT IF HE OR SHE WISHES TO LEAVE THE HOSPITAL AGAINST MEDICAL ADVICE

MICHAEL J. MORITZ, MD

Contested hospital discharge is a medicolegal issue. Every hospital has defined procedures for the process of hospital discharge that typically require the patient's or guardian's signature accepting responsibility for instructions, medications, and appropriate follow-up, along with a nurse's and/or physician's signature. When a competent patient insists on leaving the hospital before the patient's physician thinks it appropriate, the patient's departure would be "Against Medical Advice (AMA)". Most hospitals have defined policies for patients leaving AMA, which in bureaucratic fashion, often ask that the patient sign a form (an AMA form) accepting responsibility for themselves and recognizing that the discharge is not approved by the patient's physician. Most patients trying to "sign out AMA" are rational and reluctant to sign forms that absolve the hospital and their physicians of responsibility.

Thus, there are at least three ways in which the dissatisfied patient can leave the hospital.: (1) the patient signs whatever AMA forms are part of the hospital AMA discharge process and then leaves; (2) the patient refuses to sign such forms and simply leaves; or (3) in the face of the patient wanting to leave AMA but not wanting to sign forms shifting responsibility from the hospital and physicians to themselves, the physician (grudgingly) agrees to officially discharge the patient, writing the appropriate orders, signing the standard discharge forms, and so on. This third alternative is the only unacceptable one. It effectively shifts all the responsibility for postdischarge events onto the discharging physician. When pressure comes from the patient, the patient's family, nursing or ancillary staff, or others for the physician to authorize such a discharge, ignore it. Inform the parties of the second alternative, to simply leave. Discharge is an artificial process. With rare exceptions, patients in acute care hospitals are there of their own volition and are not under lock and key. When a patient leaves the hospital AMA, the patient assumes responsibility for him- or herself again, and this is true regardless of whether the patient signs a particular hospital's AMA forms.

WHAT TO DO

In an attempt to prevent "AMA confrontation," the surgeon must realize the three critical companions to disputed patient care issues are patient competency (see Chapter 153), communication, and documentation. Always maintain open, level-headed, unemotional communications. Try to find additional resources to aid in communication with the patient, such as clergy, psychiatrists and psychologists, social workers, nurses and staff, and other physicians. If there is an ethnic or language difference, try to find a suitable individual similar to the patient to enhance communications. Do not be put in the position of obstructing the patient's wishes if he or she is competent and not judged to be a harm to others, for care of the patient always and ultimately devolves to the patient. Document in the chart any and all conversations between the patient and the patient's family on one side and the physicians, nurses, and any other personnel, on the other. Document who was present, when the discussion occurred, the general concepts discussed, and the resolution. Separately document the competence of the patient as regards the entire discussion and if there was a formal evaluation by a trained professional. Document the specific risks of leaving, efforts to have the patient stay, the concern of the physician and staff for the patient's well-being, and the right of the patient to return.

The patient who leaves the hospital AMA is substituting the patient's judgment for that of the physician and assuming responsibility for their own care. This is a patient's prerogative. Ensure that the patient is aware of these simple facts, and document your attempts to so inform the patient. Do not become complicit with the patient.

One final note is that a patient leaving AMA does not terminate the physician's legal responsibility for follow-up care and this must be offered or arranged. The patient should be provided with instructions. Consultation with the hospital's legal department is advised.

SUGGESTED READINGS

Hwang SW, Li J, Gupta R, et al. What happens to patients who leave hospital against medical advice? *LMAJ* 2003:168;417–420.

The Medical and Public Health Law Site. Chapter 1-Preventive law in the medical environment—the discharge process. Available at: http://biotech.law.lsu.edu/Books/aspen/ Aspen-The-15.html. Accessed August 8, 2005.

Medical College of Ohio Hospitals. Leave from medical college hospitals against medical advice. Available at: http://www.meduohio.edu/policies/pdfs/7-10-10.pdf. Accessed January 16, 1990.

155

INVESTIGATE CARDIAC DEVICES (PACEMAKERS) BEFORE TAKING THE PATIENT TO THE OPERATING ROOM

CATHERINE MARCUCCI, MD

Cardiac devices (which were once called pacemakers) have profoundly increased in efficacy and complexity. In addition to pacemakers, there are now at least three other types of devices being implanted. Automatic implantable cardiac defibrillators (AICDs) monitor the cardiac rhythm and are capable of pacing (in response to bradyarrhythmias) and defibrillation (in response to abnormal fast or arrest rhythms). Cardiac resynchronization therapy-pacemakers (CRT-Ps) are biventricular pacers that synchronize the right and left ventricular contractions to increase cardiac output and are also capable of treating bradyarrhythmias with pacing. Cardiac resynchronization therapy-defibrillators (CRT-Ds) are biventricular pacers that synchronize the right and left ventricular contractions to increase cardiac output and are also capable of treating tachyarrhthmias (with either pacing or defibrillation).

WHAT TO DO

Surgeons usually do not have primary responsibility for management of cardiac devices intraoperatively. However, it is incumbent for the surgeon to facilitate pre-operative characterization of these devices for the anesthesiology staff to avoid day-of-surgery delays, cancelled procedures, and life-threatening device failure in the operating room. A consultation with cardiology (or, in some nonteaching hospitals, the device sales representative) for device interrogation should be obtained at least several days before an elective procedure. Patients with cardiac devices should always have a preoperative chest radiograph to confirm correct intracardiac lead placement.

There are several areas of concern in the interrogation of cardiac devices. These devices sense the cardiac rhythm electrically and this sensing is profoundly disturbed by the use of electrocautery, which is nearly ubiquitous in standard surgical procedures (except for unipolar cautery, the battery powered pen-like device used in cataract surgery and dermatologic procedures). Prior to the use of electrocautery and in consultation with surgery and anesthesiology, the cardiologist will alter the device settings so that the device, its leads, and the patient's heart will not be damaged.

In addition to actually turning off or changing the settings, the indication for device implantation (e.g., sick sinus, heart block, sudden cardiac death, heart failure, etc.) should be ascertained. This is valuable information perioperatively as it will affect the choice of resuscitative drugs (e.g., atropine, isoproteronol) while the device's functions have been altered. For pacemakers, the type of pacemaker (e.g., DDD, VVI), the paced rate, and the specific programmable features should be ascertained and documented in the chart. For AICDs and CRTs, the pacer function should be similarly charted and the frequency of use of the defibrillator or tachycardia-pacing function documented. Unless there is no chance of using unipolar cautery (e.g., cataract surgery), it is most common to adjust the pacemaker to "default" mode, such as DOO or VOO, just before the patient enters the operating room. This is usually easily done by a cardiologist in the preoperative area using portable equipment. At this time, it can also be ascertained what the underlying rhythm is and if the patient has a high percentage of paced beats. During surgery, patients with defibrillator devices generally have the defibrillator function turned off and the pacemaker function set to "default." Such patients will be closely monitored perioperatively and external or transvenous pacing and an external defibrillator used if necessary.

One final note is that after surgery and after clearance is given by the anesthesiologist, cardiology or the sales representative should be called to reset the cardiac device functions in the postoperative period.

156

INCLUDE THE ORDER "NO PROCEDURES ON _____ ARM (THE SIDE OPERATED ON)" WHEN WRITING POSTOPERATIVE ORDERS FOR MODIFIED RADICAL MASTECTOMY AND LUMPECTOMY AND AXILLARY LYMPH NODE DISSECTION

HARSH JAIN, MD

Any patient who undergoes an axillary node dissection should have "No procedures on _____ arm (the side operated on)" written in the postoperative orders with a sign stating the same posted over the patient's bed. In the early postoperative period, procedures to be avoided include phlebotomy, venipuncture, and blood pressure measurement. This is to reduce the risk of cellulitis and the occurrence of lymphedema in that arm. The same general precautions also apply to patients who have radiation of the axilla but do not apply to patients who have had a sentinel node biopsy alone, without other treatment of the axillary nodes. Long term, the need to avoid blood pressure measurement in the affected arm is not clear.

SIGNS AND SYMPTOMS

The pathophysiology concerning avoidance of procedures on the side of an axillary lymph node dissection is relatively straightforward. The lymphatic system clears fluid and large molecules that reach the interstitial space. If large molecules and fluid are not cleared because of impaired drainage (i.e., lymphatic obstruction), the oncotic pressure builds in the interstitium and results in fluid accumulation, known as lymphedema. With lymphedema, the subcutaneous space and skin become enlarged, but the deeper muscular compartment does not. The skin becomes brawny in lymphedema as a result of sclerosis of subcutaneous tissue. The easily damaged skin is a poor barrier to the ingress of bacteria into the edematous space. The accumulated fluid serves as an excellent medium for infection. Thus, the risk of cellulitis is increased; and, if this occurs, it tends to be more severe and takes longer to clear. In addition to the increased incidence of infection, other morbidities associated with lymphedema include limitation of motion, pain, weakness, and an array of psychological difficulties. Lastly, lymphangiosarcoma is an uncommon but devastating complication occurring decades after the development of lymphedema.

Although the general rule was that lymphedema after axillary dissection occurred in 10% of patients, more stringently monitored cohorts of women have documented a much higher incidence, approximately 20% at 1 year, rising to 50% at 20 years postoperatively. The incidence and degree of lymphedema are also related to the extent of interruption of the axillary lymphatics by surgery or radiation. The incidence ranged from 0% for patients who underwent partial or total mastectomy with sentinel node biopsy to 56% for patients 2 years after modified radical mastectomy with axillary node dissection and axillary radiation. The onset of lymphedema is also variable but does increase with time; new onset edema can occur as late as 15–17 years post treatment. Patients especially at risk are those who undergo both axillary node dissection and radiation therapy. Given the overall incidence of breast cancer, this problem is a significant one for a large number of patients.

Due to the consequences of edema and the lack of effective treatment for lymphedema, emphasis has been placed on prevention. Enormous effort has been expended to avoid axillary dissection, with more precise categorization of breast cancer and less disruptive axillary sampling techniques (particularly sentinel node biopsy). However, some patients will need to undergo axillary dissection or radiation and the above precautions should be followed for them.

SUGGESTED READINGS

Erickson VE, Pearson ML, Ganz PA, Adams J, Kahn KL. Arm edema in breast cancer patients. J Natl Cancer Inst 2001;93:96–111.

Harris JR, Lippman ME, Morrow M, et al. Diseases of the Breast. 2nd Ed. Philadelphia: Lippincott, Williams & Wilkins 2000:1033–1040.

Meric F, Buchholz TA, Mirza NQ, et al. Long term complications associated with breast-conservation surgery and radiotherapy. Ann Surg Oncol 2002;9:543–549.

Petrek JA, Senie RT, Peters M, Rosen PP. Lymphedema in a cohort of breast carcinoma survivors 20 years after diagnosis. Cancer 2001;92:1368–1377.

ORDER AN AMPULE OF NALOXONE (NARCAN) TO THE BEDSIDE WHEN WRITING ORDERS FOR PATIENT-CONTROLLED ANALGESIA OR IF THE PATIENT IS RECEIVING CONTINUOUS EPIDURAL NARCOTIC INFUSION

CATHERINE MARCUCCI, MD

Patient-controlled analgesia (PCA) is a commonly used and effective method of managing the postoperative pain resulting from a wide variety of surgical procedures. Commonly used medications for intravenous PCA regimens include morphine, hydromorphone (Dilaudid), and fentanyl, all powerful narcotics that will cause respiratory arrest if given in excessive doses. Accidental overdoses given via PCA pumps have occurred secondary to well-meaning family or staff members administering doses for the patient, misprogramming of the pump, and electrical malfunction of the pump. The antidote for all narcotic overdoses is the quick-acting agent Narcan (naloxone). It should be administered promptly to PCA patients in cases of unwitnessed respiratory or cardiac arrest and when a PCA patient has respiratory depression out of proportion to his medical and surgical condition.

Many hospitals use a preprinted PCA order sheet that provides a template of suggested doses, device settings, and auxiliary settings. Always check these orders to confirm that they specify an ampule of Narcan to the bedside for patients on any PCA regimen. If not, simply order "one amp of Narcan to the bedside, may be given by RN for respiratory depression" to avoid having to retrieve a dose from the pharmacy or nursing station when urgently needed. In addition to giving Narcan, the patient should receive immediate ventilatory support, either through bag mask or intubation while the narcotic antagonist is taking effect.

SIGNS AND SYMPTOMS

To briefly review, the signs and symptoms of narcotic overdose are drowsiness up to and including unresponsiveness, slurred speech, slow and labored respirations, constricted pupils (or dilated pupils in anoxic injury), muscle spasticity (especially in Dilaudid overdose), muscle flaccidity (especially in hydrocodone [vicodin] overdose), and cold clammy skin.

One final note is that care should be given in prescribing a basal rate of narcotic infusion via PCA because most overdoses on PCA are associated with this mode of narcotic delivery; the "as needed" mode is safer. Continuous narcotic infusion by epidural catheter also is associated with unexpected respiratory depression.

SUGGESTED READINGS

Brown SL, Bogner MS, Parmentier CM, Taylor JB. Human error and patient-controlled analgesia pumps. J Intraven Nurs 1997;20:311–316.
Doyle DJ, Vincente KJ. Electrical short circuit as a possible cause of death in patients on PCA machines: report on an opiate overdose and possible preventive remedy. Anesthesiology 2001;94:940.
Kwan A. Morphine overdose from patient-controlled analgesia pumps. Anaesth Intensive Care 1996;24:254–256.

USE 20 SECONDS OF ACUPRESSURE WITH YOUR FINGERTIP TO DECREASE PATIENT DISCOMFORT AT THE INSERTION SITE OF A NEEDLE

RACHAEL A. CALLCUT, MD

Perception of pain is a peripheral message transmitted at multiple levels to the central nervous system in a process termed nociception. Peripheral tissues have specialized nociceptors that sense mechanical or chemical stimuli and release neurochemicals in response. These signals are transmitted to the spinal cord via afferent pain fibers. The dorsal horn neurons of the spinal cord sense the signal and act as "gatekeepers" to potentially modulate the signal before transmitting the message to the brain via the spinothalamic and other tracts. The rostral area of the brain (thalamus, limbic system, cortex) processes the input and the patient perceives pain.

There are many strategies available to manipulate the nociceptive system at a variety of levels to interrupt or override the perception of pain. One nonpharmacologic intervention available to physicians for all patients involves acupressure with the fingertip prior to needle insertion. When mechanically stimulated, large myelinated fibers will "flood" the nociceptive pathway and partially inhibit transmission of subsequent pain stimuli. Acupressure is done with the tip of the finger at the point where the needle will enter. Firm point pressure is applied with the needle inserted immediately following release of pressure. Anecdotally, patients report that acupressure lessens both components of the "sting and burn" of local anesthetic injection. This technique is also useful when obtaining an arterial blood gas.

SUGGESTED READING

Townsend C, ed. Sabiston Textbook of Surgery. 16th Ed. Philadelphia: WB Saunders, 2001:283–284.

DO NOT ATTEMPT A RADIAL AND ULNAR ARTERY CANNULATION ON THE SAME SIDE AT THE SAME SITTING

HEATHER ABERNETHY, MD

The radial artery is the preferred site for obtaining arterial blood gases and for inserting an indwelling catheter for serial blood gases or blood pressure monitoring because it has an easily detectable pulse, lies relatively superficially, and is the nondominant hand artery in most people. Collateral flow to the hand via the ulnar artery (see *Figure 159.1*) and the presence of two palmar arches (superficial and deep, arch absent or incomplete in 15% of the population) has given physicians attempting to cannulate this artery a sense of security from ischemic complications in the event the radial artery should thrombose (physicians would simply do the Allen's test precannulation and, if cannulation was not successful, document the presence of postprocedure pulse to assure that no harm was done before moving on to another site for cannulation.) If cannulation of the radial artery for arterial access is not successful, most surgeons will use the contralateral radial artery next, and then the dorsalis pedis. Other arterial access sites used (with specific disadvantages listed) include the femoral artery (increased risk of infection), the brachial artery (inaccurate readings, lack of collaterals, median nerve injury), and the axillary artery (injury to brachial plexus and air embolism to the brain).

To increase the number of potential sites for arterial cannulation, attention has turned to the ulnar artery. It is attractive for many of the same reasons as the radial artery and has been increasingly used in pediatric intensive care and coronary angiography, with some clinicians advocating a modified Allen's test to assess patency of the radial artery as a collateral for the ulnar artery rather than vice-versa. Regardless of clinical assessment, the results of the Allen's test, or the presence of pulses, cannulation of the radial and ulnar arteries on the same hand should not be attempted at the same sitting. Transient diminution or loss of radial artery flow after (attempted) radial artery cannulation when combined with manipulation of the ulnar artery can result in hand ischemia, which can eventuate in tissue loss. Patients at high risk for this type of complication include those with peripheral vascular disease, small vessel occlusive disease, thrombophilia, heparin-induced thrombocytopenia (HIT), low cardiac output, and pressor dependence.

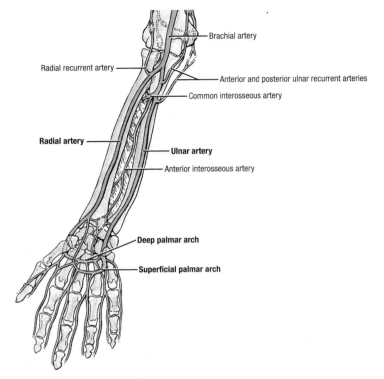

FIGURE 159.1. Arteries of the arm with the distal palmar arches.

Fluorescein dye studies and Doppler ultrasonography have shown that the Allen's test is not a reliable predictor of collateral flow or of the potential for ischemic complications. Also, the presence of a palpable pulse or bedside Doppler signal in an artery immediately after attempted cannulation is not a reliable indicator of flow (i.e., can be falsely normal) because an occluded artery may appear open with backfilling distally or brisk flow down to a complete obstruction. If there is no possible site of cannulation other than the ipsilateral ulnar artery after the radial artery has been attempted, the patient should have a duplex scan of the involved arteries to assess patency and flow and a period of 1 to 2 hours to allow arterial spasm to resolve before any attempt is made in the ipsilateral collateral circulation of the wrist.

To briefly review, the Allen's test is performed by having the patient exsanguinate the hand by making a tight fist. The examiner then uses both of his or her hands to occlude the patient's radial and ulnar arteries by squeezing each artery between the thumb and fingers. The patient then extends the fingers revealing a blanched palm. The pressure over the ulnar artery is released and the adequacy of the collateral flow is assessed by the amount of time it takes for normal color to return to the hand. Up to 7 seconds for return of original color is considered normal, 8 to 14 seconds is equivocal, and over 14 seconds is abnormal. In the Allen's test for collaterals of the ulnar artery, the pressure over the radial artery is released and length of time for return of color in the palm noted.

SUGGESTED READINGS

Cousins TR, O'Donnell JM. Arterial cannulation: a critical review. AANAJ 2004;72:267–271.

Duke J, ed. Anesthesia Secrets. 2nd Ed. Philadelphia: Hanley and Belfus, 2000:144–145.

Gellman H, Bottle MJ, Shankwiler J. Arterial patterns of the deep and superficial palmar arches. Clin Orthopedics 2001:383;41–46.

Hall JJ, Arnold AM, Valentine R, McCready RA, Mick MJ. Ultrasound imaging of the radial artery following its use for cardiac catheterization. Am J Cardiol 1996;77:108–109.

Miller RD, ed. *Anesthesia*. 4th Ed. New York: Churchill Livingstone, 2001:1169–1170.

160

MAKE THE DECISION TO INTUBATE BASED ON THE OVERALL CLINICAL PICTURE

JACK HUDKINS, MD

Specific criteria for the intubation of patients have long been discussed. The decision to intubate cannot be based solely on arterial blood gas results or pulmonary mechanical numbers, but should be made by clinical assessment of the entire patient. The old saw that the only absolute criteria for intubation is that the physician or nurse thinks the patient needs to be intubated is flippant—but perhaps not far off the mark. In making the decision to intubate, the surgeon must consider degree of respiratory distress, underlying disease process (e.g., suspected pulmonary embolism, burn to face, Ludwig's angina), and the individual's cardiopulmonary reserve (among other clinical factors), even in the setting of relatively "normal" numbers. Separate and apart from ventilation (i.e., gas exchange), accurately assessing the patient's airway and ability to protect it (i.e., mental status) is more difficult. Waiting too long to intubate often adds vomiting/aspiration/aspiration pneumonia to the patient's woes.

The criteria listed below should be used as guidelines when making the decision to intubate. The safest intubations occur earlier rather than later, in an orderly fashion, and when the patient is not in distress. The most experienced available team member should perform or supervise the procedure. In many institutions, this team member is an anesthesia professional. These staff, by far, have the most experience with intubating (especially difficult airways) and are usually more adept with fiberoptic bronchoscopes. The risks of planned intubation and mechanical ventilation are far greater if done emergently and/or by less experienced personnel.

Indications for intubation include failure to maintain an airway and failure of ventilation or oxygenation, with details listed below.

Failure to Maintain an Airway:

- Tracheal edema
- Oropharyngeal edema
- Loss of gag/cough reflex
- Glasgow Coma Scale worsening or <8
- Encephalopathy (hepatic, metabolic, post-ictal, etc.)

Failure of Ventilation or Oxygenation

- ABG: $PCO_2 > 55$, pH < 7.34, $SaO_2 < 90\%$ or $PO_2 < 60$ while breathing room air defines acute respiratory failure
- Respiratory Rate > 35 breaths per minute
- A-a gradient > 350 mmHg on 100% oxygen
- Inability to generate a negative inspiratory force of 20 mmHg
- Need for positive pressure ventilation

One final note is that a patient does not always need to be intubated in order to be ventilated. If there is a good airway and an empty stomach, use of a bag mask can be maintained (with constant monitoring of oxygen saturation, heart rate, and CO_2 retention) until an experienced airway professional can be summoned.

SUGGESTED READINGS

Marx J, Hockberger R, Walls R. Rosen's Emergency Medicine: Concepts and Clinical Practice. 5th Ed. Philadelphia: Mosby, 2002:2–4.

Pierson DJ. Indications for mechanical ventilation in adults with acute respiratory failure. Resp Care 2002;47:249–262.

161

DO NOT ATTEMPT TO ELUCIDATE ISCHEMIC CHANGES ON AN ELECTROCARDIOGRAM THAT HAS A LEFT BUNDLE-BRANCH BLOCK

LISA MARCUCCI, MD

The electrocardiogram (ECG) is one of the most ubiquitous tests in medicine, with literally millions performed each year. Although a complete discussion of the uses and characteristic patterns of this test is beyond the scope of this book, it is commonly used to detect signs of coronary artery disease by looking for the perturbations associated with ischemia and infarction.

To briefly review the wave morphology on an ECG:

1) P waves—represent electrical excitation of the atria, which causes atrial contraction.
2) QRS complex—represents electrical excitation of the ventricles, which causes synchronous ventricular contraction. The normal duration is 0.08 to 0.1 second.
3) T waves—represent the return of the ventricles from an excited state to a resting state.

Areas that are inspected for signs of ischemia or infarct on the ECG are the QRS complex, T waves, and the S-T segment. A Q wave is present in 50 to 75% of myocardial infarctions, S-T elevation is suggestive of myocardial injury, and S-T depression and/or T-wave inversion is suggestive of myocardial ischemia.

WATCH OUT FOR

With a left bundle-branch block (LBBB), electrical conduction to the left ventricle via the rapidly conducting fibers of the cardiac conducting system is delayed or fails and the right and left ventricles do not contract synchronously. The left ventricle depolarizes much more slowly via cell-to-cell conduction from the right to the left ventricle. LBBB on the ECG is manifest by an elongated QRS complex (0.11 second or greater) and distortion of the QRS complex, representing the nonsimultaneous electrical conduction of first the right and then the left ventricles. The QRS morphology may be widened or "notched" on ECG, mimicking twin mountain peaks, and the distorted QRS complex can obscure a leading Q wave. The LBBB also leads to abnormal repolarization with a distorted S-T segment and T wave, making detection of ischemic changes problematic.

Although right bundle branch block may occur in the absence of pathology, left bundle branch block is usually a consequence of significant cardiac disease, including myocardial infarction, cardiomyopathy (hypertensive and other causes), valvular disease, myocarditis, rheumatic fever, congenital heart disease, or infiltrative disease of the conducting system. LBBB is also associated with an increased mortality from myocardial infarction, leading to the American Heart Association's recommendation that reperfusion therapy be initiated in appropriate patients with an LBBB and a history consistent with acute myocardial ischemia.

SUGGESTED READINGS

Glancy DL, Khuri B. Chest pain and left bundle branch block. BUMC Proceedings 2001;14:452–454.

Sgarbossa BB, Pinski SL, Barbagelata A, et al. Electrocardiographic diagnosis of evolving acute myocardial infarction in the presence of left bundle-branch block. GUSTO-1 (Global Utilization of Streptokinase and Tissue plasminogen activator for Occluded coronary arteries) Investigators. N Engl J Med 1996;334:481–487.

Shlipak MG, Lyons WL, Go AS. Should the electrocardiogram be used to guide therapy for patients with left bundle-branch block and suspected myocardial infarction? JAMA 1999;281:714–719.

TREAT CREPITUS ASSOCIATED WITH A SOFT TISSUE INFECTION WITH A HIGH LEVEL OF CONCERN THAT MAY REQUIRE DEFINITIVE TREATMENT IN THE OPERATING ROOM

JAMES HERRINGTON, MD

Soft tissue infections range from relatively minor, superficial infections to severe, life-threatening conditions such as necrotizing fasciitis and gas gangrene, now termed necrotizing soft tissue infection (NSTI). The superficial infections involve the dermal and epidermal regions only and are not considered surgical emergencies. Examples are cellulitis, erypsipelas, furuncles, and carbuncles. These infections are treated with antibiotics and bedside incision and drainage. If discrete, fluid collections form. These infections are not typically associated with crepitus. However, the presence of crepitus, if it develops, signals a deeper infection, such as necrotizing fasciitis or gas gangrene. These are serious, life-threatening infections that require rapid recognition and urgent surgery.

The diagnosis of NSTI requires a high index of suspicion. It can occur in any region of the body but is more common in the extremities, abdominal wall, and perineum. Minor trauma, insect bites, and iatrogenic injury through medical procedures can lead to this condition. Factors that are associated with an increased risk of necrotizing fasciitis and gas gangrene are diabetes mellitus, peripheral vascular disease, malnutrition, immunosuppression, intravenous drug use, obesity, and exposure to sea water.

SIGNS AND SYMPTOMS

Necrotizing fasciitis by definition involves the fascia. Bacterial toxins likely cause the necrosis that spreads along the fascial planes. Characteristic of this condition is the ability to easily pass a finger along the fascial planes with little resistance. Overlying skin and muscle are spared early in the course but become secondarily necrotic from loss of their blood supply as the infection spreads.

In necrotizing fasciitis, high fever, cellulitis without sharp margins, and excruciating pain at the site of infection are common presenting signs. The pain is often out of proportion to the physical findings. Leukocytosis is usually present and the patient shows signs of systemic toxicity. As the condition progresses, the skin will show signs of spreading cellulitis with smooth, erythematous, shiny skin without induration. Later, bullae form, which initially contain serous fluid but progress to hemorrhagic fluid. As the infection worsens, subcutaneous fat and fascia become necrotic with loss of sensation. A foul-smelling, thin discharge is characteristically present, and the skin becomes visibly necrotic with a blue-gray coloration.

NSTI can be loosely divided into three types based on the causative organisms. Most common is type I, a polymicrobial infection that includes non–group A streptococci, other Gram-positive cocci, Gram-negative rods, and both Gram-negative and Gram-positive anaerobes. Type II is an infection caused principally by group A β-hemolytic streptococcus, with or without staphylococcus. Type III is caused by seawater-dwelling Gram-negative rods of the *Vibrio* genus and is rare. In all types, the rapidly spreading infection generates an environment where both aerobes and anaerobes generate gases in soft tissues, detectable as crepitus on examination.

SIGNS AND SYMPTOMS Gas gangrene, also known as clostridial myonecrosis, is a fulminating deep NSTI that initially involves primarily muscle and causes gas production in the soft tissues. As this deep infection requires inoculation of clostridial bacteria or spores into deep spaces, it usually follows penetrating traumatic injury or iatrogenic injury, such as surgery or placing orthopedic pins in fractures. Clostridia are obligate anaerobes, and the infection must start in hypoxic or devitalized tissue. The most common causative organism is *Clostridium perfringens*. Unlike most infections, there is relatively little inflammatory reaction and the pathophysiology of the infection is related to the exotoxins produced by the bacteria. A high index of suspicion is needed to make a prompt, life-saving diagnosis. The triad of inordinately severe pain, tachycardia out of proportion to fever, and crepitus is strongly suggestive of gas gangrene. The incubation period from the initiating event is usually short (as few as 12 hours) and the disease progresses at a fulminant pace over 24 hours. The skin quickly assumes a bronze, dark discoloration with bullae developing that will drain profuse, nonmalodorous, serosanguinous fluid. Signs of systemic toxicity quickly progress to hypotension and renal failure.

WHAT TO DO When crepitus associated with a soft tissue infection is detected, the patient should be prepared for and taken to the operating room without delay. Large-bore intravenous access is obtained and fluid resuscitation begun, even in the absence of frank hypotension. The patient should be pan-cultured and broad-spectrum (Gram-positive, Gram-negative, and anaerobic) antibiotic coverage started. If *Clostridium* is suspected, high-dose penicillin is added; if *Vibrio* is suspected, tetracycline is added.

In the operating room, the treatment is wide, radical surgical debridement to the margins of healthy-appearing tissues. Even slightly necrotic-appearing tissue must be removed. Postoperative care should be done in the intensive care unit with wounds inspected frequently for evidence of progression of infection. Very commonly, the patient is taken back to the operating room 24 to 48 hours after initial debridement for a "second look" and further debridement if necrotic tissue is evident. As an adjunctive treatment, hyperbaric treatment (even in the setting of apparently adequate initial debridement) is sometimes used to increase the oxygen content of tissue and retard or kill anaerobic bacteria.

To briefly review, crepitus or gas in the subcutaneous tissue is appreciated by the feeling of "crunching" under the skin upon palpation. If a stethoscope is pressed against the skin, a "crackling" sound is heard. Gas in the tissues is usually detectable on radiograph or computed tomography (CT) scan of the area. It can be a benign finding after laparoscopic surgery or chest tube placement.

One final note is that crepitus does not always occur in NSTI's and its absence does not rule out these conditions. The surgeon must have a low threshold for diagnosis because mortality is 20% to 30%, even with aggressive and early treatment, and increases proportionally with delay in diagnosis and treatment.

SUGGESTED READINGS

Calvet HM, Yoshikawa TT. Infections in diabetics. Infect Dis Clin North Am 2001;15:407–421.

Green RJ, Dafoe DC, Raffin TA. Necrotizing fasciitis. Chest 1996;110:219–229.

McHenry CR, Piotrowski JJ, Petrinic D, Malangoni MA. Determinants of mortality for necrotizing soft-tissue infections. Ann Surg 1995;221:558–565.

Riseman JA, Zamboni WA, Curtis A, et al. Hyperbaric oxygen therapy for necrotizing fasciitis reduces mortality and the need for debridements. Surgery 1990;108:847–850.

Do not administer sterile water intravenously to correct hypernatremia

Lisa Marcucci, MD

Correct management of electrolyte abnormalities is central to good patient care. One of the less frequently encountered electrolyte problems for surgeons is hypernatremia. Hypernatremia always reflects a hyperosmolar state and is commonly detected by lab value (serum sodium greater than 145 mEq/L and osmolality greater than 290 mOsm/L), but can present with signs and symptoms related to the central nervous system. These include lethargy leading to coma and death, weakness, irritability, seizures, and hyperreflexia.

Hypernatremia is more common in adults over 60 years of age because of decreased osmotic stimulation of thirst and decreased maximal urinary concentration (i.e., increased loss of free water). The mortality ranges from 15% to 50%, depending on the patient population. The etiology of hypernatremia in outpatients (typically presenting in the emergency room) is usually related to loss of free water in excess of sodium losses so that patients often have a deficit in extracellular volume (are dehydrated) and have variable total body sodium (deficit, normal, or excess). In contrast, inpatients usually have increased total body sodium related to overadministration of sodium-containing fluids or have inappropriately replaced free water losses (due to diuretics, perspiration, or enteric losses from vomiting, tubes, drains, fistulae, or diarrhea).

SIGNS AND SYMPTOMS

Treatment of hypernatremia is based both on the underlying cause (i.e., diabetes insipidus, osmotic diuresis, large insensible losses) and on the principle of avoiding overly rapid correction. While administering free water orally for absorption by the gastrointestinal tract is an accepted treatment, one strategy that should never be used is intravenous (IV) infusion of sterile water. Risks to the patient from using IV free water are twofold: (1) a bolus of free water risks exceeding the threshold of lowering the serum sodium concentration by more than the 0.5 mEq/L/hour, which can cause cerebral edema; and (2) IV free water may cause massive hemolysis from the abrupt fall in osmolality. Free water has an osmolality of 0 mOsm/L, and even 200 to 300 mL can lower osmolality so rapidly as to cause hemolysis, hemoglobinuria, acute renal failure, and death. Five per-cent dextrose in water or 5% dextrose in ¼-normal saline are the hyponatremic solutions of choice in correction of hypernatremia.

To briefly review hypernatremia treatment parameters:

1) The aim is to lower sodium concentration by no more than 0.5 mEq/L/hour and serum sodium should be measured frequently (at least every 4–6 hours). Maximum of 50% of the water deficit should be replaced in the first 24 hours.

2) The total water deficit is calculated using the following formula, with the concentration of sodium ([Na]) representing current serum sodium, body weight measured in kg, and total body water equal to 0.5 or 0.6 times the body weight, depending on the patient's gender:

Water deficit = normal total body water − current body water

$$= 1 - (140/[Na]) \times \text{Body Weight} \times 0.5 \text{ (women)}$$

or

$$= 1 - (140/[Na]) \times \text{Body Weight} \times 0.6 \text{ (men)}$$

3) In euvolemic hypernatremia, the treatment is water replacement either by giving free water orally or a slow infusion of 5% dextrose in water.

4) In hypervolemic hypernatremia, the treatment is removing the salt excess or diuretics and water replacement using free water orally or 5% dextrose in water.

5) In hypovolemic hypernatremia, the treatment is normal saline to correct the intravascular volume deficit, followed by half normal saline to address the hypernatremia.

SUGGESTED READINGS

Even more about sterile water. Institute for Safe Medication Practices (*ISMP*) *Medication Safety Alert!* 2003;8(6):3.

Fall PJ. Hyponatremia and hypernatremia, a systemic approach to causes and their correction. Postgraduate Med 2000;107:75–82.

Water, water everywhere but please don't give IV. ISMP Medication Safety Alert! 2003;8:1–2.

164

CONSIDER PHYSICAL RESTRAINTS ON COMBATIVE HEPATIC ENCEPHALOPATHY PATIENTS

MICHAEL J. MORITZ, MD

The use of patient restraints has become a major issue in recent years. In 2002, the Centers for Medicare & Medicaid Services added regulations regarding patient restraints to the "Conditions of Participation for Hospitals," the rules which every hospital must follow if it wishes to care for patients with Medicare or Medicaid coverage (42CFR482.13, Code of Federal Regulations). The principles outlined therein have been interpreted by the Joint Commission on Accreditation of Healthcare Organizations (JCAHO) and others and the essential elements for restraint orders include:

1) Protection and preservation of patient rights, dignity, and well being
2) Based on the patient's assessed needs and consistent with the patient's plan of care
3) Least restrictive, most effective method
4) Safe application and removal by trained, competent personnel
5) Continuous patient monitoring and reassessment during use and discontinued at the earliest possible time
6) Orders provided by licensed practitioner that are time-limited
7) Necessity, application, response, and soon as documented in the medical record

Separate from the issue of the institutional requirements for restraints is the clinical acumen needed to assess patients with delirium who may be both out of control and a danger to self or others. Both factors are key in deciding when physical restraints, as opposed to pharmaceutical sedation, are necessary. However, there are conditions known to be marked by *depressed* mental status where the patient will present with lethargy but then develop agitation or disinhibition or will fluctuate between lethargy/stupor and agitation. For these conditions, it is important to discuss restraints in terms of the elements of surprise and preparedness needed. This is not an attempt to catalog all times when this may occur, but rather to discuss the topic sufficiently to provide the background necessary for sound, clinical judgements.

One of the situations in which there can be wide swings from lethargy to agitation is hepatic encephalopathy. The classic stages of hepatic encephalopathy are described in *Table 164.1*. Most physicians' conception of progressive encephalopathy is a smoothly downward course of decreasing responsiveness. However, some patients in stage III encephalopathy will deviate from the usual course and become exceedingly agitated and uncontrollable. This is more likely to occur in adolescent and young adult patients and is more common with fulminant hepatic failure than in chronic liver disease. Such agitated stage III encephalopathy patients are notorious for spitting at and biting caregivers. Further, with their impaired liver function, there is an appropriate reluctance to use sedatives. These patients are one of the true indications for leather restraints or their more modern equivalents to protect the staff and the patient. Once the diagnosis of hepatic encephalopathy as the etiology of the agitation is known, pharmaceutical treatment of this is essential, as these patients are at increased risk for cerebral edema and intercranial hypertension. Accordingly, restraints, sedation, intubation, and mechanical ventilation are all part of their appropriate care as a prelude to a computed tomography (CT) scan of the brain and the other procedures necessary to care for their central nervous system (CNS) in the setting of liver failure. Consultation with a gastroenterologist/hepatologist is mandatory.

Delirium is distinct from hepatic encephalopathy and is a widespread problem in hospitalized patients. An in-depth discussion is beyond the scope of this book, but a few select facts merit mentioning:

1) Paradoxical reactions to central nervous system depressing drugs, classically the benzodiazepines, may result in uncontrollable

TABLE 164.1	**STAGES OF HEPATIC ENCEPHALOPATHY**	
STAGE	**INTELLECTUAL FUNCTION**	**NEUROMUSCULAR FUNCTION**
Stage I	Impaired attention, irritability, depression, personality change	Tremor, incoordination, apraxia
Stage II	Drowsiness, poor memory and computation, disordered sleep	Asterixis, ataxia, psychomotor retardation, slowed speech
Stage III	Confusion, disorientation, somnolence	Hypoactive reflexes, nystagmus, clonus
Stage IV	Stupor, coma	Poor, inappropriate, or unresponsive

delirium. A number of violent, delirious reactions to triazolam (Halcion) led to its being banned in the United Kingdom.

2) There is a lengthy list of prescription medications that may have idiosyncratic reactions and rarely cause hallucinations, agitation, and/or delirium. Drug-related but not idiosyncratic causes of delirium are the serotonin syndrome (related to drug interactions with serotonin reuptake inhibitors) and overdosage or toxicity of the monoamine oxidase inhibitors.

3) Better known agitated, delirious, withdrawal reactions from (CNS)-depressing drugs include alcohol (delirium tremens, alcoholic hallucinosis and others), benzodiazepines, barbiturates, and opiates. Toxic reactions to (CNS) stimulants have a similar hypermetabolic, hyperkinetic presentation (but without the surprise) and typical agents include the amphetamines, cocaine, methylphenidate (Ritalin and others), methylene dimethamphetamine (MDMA, or Ecstasy) and phenycyclidine (PCP).

SUGGESTED READINGS

Code of Federal Regulations, Title 42, Volume 3. (**CITE: 42CFR482.13**). Government Printing Office via GPO Access. Available at: http://frwebgate. access.gpo.gov/cgi-bin/get-cfr.cgi. Accessed July 27, 2005.

Drugs that may cause psychiatric symptoms. The Medical Letter on Drugs and Therapeutics 2002:44(1134):59–62.

Federal Register 64Fed. Reg. 36070. Code of Federal Regulations, Title 42, Volume 3. U.S. Government Printing Office via GPO Access, Cite: 42CFR482.13. http://www.access.gpo.gov/nara/cfr/cfr-retrieve.html#page1 and request 42CFR482.13. Revised October 1, 2002.

Feske SK. Neurologic emergencies: coma and confusional states: emergency diagnosis and management. *Neurologic Clinics* 1998;16:237–256.

Munoz SJ, Moritz, MJ, Bell R, et al. Factors associated with severe intracranial hypertension in candidates for emergency liver transplantation. Transplantation 1993;55:1071–1074.

165

REMEMBER THAT DIABETICS OFTEN DO NOT HAVE CHEST PAIN IN MYOCARDIAL INFARCTION AND ABSENCE OF ANGINA CANNOT BE USED TO RULE OUT SIGNIFICANT CORONARY ARTERY DISEASE

RACHAEL A. CALLCUT, MD

SIGNS AND SYMPTOMS

Coronary artery disease (CAD) is widely prevalent in the diabetic population and is the most common cause of death in people with diabetes. In addition, diabetes mellitus is an intermediate risk factor for a perioperative cardiovascular event. As many as 90% of myocardial infarctions (and the preoccurring angina) are silent in diabetics. Silent myocardial infarctions (MIs) are more common as a result of the generalized autonomic nervous system dysfunction in patients with long-standing diabetes. Thus, the index of suspicion must be elevated for less classic presentations of myocardial ischemia, including dyspnea, congestive heart failure, flash pulmonary edema, syncope, and arrhythmias. Standard workup includes 12-lead electrocardiogram, serial cardiac enzyme markers, chest radiograph, echocardiogram and continuous telemetry monitoring.

Several immediate interventions have been shown to decrease the morbidity and mortality of MI in diabetics. For those presenting with pain, relieving it is imperative. Sublingual nitroglycerin is generally not effective; however, it is appropriate to initiate therapy with administration of three doses, one every 3 minutes. Intravenous (IV) morphine is given in 4 mg boluses repeated every 5 minutes until pain is relieved. Hypotension may occur with morphine administration and is generally responsive to fluid challenges. Aspirin therapy also is initiated at presentation. Beta-blockade also has been proven to decrease infarct size, decrease arrhythmias, and increase survival. Intravenous metoprolol is commonly given in three doses of 5 mg boluses each, followed by initiation of oral dosing. Beta-blockers should not be administered if the patient has chronic obstructive pulmonary disease or asthma, pulse less than 50 beats per minute, or systolic blood pressure less than 100 mm Hg, or if the patient exhibits hemodynamic instability, heart block, or severe congestive heart failure. If contraindications do not exist, urgent cardiology consultation is warranted in order to consider patients for anticoagulant or thrombolytic therapy or for diagnostic/therapeutic catheterization.

SUGGESTED READINGS

Fauci AS, Braunwald E, Isselbacher KJ. Harrison's Principles of Internal Medicine. 14th Ed. New York: McGraw-Hill, 1998:1342–1343,2075.

Marino PL. The ICU Book. 2nd Ed. Philadelphia: Lippincott Williams & Wilkins, 1998:301–316.

Townsend C M. Sabiston Textbook of Surgery. 16th Ed. Philadelphia: W.B. Saunders, 2001:266–267.

166

REMEMBER WHEN REVIEWING DOPPLER ULTRASOUND RESULTS THAT THE SUPERFICIAL FEMORAL VEIN IS A COMPONENT OF THE DEEP VENOUS SYSTEM

PATRICK SCHANER, MD

SIGNS AND SYMPTOMS

Doppler ultrasound of the veins is a widely used test to search for the presence of deep vein thrombosis (phlebitis) that requires anticoagulation and that may result in pulmonary embolism. This test is often ordered for a patient with signs or symptoms of a suspected pulmonary embolism (pleuritic chest pain, tachypnea, tachycardia, hypocapnia, hypoxia, hypotension), deep vein thrombosis (leg swelling, calf pain, positive Homan's sign), or for a fever workup. Commonly, a preliminary reading that identifies which veins may be harboring clots is placed in the chart or reported verbally by the technician. The decision to anticoagulate a patient hinges on these results. In this setting, it is important to know the venous anatomy of the leg and the risk of pulmonary embolism for phlebitis of the relevant veins.

The venous drainage of the leg is comprised of two systems: the deep veins and the superficial veins. The two chief superficial veins are the greater and lesser saphenous veins. Other superficial veins are the superficial epigastric, superficial circumflex iliac, external pudendal veins, and surface varicosities. Components of the deep venous system include the soleal sinusoids, anterior and posterior tibial, common femoral, profunda femoral, superficial femoral, circumflex femoral, and iliac veins. The deep veins course in proximity to the major arteries (venae comitantes). Clots in the deep system put a patient at much higher risk of pulmonary embolism and usually require anticoagulation (20% of patients with clots in the superficial system also have coexisting clots in the deep system).

It is important to remember when reviewing the location of blood clots on the Doppler report that the superficial femoral vein that accompanies the superficial femoral artery is a major *deep* vein. This vein is "superficial" only relative to the profunda (i.e., deep) femoris vein but is a major deep structure despite the superficial appellation. Clots in the more proximal veins (such as the superficial femoral) have a greater risk of life-threatening embolism than those more distal and a finding of a clot here should never be dismissed as inconsequential.

SUGGESTED READINGS

April EW. Anatomy. Media, Pennsylvania: Harwal, 1984:381–382.

Ernst CB, Stanley JC, eds. Current Therapy in Vascular Surgery. St. Louis: Mosby, 1995:875–876.

Moore KL, Dalley AF, eds. Clinically Oriented Anatomy. 4th Ed. Philadelphia: J.B. Lippincott, 1999:524–526.

167

AGGRESSIVELY TREAT PHLEBITIS FROM INTRAVENOUS SITES IN IMMUNOSUPPRESSED OR HEART VALVE PATIENTS

GREGORY KENNEDY, MD, PHD

Noninfective thrombophlebitis is a relatively common occurrence in patients receiving intravenous (IV) therapy and is usually easily treated in immunocompetent patients by removing the catheter, placing warm soaks on the area, and providing a short course of narrow-spectrum antibiotics. However, in the transplant population, HIV patients and prosthetic heart valve patients, thrombophlebitis is a serious condition that must be promptly and aggressively treated. In these patients, the presence of the foreign body predisposes them to development of a bacterial infection (commonly *Staphylococcus*), resulting in a suppurative thrombophlebitis. This nidus can progress to a systemic condition including endocarditis and septic shock.

SIGNS AND SYMPTOMS

Signs and symptoms of suppurative thrombophlebitis include a tender, palpable cord, ascending lymphangitis, exudative discharge at the IV site, fever, and leukocytosis. Intravenous lines suspected of being the source of thrombophlebitis should be removed immediately and sent for culture. In addition, aerobic and anaerobic blood cultures from two peripheral sites should be obtained. An ultrasound of a suspicious site may assist in defining cephalad extension of a thrombosis. If bacteremia is confirmed, the patient should have an echocardiogram (preferably transesophageal) to evaluate for bacterial endocarditis.

The mainstay of treatment for suppurative thrombophlebitis in the high-risk patient is surgical excision of the involved vein with debridement of the involved adjacent soft tissue (if necessary) and open wound care. IV antibiotics are essential, and high-risk patients should be started on broad-spectrum antibiotics including both Gram-positive and Gram-negative coverage until culture results are available, with coverage narrowed as appropriate. In patients hospitalized for more than a few days or previously treated with antibiotics, coverage for resistant organisms is appropriate and consideration of fungal coverage may be necessary. If the patient develops endocarditis, aggressive therapy should be instituted.

SUGGESTED READING

Townsend CM. Sabiston Textbook of Surgery. 16th Ed. Philadelphia: Saunders, 2001:1385,1575.

168

ASSUME THAT IF A PATIENT IS NOT DOING WELL POSTOPERATIVELY, THERE IS AN UNDIAGNOSED COMPLICATION OF YOUR PROCEDURE UNTIL PROVEN OTHERWISE

RACHAEL A. CALLCUT, MD

Patients recover from operative procedures at variable rates and recovery is dependent on a host of patient attributes including age, ethnicity, nutritional status, obesity, perceived or real secondary gain, and comorbid conditions. However, for best care, the surgeon should always have a high index of suspicion for an undiagnosed complication in patients who do not seem to be progressing appropriately. Individual complications can have diverse presentations that make diagnosis difficult, but a diligent and thorough search must be undertaken to uncover potentially dangerous conditions. Before ascribing postoperative difficulties to comorbid conditions or to nonoperative issues, assume that the patient's problems are directly related to the surgical procedure and look there first. Some examples are as follows:

Example 1: Despite a "looks good" clinical appearance, a persistently elevated or rising white blood cell count or development of a fever should warrant a workup for postoperative infections and for deep vein thrombosis. While the patient may only have atelectasis, it is dangerous to assume that is the case and look no further. Intra-abdominal infection or anastomotic leak can present initially as leukocytosis alone with minimal physical findings, yet quickly progress to overwhelming sepsis in 24 hours. "Waiting to see what the white count does" may cause a missed therapeutic window in an impending catastrophe.

Example 2: Prolonged ileus after abdominal or bowel surgery may be indicative of any number of complications, including technical anastomotic error, anastomotic leak, intra-abdominal abscess, internal hernia, and excessive narcotic use.

Example 3: If a patient complains of excessive pain for the operation performed, a serious complication may exist. A thorough workup is required, and the patient's complaint should never be ascribed to a low-pain threshold or poor coping skills. If the pain is progressive, the urgency of the workup must be increased and ischemia, infarct, and life-threatening infection must be high on the differential diagnosis list.

In any adverse situation, look first at the surgery performed for the source of the problem.

EXAMINE THE PATIENT BEFORE SWITCHING PAIN MEDICATION WHEN A PATIENT COMPLAINS OF A LACK OF RELIEF

RACHAEL A. CALLCUT, MD

Adequate control of postoperative (post-op) pain should be a goal for every procedure. A good choice of pain medication for patients with significant incisions is the opioid hydromorphone (Dilaudid). Advantages include intravenous (including via patient-controlled anesthesia machines) or oral dosing, its relative lack of sedation and nausea, and its lack of active metabolites. The other commonly prescribed opioids (with side effects) include morphine (pruritis and nausea), fentanyl (muscle rigidity), meperidene (nausea, accumulation of epileptogenic metabolites in renal failure), oxycodone, hydrocodone, and codeine. A nonnarcotic nonsteroidal anti-inflammatory drug (NSAID) that can be used for post-op pain is ketorolac (Toradol), which works by inhibiting prostaglandin synthesis.

WATCH OUT FOR

Regardless of which pain medication is initially chosen, if patients complain of lack of pain relief or worsening pain they should be examined. It is not acceptable to ascribe this to a difference in pain tolerance among patients or a patient's belief that "it doesn't work for me" until more serious causes of pain have been ruled out. The surgeon should be alert for the presence of a new problem causing the patient's complaint of pain or coexisting markers including fever, leukocytosis, hypotension, tachycardia, anastomotic breakdown, ischemic bowel, myocardial infarction, pulmonary embolism, bladder distention, infiltrated intravenous lines, intraperitoneal or retroperitoneal bleed, limb ischemia, compartment syndrome, gastric distention, pneumonia, wound infection, and wound dehiscence (among others).

If a serious underlying cause is not found and the pain medication is changed, the patient should be followed up to insure that the change is effective and to monitor development of side effects (e.g., bleeding and renal insufficiency with prolonged use of ketorolac).

DO NOT DISCOUNT A PATIENT'S COMPLAINT OF NECK OR BACK PAIN

MICHAEL J. MORITZ, MD

Two illustrative cases:

Case 1: A transplant recipient with a long, debilitating posttransplant course, including myocardial infarction, necrotizing *Pseudomonas* pneumonia, and iliofemoral deep venous thrombosis returned for their first office visit still wheelchair-bound and complaining of posterior neck pain. On the second visit, a rehabilitation consultation was requested and spine films were obtained; the reading was degenerative joint disease. When admitted for worsening neck pain, a computed tomography (CT) scan revealed cervical osteomyelitis. Conservative therapy was pursued until spinal instability mandated surgery. Cultures grew *Pseudomonas*.

Case 2: A hemodialysis patient with a right thigh dialysis graft presented with posterior lumbar pain of less than 2 weeks duration. Plain films were diagnostic for osteomyelitis. Blood cultures were positive for group B streptococci. She had had routine dental work 2 weeks before the onset of symptoms and 4 weeks before hospital admission. After six weeks of intravenous antibiotics, her sedimentation rate had fallen considerably, her pain was much better, and her leukocytosis was gone. She was prescribed oral antibiotics to complete one year of therapy.

Absent prior spinal surgery, vertebral osteomyelitis and diskitis are infections that are usually spread hematogenously. Hence, any patient with bacteremia (documented or not) is at risk for acquiring this infection, particularly immunocompromised patients. Patients typically present with pain in the involved area that is subacute in onset over days to several weeks. Patients may or may not have low-grade fever. Underlying medical conditions associated with hematogenous osteomyelitis include dialysis-dependent renal failure, HIV infection, cancer chemotherapy, chronic immunosuppression (solid organ transplant, autoimmune disease), cirrhosis, alcoholism, and diabetes.

The literature is conflicting on the relative incidence of lumbar, thoracic, and cervical spine osteomyelitis with more recent series having similar proportional involvement of the three areas and older publications favoring lumbar predominance. As the neurologic consequences of delayed diagnosis are greatest for cervical spine disease, its relative incidence should not diminish its place in the differential diagnosis of spine (i.e., back or neck) pain.

Most patients with spinal osteomyelitis and diskitis will have a single organism causing infection. *Staphylococcus aureus* is the most common pathogen, followed by other skin organisms (coagulase-negative staphylococci, streptococci). Aerobic Gram-negative rods account for 30% of infections. Uncommon pathogens such as fungi are responsible for a small proportion of cases. Intravenous drug abusers have a different spectrum of pathogens, including *Serratia marcescens*, *Pseudomonas aeruginosa*, coagulase-negative staphylococci, and *Candida* species. The microbiologic diagnosis can be made from positive blood cultures in three-fourths of patients; the remainder will require an invasive procedure, usually CT-guided needle biopsy of the involved area.

WHAT NOT TO DO

It is paramount that inpatients who complain of steadily worsening back pain should not have their complaints ascribed to the well-known shortcomings of hospital mattresses. Pain from spinal osteomyelitis will typically not improve with rest, unlike most other etiologies of back pain. Plain films of the symptomatic area should be obtained first and may be normal early in the course. As the infection spreads from the disk space to adjacent vertebral bodies, end-plate erosion will be seen, followed by loss of the disk space and destruction of the vertebral body or bodies. CT and/or magnetic resonance imaging (MRI) of the spine will usually follow, based on inconclusive films with persistent or worsening symptoms or on suggestive films requiring greater anatomic definition. Most patients will have both bony involvement (less than 5% have only disk involvement) and disk involvement (diskitis absent in 10% of patients). Cord compression will be present in almost 50%, a paraspinal mass or abscess will be present in almost 50%, and the posterior spinal elements will be involved in one-third of individuals.

WHAT TO DO

Treatment starts with empiric antibiotics based on likely pathogens and with adjustment based on definitive culture and sensitivity results. The majority of patients will respond to appropriate antibiotics and a minority will require surgery, whether emergently or because of failure to respond to antibiotics. Surgery is indicated based on the level and extent of vertebral destruction, the level and extent of cord compromise, the degree of spinal (kyphotic) deformity, and the instability of the spine. Surgery can be performed via the anterior and/or posterior approach, based on anatomic considerations. The goals of surgery are drainage of infection, debridement of infected material, and spinal reconstruction/stabilization with bone with or without placement of instrumentation. All patients will require a minimum of 6 weeks of antibiotics (at least 6 weeks from the time of surgery for surgical patients).

In today's world with numerous complex, immunocompromised patients at risk for silent hematogenous spread of infection to the spine, persistent complaints of back pain must be taken seriously, at least seriously enough to order and check the appropriate radiologic studies.

SUGGESTED READINGS

Fernandez M, Carrol CL, Baker CJ. Discitis and vertebral osteomyelitis in children: an 18-year review. Pediatrics 2000;105:1299–1304.

McCutchen TM, Cuddy BG. Intervertebral disk space infection. Neurosurg Q 2001;11:209–219.

Rakel RE, Boyle ET, eds. Conn's Current Therapy 2002. 54th Ed. Philadelphia: WB Saunders, 2002:1011–1016.

Rezai AR, Woo HH, Errico TJ, Cooper PR. Contemporary management of spinal osteomyelitis. Neurosurgery 1999;44:1018–1025.

BE ALERT FOR ABDOMINAL SEPSIS IN THE MORBIDLY OBESE PATIENT

ADRIAN LATA, MD

SIGNS AND SYMPTOMS

Recognition of an abdominal catastrophe in the morbidly obese patient is a difficult task. There are at least three barriers to detection and diagnosis of abdominal complaints in these patients: (1) obese patients have a blunted physiologic response to peritonitis with diminished or altered symptoms and signs; (2) obese patients are more difficult to examine and localizing abdominal problems is very difficult; and (3) obtaining imaging studies is more difficult because increasing physical bulk diminishes the accuracy of both ultrasound and abdominal plain radiographs and computed tomography (CT) scanning will be unobtainable if the patient exceeds the weight limit of the table. Regarding the blunted symptoms and signs of peritonitis, such patients have fewer abdominal complaints and findings on examination and may not have peritoneal signs (e.g., guarding, rebound tenderness) despite the presence of peritonitis. Regarding altered findings, the classic example is abdominal sepsis that presents as shortness of breath, tachypnea, and/or hypoxia often accompanied by tachycardia; these symptoms mimic the presentation of pulmonary disorders to which these patients are also susceptible, including pulmonary embolism, pneumonia, and atelectasis.

After surgery for morbid obesity, the complication of an anastomotic or staple-line leak is extremely serious and may be life-threatening. The incidence of this complication is 2% in open gastric bypass and has been reported as 3% in laparoscopic cases. Because clinical signs can be subtle, the presentation can be delayed until signs of severe sepsis are evident. The clinician must be alert to earlier, subtle indications that something is amiss, including: a patient who is not progressing favorably, symptoms or signs of a pulmonary problem, marked anxiety, respiratory distress, pain elsewhere (back, pelvis, shoulder), tenesmus, hiccups, or urinary frequency. The patient may admit to a feeling of impending doom. Tachycardia may be the best early indicator of an anastamotic leak. If tachycardia does not respond to increased fluid infusion or a slight increase in analgesia, the patient should have an immediate Gastrograffin contrast study to visualize the anastomoses.

As mentioned above, examination in the morbidly obese may be unhelpful, although palpation away from the surgical wound may reveal rebound tenderness. The leukocyte count is often elevated but can be normal. A left pleural effusion is common on chest radiographs, but a patient with atelectasis and a pleural effusion has a leak until proven otherwise.

Because of the high index of suspicion needed in morbidly obese patients, radiographic contrast studies using water-soluble agents (such as Gastrograffin upper gastrointestinal [GI] series or CT scan with oral Gastrograffin) may be indicated even when few clinical signs are present. Contrast studies are relatively accurate in diagnosing a leak at the gastrojejunostomy or the proximal gastric pouch and are much less accurate in diagnosing problems at the enteroenteric anastomosis or the excluded stomach. Computed tomography of the chest, abdomen, and pelvis will also be part of the diagnostic workup in many patients, particularly those with pulmonary or pelvic complaints. Chest CT with contrast should be performed as part of the workup for pulmonary embolism. If the chest CT is nondiagnostic, a pulmonary angiogram may be needed to diagnose a pulmonary embolism.

WHAT TO DO

If patient has a suspected leak based on clinical signs and the Gastrograffin study is nondiagnostic, laparotomy is the best course of action. Because failure to recognize a leak may result in the patient's death, exploratory laparotomy should be performed empirically in patients with progressive tachypnea and tachycardia in whom pulmonary embolism has been ruled out. In patients who are rapidly deteriorating, exploratory laparotomy should be undertaken without GI radiographs. If a leak is discovered at laparotomy, the defect should be closed if possible (although the closure is likely to leak again), the area widely and extensively drained, and consideration given to appropriate diversion and placement of tubes (gastrostomy and/or jejunostomy, either anterograde or retrograde). Even with the skin left open, deep wound infections that may be severe are common sequelae of peritonitis in these patients. Reexploration is not a benign procedure in the morbidly obese patient, but it is better to use caution than to miss a potential disaster.

SUGGESTED READINGS

Arteaga JR, Huerta S, Livingston EH. Management of gastrojejunal anastomotic leaks after Roux-en-Y gastric bypass. Am Surg 2002;68:1061–1065.

Brolin, RE. Gastric bypass. Surg Clin North Am 2001;81:1077–1095.

Byrne, TK. Complications of surgery for obesity. Surg Clin North Am 2001;81: 1181–1193.

Marshall JS, Srivastava A, Gupta SK, Rossi TR, DeBord JR. Roux-en-Y gastric bypass leak complications. Arch Surg 2003;138:520–523.

Sugerman, HJ, DeMaria, EJ. Gastric surgery for morbid obesity. In: Baker RJ, Fischer JE, ed. Mastery of Surgery. 4th Ed. Philadelphia: Lippincott Williams & Wilkins, 2001:1032.

172

CONSIDER AN ADDISONIAN STATE IF IT "LOOKS LIKE SEPSIS AND SMELLS LIKE SEPSIS" BUT YOU CANNOT IDENTIFY ANY OFFENDING MICROBES

RACHAEL A. CALLCUT, MD

Patients in the intensive care unit (ICU) with respiratory and/or cardiovascular failure may remain refractory to treatment despite aggressive resuscitation efforts (including adequate volume resuscitation, thorough search for infectious etiologies that may encompass an empiric trial of antibiotics for fungi and pseudomonads, and a thorough workup for cardiopulmonary disease). In this situation, consideration should be given to relative adrenal insufficiency as an underlying cause of the "septic picture." This occurs in patients under physiologic stress when the hypothalamic-pituitary-adrenal axis is unable to respond with an appropriate increase in cortisol production, leaving the patient susceptible to adrenal insufficiency. It has been reported to cause clinically significant symptoms in 1% to 6% of critically ill surgical ICU patients.

In addition to primary Addison's disease, there are many conditions that predispose a patient to developing relative adrenal insufficiency under physiologic stress. These conditions include: septic shock, chronic steroid usage (transplant patients, asthmatics, etc.); infiltrative diseases such as sarcoidosis, amyloidosis, adrenal metastases, and tubercular involvement of the adrenal glands; and HIV. In susceptible individuals, an Addisonian state may develop after major operations such as repair of abdominal aortic aneurysm, coronary artery bypass grafting, or the Whipple procedure, or after relatively minor surgical procedures.

To make the diagnosis, the surgeon must have a high index of suspicion because almost all of the signs and symptoms are nonspecific. The diagnosis is made by measuring serum cortisol levels. Adrenal insufficiency is diagnosed if the patient has a random serum cortisol less than 20 μg/dL or the cortisol level fails to increase > 9 μg/dL when tested 30 and 60 minutes after adrenal stimulation with a supraphysiologic dose of 250 μg of corticotropin (adrenocorticotropic hormone, or ACTH). However, ICU patients with some degree of adrenal insufficiency may respond to this supraphysiologic ACTH dose and use of the low-dose corticotropin stimulation test

(1 to 2 μg ACTH) is more sensitive (with the same outcome parameters). Treatment protocols vary, but most surgeons use 150–300 mg/day of hydrocortisone in three divided doses for 48 hours with a taper over the next 5 to 10 days. Because confirming the diagnosis by cortisol testing can take days, the clinical situation may warrant beginning a therapeutic trial of steroids while awaiting the testing results. If the patient relapses during the taper, the initial dose should be repeated with a slower taper. If there is no improvement with steroids after 48 hours, most clinicians will discontinue steroid use.

SIGNS AND SYMPTOMS To briefly review, in the surgical ICU, patients at higher risk of adrenal insufficiency include those with pressor-dependent hypotension, ventilator dependence, and older age (more than 55 years). The clinical findings of an Addisonian state include hypotension, respiratory failure and inability to wean from the ventilator, fever, tachycardia, depressed mental status, abdominal pain, nausea, vomiting, lethargy, and weakness. Laboratory findings of classic Addison's disease are infrequently present but include hyponatremia, hyperkalemia, eosinophilia, lymphocytosis, hypoglycemia, and hypercalcemia.

SUGGESTED READINGS

Rivers EP, Gaspari M, Saad GA, et al. Adrenal insufficiency in high-risk surgical ICU patients. Chest 2001;119:889–896.

Shenker Y, Skatrud JB. Adrenal insufficiency in critically ill patients. Am J Resp Crit Care Med 2001;163:1520–1523.

Zaloga GP, Marik P. Hypothalamic-pituitary-adrenal insufficiency. Crit Care Clin 2001;17:25–41.

173

Do not put adhesive tape on a patient with fragile skin

Michael J. Moritz, MD

Adhesive tape is as ubiquitous in medicine as stethoscopes and tongue depressors. Experienced patients fear tape almost as much as they do needles. Adhesive tape is cheap and readily available and can be fashioned to every shape and situation, hence it is used everywhere and for everything. The fact that there are innumerable types of adhesive tape is testimony to the fact that each type of tape has significant shortcomings. There is no tape to which someone is not allergic.

Two of the minor problems with tape are avulsion of hair and cross-contamination of patients with bacteria and other pathogens. Removal of any kind of adhesive from skin will take the patient's hair off. This is painful but does not cause lasting disfigurement. Rolls of adhesive tape in hospitals are frequently colonized on their outer layers with pathogenic bacteria, thus presenting a source of cross-contamination of patients. Discarding the outer layers or "assigning" tape to a single patient can avoid this problem.

The worst problem with tape is its adhesiveness; it does not know when to let go. Removing tape can easily remove the outer layers of the epidermis, the equivalent of a partial thickness burn. Tape burns, as they are called, are often deep into the epidermis, slow to heal (related to the factors enumerated below), painful for an extended period of time, and leave quite noticeable scars.

WATCH OUT FOR

Patients susceptible to tape injury are those with fragile skin. Age, location on the body, disease process, and medications all contribute to the risk. Children and elderly patients who have thinner, more fragile skin are at greater risk. Areas of the body that are particularly susceptible are those with thinner epidermis, such as the face (particularly the eyelids and periorbital area), the dorsum of the hand, the anterior-medial forearm, and the shin. Numerous conditions are associated with skin fragility, including amyloidosis, collagen disorders (e.g., Ehlers-Danlos syndrome), cirrhosis, peripheral vascular disease, and prior radiation therapy. Medications associated with increased skin fragility include corticosteroids and chemotherapeutic agents. Patients with diabetes represent an interesting group because they have thicker skin than do patients without diabetics, at least in part because of the accumulation of glycosylated proteins. However, this thicker skin is not tougher; when they have other disorders, such as peripheral vascular disease, their skin can be quite fragile and incredibly slow to heal.

The solution is to avoid the use of tape on the skin whenever possible. For most indications, there are superior methods of securing catheters, dressings, tubes, and so on. Circumferential bandages, binders, netting, and other devices often provide superior fixation without the troubles of adhesive tape. On extremities, dressings are better held in place with a circumferentially wrapped bandage. For the abdomen, an abdominal binder holds dressings in place and protects tubes from the patient's hands. On the head and face, a variety of dressings similar to sweatbands hold dressings without tape on awkward surfaces such as the ear and the scalp. Tape should always be no better than a second choice. Commercial packets of a solvent-based adhesive remover are available in the operating room and remove tape easily. Nail polish remover works well, but is flammable and should not be used in the hospital.

SUGGESTED READINGS

Paron NG, Lambert P.W. Cutaneous manifestations of diabetes mellitus. Primary Care 2000;27:371–383.

Redelmeier DA, Livesley NJ. Adhesive tape and intravascular-catheter-associated infections. J Gen Intern Med 1999;14:373–375.

174

DO A THOROUGH HEAD AND NECK EXAMINATION WHEN AN ANTERIOR NECK MASS IS DISCOVERED, AND DO A FINE-NEEDLE ASPIRATION OF THE MASS AS THE FIRST TISSUE DIAGNOSIS PROCEDURE

MICHAEL J. MORITZ, MD

WHAT NOT TO DO

The workup of an anterior neck mass is a well-delineated paradigm with relatively few pitfalls. One of the most serious errors to avoid is the excisional biopsy of an enlarged lymph node that contains metastatic carcinoma from a head and neck primary that violates the incisions used for surgical dissection of the lymph nodes of the neck (i.e., a neck dissection). This error can significantly alter the treatment choices for a patient and jeopardize the patient's treatment outcome. If the surgeon remembers and avoids this error, then the remainder of the workup is straightforward.

The relative frequency of etiologies of anterior neck masses is affected by age, generally divided into younger than and older than 40 years of age. If the patient is less than 40 years, inflammatory lesions predominate, followed by congenital and then neoplastic etiologies. Neoplasms are most commonly lymphoma, followed by thyroid carcinoma and sarcomas. Over age 40, neoplastic lesions predominate, with inflammatory and congenital etiologies less likely. In this population, approximately 30% of anterior neck masses will be metastatic adenopathy from head and neck tumors, and 20% will be a malignancy of another type; thus approximately 50% will have a neoplastic etiology.

As a result of these differing etiologies, the initial treatment varies. In appropriate patients (i.e., children and young adults) with a small (less than 2 cm) node thought to be inflammatory, a short course of empiric antibiotics with follow-up within 2 to 3 weeks is appropriate; failure of the mass to shrink or resolve prompts further workup.

WHAT TO DO

The workup of an anterior neck mass begins with a thorough history. The time course of the mass, associated symptoms, prior radiation, and personal habits (i.e., tobacco and alcohol use) are key facts to be elicited. Prior trauma, surgery, or radiation will alter the normal lymphatic drainage of the neck as may issues of disease recurrence.

The physical examination of the head and neck includes the scalp, the ears, digital examination of the available oropharyngeal surfaces and neck areas, and visualization of all mucosal surfaces of the aerodigestive tract above the thoracic inlet using panendoscopy.

If the diagnosis remains elusive, the next step is needle aspiration biopsy of the mass. Benign lesions are managed appropriately. Malignant lesions will be divided into (1) lymphoma, for which excision is indicated for pathologic confirmation and further classification, and (2) metastatic, for which repeat complete endoscopy (panendoscopy) under anesthesia with biopsies of anatomically high-risk areas is performed.

In the uncommon circumstance (less than 5% of anterior neck masses) where physical examination including endoscopy with biopsies fail to reveal the source of an anterior neck mass with a malignant diagnosis on needle aspiration biopsy, then an excisional biopsy is performed. It is done through an incision compatible with a neck dissection because a common operative strategy is to perform the neck dissection at the same procedure if the frozen section diagnosis is squamous cell (epidermoid) carcinoma or melanoma. If the frozen section is lymphoma or adenocarcinoma, then the procedure is terminated with the excisional biopsy. If the frozen section is indeterminate or inflammatory, a portion is sent for culture (particularly acid-fast bacteria and fungi). Excisional biopsy of an anterior neck mass is therefore a late step in an extensive workup. The surgeon should be prepared to perform the appropriate neck dissection if metastatic epidermoid carcinoma is found.

One final note is that a surgeon may be appropriately asked to perform an excisional biopsy of a neck mass if the patient likely has lymphoma; that is, if multiple areas of adenopathy are found on examination or imaging in the setting of appropriate constitutional symptoms.

SUGGESTED READING

McGuirt WF. The neck mass. Med Clin North Am 1999;83:219–234.

STAY UP-TO-DATE ON THE LATEST ADVANCED CARDIAC LIFE SUPPORT (ACLS) PROTOCOLS

LISA MARCUCCI, MD

The American Heart Association published new advanced cardiac life support (ACLS) guidelines in 2001, which included a new case-based approach. In conjunction with the new guidelines, the ACLS course was modified to emphasize the essential components of the resuscitation of those suffering life-threatening cardiac arrhythmias, respiratory arrests, and acute ischemic strokes. In addition, immediate post resuscitation care, ethical, and legal issues were all added to the curriculum. Health care providers are required to participate in a refresher course of their skills every two years. You can review the most recent changes to ACLS protocols at www.americanheart.org/cpr.

SUGGESTED READING

Cummins R, ed. ACLS Provider Manual. American Heart Association. 2001.

ALWAYS ASK FOR HELP IF YOU ARE UNCERTAIN OF THE BEST COURSE OF ACTION

MICHAEL J. MORITZ, MD

This truism should be a constant presence for all health care providers, regardless of position, experience, or lack thereof. It is rare that there is no one with whom to consult who doesn't have either greater experience or a different, potentially valuable perspective on a problem. There are two important corollaries to this truism: (1) never let a phone call stand in the way of the help that you may need; and (2) never let the time of day (or night) stand in the way of the help that you may need. Note the phrasing "help that you *may* need." This is a reminder to ask for help when unsure; do not wait until until the trouble has progressed beyond your capabilities before recognizing the gravity of the situation.

For relatively junior providers, there are both more resources available (i.e., more relatively senior individuals) and more potential dangers due to their limited information base and experience base. For more senior individuals, there are the risks of hubris, overconfidence, and the perception that, as the experienced resource, it is unbecoming to seek another perspective. The rarest problem is the unavailability of someone to call. With the generous supply in this country of medical schools and subspecialists and universal access via the Internet to a host of medical resources, there are few instances where help is hard to find.

Patients become ill at inconvenient times. They appear to delay seeking medical attention until nights, weekends, and holidays. Patients don't make patient care easy. Regardless, excellence in patient care is our rallying cry and part of giving quality care is seeking help when circumstances so warrant. If we, as caregivers, keep the patient's well-being uppermost in mind, then issues of not wanting to call for help for whatever reason will be diminished. In conclusion, good patient care will drive us as practitioners to seek appropriate counsel. Always keep this in mind; do not fail to ask for help if you are uncertain of the best course of action.

EMERGENCY DEPARTMENT

OPERATING ROOM

MEDICATIONS

LINES, DRAINS, AND TUBES

WOUNDS

BLEEDING

GASTROINTESTINAL TRACT

WARDS

INTENSIVE CARE UNIT

LABORATORY

177

DO NOT ATTEMPT TO WEAN A PATIENT ON A VENTILATOR WITH AN ABDOMINAL BINDER IN PLACE

LISA MARCUCCI, MD

At the risk of being glib, a significant amount of care given in critical care units revolves around which patients should be put on ventilators, how long they should be on them, and what is the best and fastest way to get patients off them. To this end, a burgeoning research effort has focused on different criteria for intubation, the use of noninvasive ventilation, treatment protocols for acute lung injury and adult respiratory distress syndrome, weaning modalities, extubation protocols and the like. The accumulating evidence has shown that the comorbidities of intubation/tracheostomy and mechanical ventilation are significant, from the well-described tracheal sequelae to ventilator-associated pneumonia and diaphragmatic dysfunction. This dysfunction of the diaphragm during mechanical ventilation is ubiquitous in patients and worsens in sepsis and after some specific types of surgery (e.g., cardiac). Generally speaking, the quicker a patient can get off mechanical ventilation, the better.

WATCH OUT FOR

One simple thing that should always be checked while ventilation and weaning decisions of greater complexity are being contemplated and implemented is the presence of a circumferential abdominal binder or other partially circumferential abdominal restrictive device (e.g., bogata bag, Vacuum assisted closure (VAC) dressing) on the patient. These mechanical supports are generally intended to keep abdominal contents intra-abdominal or to buttress a weak abdominal wall. They necessarily exert inward pressure on the abdominal contents, which is transmitted throughout the abdominal cavity including the cephalad boundary of the diaphragm. Depending on body habitus and "tightness" of the device, this transmitted pressure (to an already mechanically-dysfunctional diaphragm) may cause sufficient restriction of movement to interfere with proper lung expansion, thus hampering weaning and extubation attempts. Thus, if at all possible, abdominal binders should be removed when weaning is attempted. If weaning is not progressing and other causes have been eliminated, careful consideration to the contribution a partially circumferential abdominal restrictive device might be making must be undertaken.

SUGGESTED READINGS

Betters JL, Criswell DS, Shanely RA, et al. Trolox attenuates mechanical ventilation-induced diaphragmatic dysfunction and proteolysis. Am J Resp Crit Care Med 2004; 170:1179–1184.

Kuniyoshi Y, Yamashiro S, Miyagi K, et al. Diaphragmatic plication in adults with diaphragm paralysis after cardiac surgery. Ann Thorac Cardiovasc Surg 2004; 10:160–166.

Nin N, Cassina A, Boggia J, et al. Septic diaphragmatic dysfunction is prevented by Mn(III)porphyrin therapy and inducible nitric oxide synthase inhibition. Intensive Care Med 2004; 30:2271–2278.

STRONGLY CONSIDER THE USE OF SMALLER TIDAL VOLUMES WHEN VENTILATING PATIENTS WITH ACUTE LUNG INJURY OR ACUTE RESPIRATORY DISTRESS SYNDROME

LISA MARCUCCI, MD

Optimum ventilation of patients with acute lung injury and/or acute respiratory distress syndrome is, in part, based on not contributing to the already existing damage. To this end, a considerable amount of work has been done in developing "lung protective" ventilation paradigms that decrease barotrauma by decreasing overdistention of the lung on inspiration, decreasing repeated opening and closing of small bronchioles, and lowering mechanical stress at the margins between aerated and atelectatic lung segments.

Any lung protective paradigm must balance the advantages of mechanical stretching of the lung versus the need for adequate gas exchange. Several recent studies have shown that using lung protective protocols can reduce mortality significantly. The current protocols use the following guidelines:

1) Lower tidal volumes (6 to 7 mL/kg) are more protective than the tidal volumes used in conventional ventilation (10 to 15 mL/kg).

2) Higher frequency ventilation is used to increase minute ventilation, with careful consideration of the risk of creating excessive air trapping and an unacceptable level of intrinsic positive end-expiratory pressure.

3) Plateau airway pressures should not exceed 30 to 35 mm Hg (the normal maximum transalveolar pressure at total lung capacity).

4) Abnormal blood gas readings at the following extremes are not desirable but tolerable: pH of 7.2, PCO_2 of 60 to 65, and PO_2 of 55.

5) Prone positioning of patients can improve alveolar recruitment, but may not affect overall outcome.

SUGGESTED READINGS

Krishnan JA, Brower RG. High-frequency ventilation for acute lung injury. Chest, 2000;118:795–807.

MacIntyre NR. Setting the frequency-tidal volume pattern. Resp Care 2002;47:266–274.

Petrucci N, Iacovelli W. Ventilation with smaller tidal volumes: a quantitative systematic review of randomized controlled trials. Anesth Analg 2004;99 193–200.

Young MP, Manning HL, Wilson DL, et al. Ventilation of patients with acute lung injury and acute respiratory distress syndrome: has new evidence changed clinical practice. Crit Care Med 2004;32:1260–1265.

ALLOW A SEDATED PATIENT TO AWAKEN EVERY 24 HOURS

MICHAEL J. MORITZ, MD

The trend in patient care has swung towards ensuring patient comfort. For intensive care unit (ICU) patients, particularly those on mechanical ventilation, sedation and analgesia are important adjuncts to patient care. Analogous to patient-controlled analgesia which provides a steady baseline dose of intravenous narcotic and better analgesia than intermittent as-needed dosing, the standard in most ICUs has become protocol-driven continuous infusion of sedatives. Often, sedatives and analgesics are given in combination; for example, sedation using a benzodiazepine (e.g., midazolam or lorazepam) or barbiturate (e.g., propofol) may be used in addition to analgesia using a narcotic (e.g., fentanyl). In addition to simple comfort, sedation and analgesia are helpful in avoiding agitation-driven dislodgement of tubes and catheters and are vital in patients requiring high levels of ventilatory support or nonconventional modalities of ventilation (e.g., permissive hypercapnia or high-frequency ventilation). However, continuous sedation can lead to unforeseen oversedation. Although the drugs used have rapid onsets and short half-lives, when used as continuous infusions the tissues become saturated and disposition kinetics are altered. In addition, scales to document the level of sedation and analgesia are subjective and not well standardized and again can lead to oversedation.

WHAT TO DO

Emergence from sedation after drug discontinuation varies considerably as a function of the depth of sedation maintained, the duration of the infusion, and the patient's size and body composition. To keep the emergence time from sedation in the appropriate ICU patients rapid and predictable, (see below) the following strategies should be used: (1) titrate the infusion rate to maintain a light level of sedation at all times (i.e., patient asleep but arousable and responsive to commands); (2) frequently reassess the patient's depth of sedation and adjust the infusion every 3 to 4 hours for the first 24 hours, and then at least daily thereafter; (3) suspend sedative infusions daily to allow the patients to emerge to a light level of sedation, and then resume the infusion at the minimal rate required; and (4) in morbidly obese patients, dose the sedative based on ideal (not actual) body weight (as drugs accumulate in adipose tissue).

In medical ICU patients, analgesia plus sedation (compared to sedation alone) is associated with longer time on mechanical ventilation. Interruption of sedation once a day in medical ICU patients has been shown to lead to shorter ICU stays and a lower rate of complications of critical illness for 6 of the 7 complications studied; ventilator-associated pneumonia, barotrauma, bacteremia, venous thromboembolic disease, cholestasis, and sinusitis. It seems reasonable to assume that surgical ICU patients would similarly benefit from daily interruption of sedation.

There are several groups of patients where intermittent interruption of the sedation may not be desirable. These include: patients in barbiturate coma secondary to severe head injury or severe hepatic encephalopathy; patients with severe respiratory failure acute respiratory distress syndrome (ARDS) on maximal ventilator support; patients with a borderline abdominal compartment syndrome; and patients with an open abdominal or chest wall.

SUGGESTED READINGS

Barr J, Egan TD, Sandoval NF, et al. Propofol dosing regiments for ICU sedation based upon an integrated pharmacokinetic-pharmacodynamic model. Anesthesiology 2001;95:324–333.

Schweickert WD, Gehlbach BK, Pohlman AS, et al. Daily interruption of sedative infusions and complications of critical illness in mechanically ventilated patients. Crit Care Med 2004;32:1272–1276.

Szokol JW, Vender JS. Anxiety, delirium, and pain in the intensive care unit. Crit Care Clin 2001;17:821–842.

180

Maintain tight glucose control in the intensive care unit

Michael J. Moritz, MD

Hyperglycemia and insulin resistance are common in critically ill patients even if they did not have diabetes before their illnesses. Hyperglycemia in the intensive care unit (ICU) setting has been shown to be associated with an increased mortality and restoration of normoglycemia using intensive insulin therapy has decreased mortality for the following populations: myocardial infarction, burn, and stroke. Specifically, in the surgical ICU setting, the use of intensive insulin therapy to achieve normoglycemia has resulted in a lower incidence of nosocomial infections.

The most compelling study by van den Berghe et al. showed that, for hyperglycemic patients in the surgical ICU setting on the ventilator, intensive insulin therapy to achieve normoglycemia (80 to 110 mg/dL = 4.4 to 6.1 mmol/L) resulted in a 43% reduction in mortality (8% compared to 4.6%) when compared to patients treated with sliding scale insulin with the aim of achieving a glucose level between 180 and 200 mg/dL (10.0 to 11.1 mmol/L). The lowered mortality was largely accounted for in the group with an ICU stay of more than 5 days whose mortality from multiple organ failure was lowered. Additional outcomes associated with normoglycemia included fewer bacteremias, reduced requirement for hemodialysis, fewer transfusions, and shorter duration on the ventilator and in the ICU. Although their ICU population was skewed towards postoperative cardiac surgery patients, the longer-ICU-stay population in whom the mortality reduction was more striking, and therefore a better balanced group.

Accordingly, the currently available evidence favors aiming for *normoglycemia* (blood glucose level of less than 110 mg/dL = 6.1 mmol/L) through intravenous insulin infusion in adult surgical ICU patients. It has not been proven that the same improved outcomes will be found in nonadult or nonsurgical ICU patients. The use of intensive insulin infusion can result in hypoglycemia either from excess insulin or from improvement in the patients' conditions (with a fall in insulin resistance). Many ICU's counteract this risk of hypoglycemia by also placing the patient on an infusion of dextrose during insulin administration. Frequent blood glucose monitoring (on the order of hourly) is an important part of the treatment protocol in insulin infusion to avoid hypoglycemia.

SUGGESTED READINGS

Coursin DB, Connery LE, Ketzler JT. Perioperative diabetic and hyperglycemic management issues. Crit Care Med 2004;32:S116–125.

van den Berghe G, Wouters P, Weekers F, et al. Intensive insulin therapy in the surgical intensive care unit. N Engl J Med 2001;345:1359–1367.

EMERGENCY DEPARTMENT

OPERATING ROOM

MEDICATIONS

LINES, DRAINS, AND TUBES

WOUNDS

BLEEDING

GASTROINTESTINAL TRACT

WARDS

INTENSIVE CARE UNIT

LABORATORY

181

Obtain a Pregnancy Test on Every Female Between the Ages of Ten and Fifty Years

Gregory Kennedy, MD, PhD

Research has shown that history is not a reliable indicator of pregnancy in women of childbearing age. In addition, many women do not give reliable information when they tell their surgeon they have had a hysterectomy. To avoid possible injury to the developing fetus from teratogenic drugs (or to accurately detail risks in an emergent surgery or procedure), all women between the ages of ten and fifty years must have a pregnancy test on admission to the hospital or before any invasive procedure or radiologic test using dye or radiation (including magnetic resonance imaging) is performed. The best method to determine pregnancy status is to check for the presence of human chorionic gonadotropin (hCG). This substance is produced by the placental trophoblastic tissue in the placenta. The β-subunit should be tested for because there are many false positives if the presence of whole hCG only is investigated; the test for whole hCG will pick up the presence of thyroid stimulating hormone, luteinizing hormone, and follicular stimulating hormone. Both the urine and blood can be tested for β-hCG.

If a pregnancy test has been included in a preoperative evaluation, the test should be repeated on the morning of surgery to insure that an early pregnancy was not missed with the first test. Pregnancy cannot be detected until the blastocyst implants, which may occur up to 7 days after conception. The results of a home pregnancy test kit should not be substituted because the sensitivity and specificity of these tests cannot match the results available in a clinical laboratory.

Pregnancy tests can be positive in the absence of conception. For example, hCG is a tumor marker for trophoblastic tumors such as hydatidiform mole, choriocarcinoma, embryonal cell cancers, and teratomas. On occasion, nontrophoblastic tumors such as carcinomas of the pancreas, stomach, breast, colon, small intestine, kidney, and malignant melanoma tumors may secrete hCG. Some fertility drugs (Profasi, Pregnyl, and Novarel) use hCG and will give a false positive pregnancy test result if they have been used in the preceding 14 days. If a pregnancy test comes back positive and the patient insists there is no possibility of pregnancy, further workup to elicit one of the above causes is mandated.

SUGGESTED READINGS

Bennington JL, Brecher G, Lee WS, eds. Dictionary and Encyclopedia of Laboratory Medicine and Technology. Philadelphia: Saunders, 1984.

Wilcox AJ, Baird DD, Dunson D, McChesney R, Weinberg CR. Natural limits of pregnancy testing in relation to the expected menstrual period. JAMA, 2001;286:1759–1761.

DO NOT USE A HEMOCCULT TEST KIT TO TEST FOR THE PRESENCE OF BLOOD IN GASTRIC CONTENTS

RACHAEL A. CALLCUT, MD

Upper gastrointestinal (GI) bleeding is a common and serious disorder with a significant mortality. Prompt diagnosis is important in successfully treating this condition. It has been estimated that 10% of upper GI bleeding occurs without visualization of gross blood in the nasogastric tube aspirate, requiring chemical testing for the presence of blood to confirm the diagnosis. This is most correctly done with a Gastroccult test kit. A Hemoccult test kit should not be used in this situation because the acidic pH of the gastric aspirate (pH of 1 to 4 in most patients) will cause false results. If a Gastroccult test kit can not be located, a urine dipstick may be substituted to screen for presence of red blood cells in the aspirate.

Gastroccult kits should be stored at room temperature and samples should be tested within four days of application of the gastric aspirate to the test slide. A blue color change on the slide once the Gastroccult solution is applied indicates a positive test for blood.

SUGGESTED READING

Gastroccult package insert. Beckman Coulter, Inc., Fullerton, CA, 2002.
Available at: http://usuhs.mil/med/milmedlectgibleed.ppt. Accessed July, 2005.

183

DO NOT DISREGARD AN EVEN SLIGHTLY ELEVATED PARTIAL THROMBOPLASTIN TIME (PTT) WHEN THE PROTHROMBIN TIME (PT) IS NORMAL

LISA MARCUCCI, MD

The consensus on preoperative laboratory screening is moving toward fewer tests being performed. Although the yield is low, preoperative coagulation studies can be vitally important. When ordered, these tests must be correctly interpreted for good care. Any abnormality of the partial thromboplastin time (PTT) in the setting of a normal prothrombin time (PT) cannot be dismissed as a lab error or "the tube wasn't completely filled" because it can be a marker for an underlying coagulation factor disorder that can cause fatal bleeding.

PTT measures the coagulation ability of the intrinsic pathway and, to a lesser extent, the common pathway in the clotting cascade. Factors in the intrinsic pathway include VIII, IX, XI, XII, and prekallikrein. Factors in the common pathway include fibrinogen, II, V, VII, and X. Anticoagulation with heparin (including the low–molecular-weight heparins if used in sufficiently high doses), hirudin, danaparoid, and argatroban cause a prolonged PTT in the setting of a normal PT. However, a prolonged PTT with normal PT in the absence of these drugs must prompt further laboratory investigation using mixing studies.

WHAT TO DO

Virtually every laboratory has a protocol for performing a PTT mixing study. For PTT mixing studies, the patient's serum is mixed with pooled serum of normal controls and then incubated for 1 to 2 hours at an elevated temperature. The PTT is measured twice after mixing—before and after incubation. There are three possible outcomes of this test:

1) **The PTT of the mixture is normal on initial mixing and remains normal after incubation.** This suggests that the patient's abnormal PTT is due to a deficiency of factor VIII, IX, XI, XII, or prekallikrein because the pooled serum provides the missing factor. Specific assays for factors VIII, IX, XI, and XII are then performed to find out which factor is deficient. Assays for prekallikrein are not performed because deficiency of this factor causes an increased PTT but is extremely rare and does not cause

abnormal bleeding. Treatment is repletion of the missing factor before a surgery or invasive procedure.

2) **The PTT is immediately prolonged on mixing and remains prolonged after incubation.** This suggests the presence of a coagulation inhibitor in the patient's serum. The most common inhibitor causing this mixing study outcome is lupus anticoagulant and assays for this should be performed. If this is negative, specific assays for inhibitors for factors IX, XI, and XII are done. Inhibitors are antibodies against the individual factors and are detected by testing for their unique molecular composition. The presence of lupus anticoagulant often causes an increased PTT but is paradoxically associated with thrombosis, not bleeding, and may require preoperative anticoagulation.

3) **The PTT of the mixture is initially normal (or signficantly shorter than the patient's PTT) and then becomes prolonged after incubation.** This strongly suggests the presence of a factor VIII inhibitor. A factor VIII assay should be performed and, if this factor is decreased, then a factor VIII inhibitor assay (Bethesda assay) should be performed. The larger the amount of inhibitor present, the higher the risk of severe bleeding. Each Bethesda unit connotes reduction in functional factor VIII of 50% (i.e., 3 Bethesda units contain only 12.5% functional factor VIII).

Treatment of acquired factor VIII inhibitor is difficult and is aimed at reversing the coagulopathy and eliminating the inhibitor. Substances used to stop active bleeding include desmopressin acetate (DDAVP), factor VIII bolus/infusion, prothrombin complex concentrates (which bypass factor VIII), recombinant factor VIIa (very expensive), and repletion of ongoing loss of blood components. Treatment protocols aimed at eliminating the underlying inhibitor use corticosteroids, plasmapheresis, intravenous immunoglobulin, and (in resistant cases) cyclophosphamide.

SIGNS AND SYMPTOMS

Clinically, acquired factor VIII inhibitor can present as spontaneous muscle and soft tissue hematoma, hematuria, severe epistaxis, or a fatal bleed with even mildly invasive procedures such as cystoscopy or bronchoscopy. As these inhibitors are *acquired*, lack of a previous bleeding diasthesis does not rule out their presence at the time of the prolonged PTT. Most often their etiology is idiopathic, but factor inhibitors are associated with several conditions as listed below:

autoimmune—systemic lupus erythematosis, rheumatoid arthritis, ulcerative colitis, psoriasis, and pemphigus vulgaris.

pregnancy—can appear at term or just after delivery, sometimes with spontaneous disappearance 12 to 18 months postpartum; most likely to occur in the first pregnancy.

malignancy—lymphoproliferative disorders, plasma cell dyscrasias, and solid tumors.

drugs—sulfa, penicillin, phenytoin, and especially animal derived, non-autologous fibrin glue. This type of fibrin glue is made from the mixing of several components of bovine serum of which remnants of bovine factor VIII may survive. Two percent of patients receiving fibrin glue develop acquired factor VIII inhibitor because of this exposure to bovine factor VIII.

SUGGESTED READINGS

Au WY, Lam CC, Kwong YL. Measuring acquired factor 8 inhibitor. *Haemophilia*, January 2004;10(1):98.

Pentale N, Fulgaro C, Guerra L. Acquired factor 8 inhibitor. *Blood*, October 5, 1997; 90(8):3233.

http://www.medicine.northwestern.edu, Accessed July 2004.

http://www.mgh.harvard.edu/labmed/lab/coag/handbook/co003400.htm, Accessed July 2004.

REMEMBER THAT URINE ELECTROLYTES, COMMONLY USED AS AN INDICATOR OF INTRAVASCULAR VOLUME, ARE SIGNIFICANTLY ALTERED AFTER DIURETICS ARE GIVEN

MICHAEL J. MORITZ, MD

Urine electrolytes reflect many patient variables, including: volume status (i.e., hypovolemia, normovolemia, hypervolemia); the ability of the renal tubules to function appropriately (i.e., the presence or absence of acute tubular necrosis, or ATN); and the presence or absence of a salt-losing state (i.e., the syndrome of inappropriate antidiuretic hormone secretion [SIADH], salt-wasting [cerebral or renal], and adrenal insufficiency). Urine electrolytes are best measured on a random, or spot, urine specimen. Measuring the 24-hour urinary loss of electrolytes is time consuming, reflects total intake (in a steady state), and is not useful in the acute setting. Spot urine electrolytes can be expressed simply as the concentration in urine (in mEq/L) or can be normalized by the excretion of creatinine as fractional excretion (FE). In formula form, the FE of analyte x is expressed as:

$$FE_x = 100 \times (U_x/P_x) / (U_{cr}/P_{cr})$$

where U_x and U_{cr} are the urinary concentrations of x and creatinine, and P_x and P_{cr} are the respective plasma concentrations.

The most common clinical use of urine electrolytes is in the diagnosis of the cause of oliguria to distinguish hypovolemia (a prerenal state) from intrinsic renal dysfunction, typically ATN. The distinctions between the two diagnoses are shown in *Table 184.1*.

WATCH OUT FOR

With urine electrolytes, values that are distinctive have significant diagnostic utility, whereas those that are near the boundary are of little or no diagnostic value. In prerenal states, the FE_{Na} is typically less than 1, whereas in ATN, SIADH, or a salt-losing state, the FE_{Na} is greater than 1 and often greater than 3. Additionally, there are conditions in which the diagnostic accuracy of urine electrolytes in distinguishing these two states is poor. These conditions include: (1) purely glomerular diseases such as poststreptococcal glomerulonephritis, in which tubular function and renal blood flow are unaffected but the decrease in glomerular filtration

TABLE 184.1	USING URINE ELECTROLYTES TO DIAGNOSE A PRERENAL STATE FROM INTRINSIC RENAL DYSFUNCTION		
ANALYTE	PRERENAL STATE	PARENCHYMAL DISEASE (RENAL DISEASE)	
Urine sodium (mEq/L)	<20	>40	
FE_{Na}	<1	>1	
Urine osmolality (mOsm/L)	>500	<350	

leads to an inappropriately low urine sodium; (2) radio-iodinated contrast nephropathy; (3) severe metabolic acidosis due to vomiting, where the urinary bicarbonate increases with an accompanying increase in cations, including sodium (in this state, urinary chloride or FE_{Cl} better reflect the intravascular volume); and (4) use of hypertonic saline solutions. Of note, the low urine sodium and low FE_{Na} accurately reflect inadequate circulating volume in states with total body salt and water excess but contracted intravascular volume such as cirrhosis, congestive heart failure, and nephrotic syndrome.

All diuretics increase urine volume, sodium excretion, and loss of other electrolytes and this renders urine electrolyte testing useless as a measure of volume status. The amount of disturbance that occurs is a function of the site of action of the diuretic. For example, the loop diuretics furosemide (Lasix) and bumetanide (Bumex) are potent inhibitors of sodium and chloride absorption in the loop of Henle, producing an increase in both the clearance of free water and the fractional excretion of sodium (FE_{Na}). The FE_{Na} can rise from 20% to 25%, producing urine with urine sodium of around 70 mEq/L, akin to half normal saline (0.5N physiologic saline solution = 72 mEq/L of sodium and chloride). The potency of these drugs is such that they will produce a diuresis irrespective of the volume status (i.e., even in a volume-contracted state) and despite renal dysfunction. Use of loop diuretics in the volume-contracted state in the presence of (near) normal renal reserve will typically overpower the endogenous responses to hypovolemia (increased antidiuretic hormone [ADH] secretion, increased aldosterone secretion, activation of the renin-angiotensin system), and will increase urine output and sodium loss in the urine, exacerbating the hypovolemic state.

One final note is that urine electrolytes are inaccurate for up to 36 hours after loop diuretics have been administered.

SUGGESTED READINGS

Goldman L, Bennett JC, eds. Cecil Textbook of Medicine. 21st Ed. Philadelphia: WB Saunders, 2000:529.

Kamel KS, Ethier JH, Richardson RM, Bear RA, Halperin ML. Urine electrolytes and osmolality: when and how to use them. Am J Nephrol 1990;10:89–102.

185

MAKE SURE THAT THE LABS DRAWN FOR TACROLIMUS AND CYCLOSPORIN LEVELS ARE TIMED APPROPRIATELY

MICHAEL J. MORITZ, MD

The relationship between drug dosing, drug levels, and drug effects is complex and varies amongst different pharmaceuticals. To briefly review pharmacokinetic terminology: C is the abbreviation for concentration, equivalent to level; C_0, the level at time zero (right before taking the next dose), is synonymous with C_{min}, the minimum or trough level; C_{max} is the maximum or peak level; Cx is the level at x hours after drug ingestion; AUC is area under the curve, a better measure of drug exposure than blood levels.

With the calcineurin-inhibitor immunosuppressants cyclosporine and tacrolimus, AUC correlates best with the desired immuno-suppressive effect. Thus, a higher AUC leads to a lower incidence of acute rejection. Unfortunately, measurement of a true AUC requires multiple blood levels over the 12-hour period following dosing and is both expensive and inconvenient. Therefore, for clinical use the custom is to use a single measured level that is proportionate to the AUC as a marker for measuring drug exposure. Studies in tacrolimus-treated patients have shown that C_{min}, the trough level, is reasonably propor-tionate to AUC. Adjusting the trough level to the desired range should result in adequate drug exposure to minimize the incidence of rejection.

Studies in patients treated with cyclosporine-modified USP (the second generation formulation of cyclosporine, also know by the trade name Neoral) have shown good correlation between higher AUC and lower rejection rate. In contrast, the correlations between C_{min} and AUC and between C_{min} and rejection rate are poorer. However, there is a better relationship between the AUC and the level measured 2 hours postdose, the C_2 level. The relationship between C_2 level and the incidence of rejection has been investigated early posttransplant in a variety of solid organ recipients and there does appear to be a bet-ter correlation between the incidence of rejection and C_2 compared to C_{min}. Accordingly, there is increasing interest in switching from C_{min} monitoring to C_2 monitoring for cyclosporine dosing, although the logistics in drawing blood 2 hours after taking an oral dose are problematic in both outpatients and inpatients, and interpatient variables related to differences in gastric emptying have not been adequately investigated.

With both cyclosporine and tacrolimus, certain side effects directly relate to blood level and thus peak in severity approximately 1 hour after an oral dose; these include hypertension, headache, and tremulousness. In contrast, nephrotoxicity has not been correlated with a particular pharmacokinetic parameter.

The window for accurately drawing a C_{min} has been well defined as within the 2-hour window from C_{10} to C_{12} (C_{12} is the same as both C_{min} and C_0 for twice daily drugs). The window for a C_{min} is broad because the slope of the pharmacokinetic curve is relatively flat during this interval. The window for accurately drawing a C_2 level is only 30 minutes (15 minutes before and after the 2-hour mark), which will provide a 10% margin of error.

Pharmacokinetics in human beings is relatively imprecise. The timing and composition of meals alters drug bioavailability. Intestinal absorption changes over time, as does intestinal first-pass metabolism. Drug interactions are numerous and may change over time. The susceptibility of the relevant components of the immune system to the immunosuppressant drugs is variable within an individual and between individuals. Numerous other factors affect drug levels, drug exposure, and the effectiveness of the drug. To minimize these effects, blood drawing for drug levels must keep constant as many factors as possible; specifically, drug levels must be done while fasting and with a constant time relationship to the prior dose (whether a trough level or a timed level).

SUGGESTED READINGS

Canadian Neoral Renal Transplantation Study Group. Absorption profiling of cyclosporine microemulsion (Neoral) during the first 2 weeks after renal transplantation. Transplantation, 2001;72:1024–1032.

International Neoral Renal Transplantation Study Group. Cyclosporine microemulsion (Neoral) absorption profiling and sparse-sample predictors during the first 3 months after renal transplantation. Am J Transplantation 2002; 2:148–156.

Undre, N.A. Pharmacokinetics of tacrolimus-based combination therapies. Nephrol Dial Transplant 2003;18:i12–15.

Undre NA, van Hooff J, Christiaans M, et al. Low systemic exposure to tacrolimus correlates with acute rejection. Transplantation Proc 1999;31:96–98.

KNOW THE RISKS OF DISEASE TRANSMISSION AND THE UNIVERSAL DONOR AND RECIPIENT TYPES FOR TRANSFUSION (THE UNIVERSAL DONOR FOR RED CELLS IS "O" NEGATIVE AND FOR FRESH FROZEN PLASMA [FFP] IS "AB" POSITIVE)

MICHAEL J. MORITZ, MD

WATCH OUT FOR

Each year in the United States, about 12 million units of blood are donated and converted into about 20 million units of blood products and about 4 million patients are transfused. Upon this background, interpreting the risk of known transfusion-transmitted infections can be kept in context. Nucleic acid amplification testing (NAT) became the standard test for hepatitis C and HIV in 2002 and West Nile virus in 2003, with dramatically improved sensitivity and decreased risk—now less than 1 in 2 million for both hepatitis C and HIV, and less than 1 in 1 million for West Nile virus (expressed as infections transmitted per single unit transfusion). The risk of hepatitis A is less than 1 in 1 million, and for hepatitis B is 1 in 200,000. The other major human retrovirus (other than HIV) is HTLV-1 (T-cell lymphotropic virus type I), with a transfusion risk of 1 in 3 million. In the Herpesvirus family, transmission of cytomegalovirus (CMV) and human herpesvirus 8 is dependent on circulating leukocytes, and the risk has fallen with leuko-reduced transfusions. Bacterial contamination is thought to occur in 1 to 2 units per million. Cruetzfeldt-Jakob disease (CJD) has not been reported to have transfusion as a vector, whereas variant CJD (bovine spongiform encephalopathy [BSE] or mad cow disease) may have been transmitted by transfusion in one case in the United Kingdom. The risk of malaria, Chagas' disease, and leishmaniasis is low, but serum screening is not routinely performed. The risk of acquiring transfusion related tickborne disease (especially the controversial Lyme disease and the related infections of babesiosis, ehrlichiosis, and *Bartonella*) is unknown but may be significant as a result of the following factors: presence in the blood of the causative organisms; non–serum-based screening; long periods of asymptomatic infection; greatly increased incidence in the last 20 years (although the clinical syndrome of Lyme was first described over 90 years ago as Afzelius disease); and significant misdiagnosis of Lyme disease as multiple sclerosis, chronic fatigue syndrome, and fibromyalgia (controversial).

The ABO blood groups were originally described by Karl Landsteiner in 1930. The A and B antigens are present not only on red cell membranes, but on the membranes of many cell types and in soluble form in tissue fluids as well. Biochemically, the A and B antigens are well-characterized oligosaccharides. Genetically, the A and B antigens comprise genes for two different glycosyltransferases that modify the H oligosaccharide by adding the terminal sugar moiety. The absence of both the A and B genes (and corresponding glycosyltransferases) leaves the H oligosaccharide unmodified, which is also called the blood group O oligosaccharide. On cell membranes the oligosaccharides are linked to lipids or proteins (glycolipids or glycoproteins). The A and B antigens are widely distributed in nature; hence shortly after birth, the corresponding antibodies (to the antigens intrinsically lacking) are produced by the infant.

In contrast, many other red cell groupings such as Rh, Kell, Duffy, and Kidd antigens occur only on hematopoietic cell lines. Antibodies against these antigens only occur after exposure to foreign antigens, usually via pregnancies or incompatible blood transfusions. In other words, only the ABO blood groups provoke "naturally occurring" antibodies.

In the blood bank, determining the phenotype of an individual is done by testing for both the antigens present on red cells and the invariably present corresponding antibodies in serum. *Table 186.1* lists the rules that define the ABO blood types and the compatible transfusions for red cells (packed red blood cells, whole blood).

TABLE 186.1	RULES DEFINING THE ABO BLOOD TYPES AND THE COMPATIBLE TRANSFUSIONS FOR RED CELLS (RBCs)		
RED CELL ANTIGENS	**SERUM ANTIBODIES**	**ABO BLOOD TYPE**	**COMPATIBLE RBCs**
A	Anti-B	A	A or O
B	Anti-A	B	B or O
AB	None	AB	All (AB, A, B, or O)
O	Anti-A & anti-B	O	O

Type O, lacking the A and B antigens on the cells, is the universal red cell donor. Type AB, lacking anti-A and anti-B antibodies in the serum, is the universal red cell recipient and can accept any type of red cells.

The rules for fresh frozen plasma (FFP) transfusion are the opposite, with type AB the universal donor plasma. Individuals with type AB lack anti-A and anti-B antibodies. To avoid confusion with the critically important RBC transfusion rules and because FFP is frozen (and hence not usually in scarce supply), FFP is generally used in a type-specific fashion (e.g., A to A).

SUGGESTED READINGS

Fiebig EW, Busch MP. Emerging infections in transfusion medicine. Clin Lab Med 2004;24:797–823.

Salmon C, Carton JP, Rouger P, eds. The ABO System. In: The Human Blood Groups. Chicago: Year Book Medical Publishers, 1984:94–140.

Page numbers in italics denote figures; those followed by a t denote tables.

A

A antigens, in ABO blood groups, 436, 436t

AB antigens, in ABO blood groups, 436, 436t

ABCDE mnemonic, for melanoma diagnosis, *165*, 165–166

ABC's (airway, breathing, circulation), for beta-blocker toxicity, 241

Abdomen
acute, 339
drain placement, for bleeding varices, 124
pulsatile mass of, with ruptured abdominal aortic aneurysm, 2, 5

Abdominal aorta
aneurysm of (*see* Abdominal aortic aneurysm (AAA))
cross-clamping for bleeding control, 84
endovascular stents for, 315–316, 344
renal artery use, 139
infrarenal reconstruction of, 343–344
traumatic hematoma of, 82, *83*

Abdominal aortic aneurysm (AAA)
endovascular stents for, 315–316, 344
renal artery use, 139
repair of
bowel movement w/in first 24 hrs, 343–344
hemostasis challenges with, 140
left renal vein exposure for, 136
ruptured, 2–4
differential diagnosis of, 2, 5–6
incidence of, 2
mortality rate, 2, 5
senior staff notification, 3–4
signs and symptoms, 2–3, 5
stable patient management, 3
unstable patient management, 2–3, 6

Abdominal arterial fistula, 315–316

Abdominal binder
ventilator weaning contraindication, 412
for wound dehiscence, 307

Abdominal compartment syndrome, 124

Abdominal examination
for midgut volvulus, in infants, 91
serial, for ischemic colitis diagnosis, 343

Abdominal pain
aortic dissection and, 6
ruptured abdominal aortic aneurysm and, 2, 5

Abdominal sepsis (*see* Peritonitis)

Abdominal surgery
cirrhosis contraindication, 345–346
multiple, fungal infection prophylaxis for, 210
persistent tachycardia and tachypnea following, 354–355
wound dehiscence factors, 169–170, 307–308

Abdominal wall injury, 71–72

ABO blood groups, 436
compatible transfusion rules, 436, 436t

Abscess(es)
breast
lactation-related, 93–94
recurring subareolar, 94
cellulitis versus, 34
drains for, malfunctioning workup for, 259
groin, emergency room management of, 29
incision and drainage of
emergency room cautions per anatomical type, 29
technique for, 34–35
perirectal, 31–33, 32t (*see also specific type*)
post-abdominal surgery, 355

teeth, Ludwig's angina with, 87–88
wound infections as, 300–301
Acanthamoeba keratitis, chlorhexidine
treatment of, 107
Acetabular fracture, mechanisms of, 67
Acetaminophen
allergic reaction to, 177
overdose, *N*-acetylcysteine for, 220
Acetylcholine, physiologic effects of,
238–239
N-Acetylcysteine (NAC)
for acetaminophen overdose, 220
for iodine contrast nephrotoxicity,
219–220
Acid-base disturbances
digoxin toxicity amplified with, 240
metformin-associated, 223
physiology of, 223
urine electrolyte alterations with, 431,
431t
Acidophilus, for patients on antibiotics,
192
Actinomycin D (Cosmegen), inadvertent
extravascular administration of,
174
Activated clotting time (ACT), for
protamine administration, 233
Activated partial thromboplastin time
(aPTT), for protamine
administration, 233
Acupressure, for needlestick pain, 366
Acute abdomen
corticosteroids causing, 339
diagnostic workup for, 339
Acute respiratory distress syndrome,
ventilation protocols for, 414
Acute tubular necrosis (ATN), urine
electrolyte alterations with,
430–431
Addisonian insufficiency
diagnostic strategies, 401–402
ICU patient risks for, 401–402
signs and symptoms of, 402
Adenomas, colorectal, rectal exam
detection of, 333
Adhesions
enterotomy repair and, 130–131
intestinal, barium contrast studies
causing, 338

Adhesive tape, fragile skin
contraindication, 403–404
Adolescents, liver injuries with CPR, 326
Adrenal insufficiency, urine electrolyte
alterations with, 430–431
Adrenal vein, left renal vein relationship
to, 135–136
Adrenergic drugs, oxazalidinones
cautions, 201
Advanced cardiac life support (ACLS),
407
Advanced Trauma Life Support
(ATLS), 81
Adverse drug reactions
definitions of, 177
manifestations of, 177–178
side effects versus, 177–178
Aerodigestive tract, panendoscopy of, for
mass evaluation, 402
Afterload, 293
verapamil effects on, 229
Afzelius disease, blood transfusion
screening for, 435
"Against Medical Advice" (AMA),
discharge policies, 362–363
Agitation
depression fluctuating with, 383–384
drug-related etiologies of, 384–385
in ICU patients, control strategies,
415–416
Air embolism
from central venous catheters, 277,
287
positioning prevention of, 286–287
signs and symptoms of, 287
treatment of significant, 287
Airway management (*see also*
Endotracheal intubation)
for facial fractures, 61
for hemorrhaging tracheostomy, 316
inhalation injury and, 45–46
for Ludwig's angina, 87–88
Airway pressures, plateau, acute lung
disorder recommendations, 414
Alanine aminotransferase (ALT), for
intra-abdominal trauma, in
children, 325
Albuterol, leukocytosis associated with,
243

Alcohol consumption
  delirious withdrawal reaction to, 385
  heavy (*see also* Intoxicated patient)
    cirrhosis related to, 323
    gastritis related to, 323
Alcohol overdose, rhabdomyolysis with, 89
Allen's test, for radial artery patency, 371–372
  reliability limitations, 372
Allergies
  fish, protamine administration risks and, 233
  latex, 293
  medication, verbal orders and, 177–178
  milk, Lactinex cautions, 193–194
Aloe vera, for frostbite, 50
Alpha$_1$-proteinase inhibitor (Prolastin), leukocytosis associated with, 243
Alpha-blockers, erectile dysfunction agents and, 213
American Heart Association
  ACLS guidelines, 407
  reperfusion therapy recommendations, 377
Amicar, rhabdomyolysis related to, 89
Amikacin
  peak and trough levels for, 195, 197t
  properties of, 196
  toxic side effects of, 196
Aminoglycosides
  cirrhosis contraindication, 187
  class properties of, 196
  every 8 hours dosing of, 196, 197t
    serum monitoring, 197
  once-a-day dosing of, 196, 197t
    creatinine clearance and, 197, 198t
  for *P. aeruginosa* infections, 204–205
  peak and trough levels for, 195, 197
    renal function and, 197, 198t
  pharmacokinetic dosing of, 197
  toxic side effects of, 190, 190t, 196
Aminophylline, for beta-blocker toxicity, 242
Amiodarone, rhabdomyolysis related to, 89
Amoxicillin plus clavulanate (Augmentin)

for bite wounds, 37
for facial lacerations, 56
for vancomycin-resistant enterococci, 200
Amphetamines, delirious reactions to, 385
Ampicillin
  for bite wounds, 36–37
  for overwhelming postsplenectomy sepsis, 208
Ampicillin-sulbactam (Unasyn)
  cytologic side effects of, 245
  for vancomycin-resistant enterococci, 200
Amputation(s), traumatic
  emergency room management of, 38
  replantation preparation, 38–39
  saline preservation procedure for, 38, 40
Amsterdam criteria, for familial colorectal cancer, 333
Amylase
  in acute abdomen, 339
  intra-abdominal trauma impact on, in children, 325
Anaerobic bacteria
  in bite wounds
    animal, 37
    human, 36
  in Ludwig's angina, 87
  in necrotizing soft tissue infection, 304, 379
    surgical considerations, 380
  in perirectal abscess, 31, 33
Analgesics/analgesia
  for deep abscess incision and drainage, 34
  of ICU patients
    continuous infusion protocols, 415
    emergence time strategies, 415
    for mechanical ventilation management, 415–416
  patient-controlled (*see* Patient-controlled analgesia (PCA))
  post-abdominal surgery, 354–355
  prodrug coadministrations, 214
  reversal agents for, 238t, 239

Anaphylaxis/anaphylactoid reaction
  in adverse drug reactions, 177, 220
  with intravenous vitamin K, 227–228,
    241
  protamine risk for, 233
Anastomosis
  leaking
    enterocutaneous fistulae with, 130
    in gastric bypass patients, 398–399
    postoperative signs of, 355
  postoperative complications of, 392
  stapling devices for, 140–141
  surgical, NG tube cautions with, 253
  urinary, suture for, 147
  vascular, for hemodialysis access, 267
Anesthesia
  DVT prophylaxis before induction,
    106
  general, for deep abscess incision and
    drainage, 34
  local (*see* Local anesthetic)
Anesthesia consult
  for implanted cardiac devices, 364–365
  for perioperative beta-blocker
    selection, 217
Anesthesiologist
  addressing properly, 172
  endotracheal intubation expertise,
    374–375
  inform of all injections, 114
  permission to move intubated patient,
    116
Anesthetized patient, lateral decubitus
    positioning of
  general rules for, 111
  nerve injuries in, 111
  specific recommendations for,
    111–113
Aneurysm(s)
  abdominal aortic
    differential diagnosis of, 5–7
    postoperative complications of,
      343–344
    ruptured, 2–4, 5
  mycotic
    antibiotic therapy for, 29–30
    diagnosis of, 29
    differential diagnosis of, 29
    surgical treatment of, 29
  thoracic aortic, 6

Angina
  absence in diabetics, 386
  Ludwig's, 87–88
  perioperative, prophylactic beta-
    blockers for, 216
  Viagra cautions, 213
Angiodysplasia, bleeding from, 312–313
Angiography
  arterial (*see* Arteriography)
  of pelvic hemorrhage, 67
  pulmonary, for embolism workup, 399
  for retroperitoneal hematoma, 84
  of seat belt-related trauma, 171
Animal bites
  emergency room management of,
    36–37
  rabies prophylaxis for, 52
  snake, rhabdomyolysis with, 89
Ankle-brachial index, in popliteal artery
    injury screening, 28
Anorectal abscess (*see* Perirectal
    abscesses)
Antacids, for "stress gastritis"
    prevention, 323
Antecubital fossa, abscess of, emergency
    room management of, 29
Anterior neck mass, workup guidelines,
    405–406
Anterior-posterior (AP) radiographs
  chest, for blunt sternal trauma, 65–66
  pelvic, for fall injuries, 67
Anthracyclines, inadvertent
    extravascular administration of,
    174
  antidote for, 175
Anti-A antibodies, in ABO blood
    groups, 436, 436t
Antiarrhythmic agents
  digoxin mechanisms, 240
  verapamil mechanisms, 229–230
Anti-B antibodies, in ABO blood groups,
    436, 436t
Antibiotic ointment
  for burns, of dorsal foot, 43
  for central venous catheter site, 265
Antibiotics
  allergic reaction to, 177
  for amputation reimplantation, 39
  antidepressant cautions, 215
  for bite wounds, 36–37

for breast inflammatory disorders, 93, 96
for frostbite, 50
for IV site thrombophlebitis, 390–391
Lactinex for patient on, 192
contraindications to, 193–194
for Ludwig's angina, 88
for mycotic aneurysm, 30
for necrotizing soft tissue infection, 304
for overwhelming postsplenectomy sepsis, 208
prophylactic, 209
for *P. aeruginosa* sepsis, 205
for perirectal abscess, 33
probiotic therapy for patient on, 192–194
prophylactic
for facial lacerations, 56
for open fractures, 17–18
resistance to, 199 (*see also specific agent or pathogen*)
for ruptured abdominal aortic aneurysm, 3
severe and irreversible side effects of, 189–191, 190t
for soft tissue infections, 378
for vancomycin-resistant enterococci, 200–201
for vertebral osteomyelitis, 396–397
for wound infection, 301
Antibodies
in ABO blood groups, 436, 436t
in heparin-induced thrombocytopenia, 225–226
Antibody assays, for clotting factor deficiencies, 428
Anticholinergics
for facial lacerations, 56
physiologic effects of, 237–238, 238t
Anticoagulation therapy
for deep vein thrombosis, 388
for diabetic myocardial infarction, 386
heparin-induced thrombocytopenia and, 105, 225–226
long-term, perioperative management of, 318–319
PTT results with, 427

retroperitoneal bleeding related to, 320
reversal of, 321
reversal for invasive procedures, 233
warfarin management, 318–319
Anticonvulsants
IV administration cautions, 231–232
reversal agents for, 238t, 239
Antidepressants
MAOI compounds, 215
St. John's wort as, 184
tricyclic, 215
Antidotes
for atropine, 238, 238t
atropine as, 237, 238t
for benzodiazepine toxicity, 238t, 239–240
for beta-blocker toxicity, 238t, 241–242
for digoxin toxicity, 238t, 240–241
for heparin, 238t, 239
for narcotic toxicity, 238t, 239
for overcoagulation, 233, 321
vitamin K, 227–228, 238t, 241
warfarin management, 318–319
pharmacological properties of, 237
for poisons, 237
Antiemetics, caution with NG tube malfunctioning, 253–254
Antigens, in ABO blood groups, 436, 436t
Antihistamines
for adverse drug reactions, 178
for IV vitamin K pretreatment, 227–228
Antimesenteric fat
anomalous, 128
normal, 128
pathologic, 128
Antiplatelet drugs
perioperative bleeding risks, with anticoagulation history, 318–319
retroperitoneal bleeding related to, 320
Antiretroviral therapy, bloodborne pathogen transmission and, 98
Antithrombin III deficiency, deep vein thrombosis risks, 105
Anxiolytics, reversal agents for, 238t, 239

Aorta
  abdominal
    aneurysm of (*see* Abdominal aortic
      aneurysm (AAA))
    bowel movement w/in first 24 hrs
      of repair, 343–344
    cross-clamping for bleeding
      control, 84
    endovascular stents for, 139,
      315–316, 344
    infrarenal reconstruction of,
      343–344
    traumatic hematoma of, 82, *83*
  left renal vein relationship to, 135
  thoracic
    aneurysm of, 6
    dissection of, 5–7
    traumatic injuries of, 8–9, 10, 65–66
Aortic aneurysm
  abdominal (*see* Abdominal aortic
    aneurysm (AAA))
  thoracic, 6
Aortic compressor, for bleeding control,
  84
Aortic disruption, traumatic, 8–9, 10, 65
Aortic dissection
  diagnostic workup for, 6–7
  medical management of, 6
  mortality rate, 7
  pathology of, 5–6
  ruptured abdominal aortic aneurysm
    versus, 5
Aortic valve
  aortic dissection effects on, 6
  blunt chest trauma and, 10
Aortoduodenal fistula, 315–316
Aortoenteric fistulae, 312
  diagnosis of, 315–316
  signs and symptoms of, 315
  treatment of, 316
Aortography, for traumatic injuries, 8,
  66
Aplastic anemia, chloramphenicol side
  effect, 189, 190t
Appendectomy, laparoscopic, 151–152
Appendices epiploicae, 128
Appendicitis
  avulsion of, 152
  computed tomography predictive
    value, 341, *342*

pathologic progression of, 151
  signs and symptoms of, 342
Appendix, distinguishing landmarks of,
  128
Area under the curve (AUC), in
  pharmacokinetics, 433
Argatroban, PTT results with, 427
Argon beam coagulation, for traumatic
  hepatic hemorrhage, 122
Arm abduction, deltoid numbness with,
  14–15
Arrhythmias
  ACLS protocols, 403
  digoxin-associated, 240
  with implanted cardiac devices,
    364–365
  intraoperative etiologies of, 114
  myocardial contusion and, 12
  perioperative, prophylactic beta-
    blockers for, 216
  pulmonary artery catheter-induced,
    290–292, 295
  verapamil-associated, 229–230
  Viagra cautions, 212
Arterial blood, discriminating from
  venous blood, 279–281
Arterial blood gas
  acute lung disorder protocols, 410
  Allen's test precannulation, 371–372
    reliability limitations, 372
  endotracheal intubation indications
    based on, 375
  pain control for obtaining, 370
  radial versus ulnar artery sticks for,
    371–372, *372*
  sites for obtaining, 371
Arterial fistula
  abdominal, 315–316
  aortoenteric, 312, 315–316
  signs and symptoms of, 315
  tracheobrachiocephalic, 316–317
  venous, as puncture complication, 281
Arteriography
  for embolization therapy (*see*
    Embolization)
  for great vessel trauma, 9
  iodine contrast nephrotoxicity with,
    219–220
  mycotic aneurysm evaluation, 29
  for popliteal artery injury, 27–28

postoperative, for intra-abdominal trauma, in children, 326
Arteriovenous fistula, as puncture complication, 281
Arteriovenous malformations, 312
Artery(ies) (*see also specific arteries*)
 of arm, with distal palmar arches, *372*
 cannulation for blood gas (*see* Arterial blood gas)
 hemodialysis access techniques, 267
 of hepatobiliary tree, 117
 inadvertent puncture of, 274, 279
  complications with, 281, 288
 injuries of
  with abdominal trauma, 82–84, *83*
  with central line placement, 274, 279, 281, 288
  in facial lacerations, 55
  hard signs of, 27
  in liver trauma, 122–124
 ligation of, for mycotic aneurysm, 29
 localized dilation of, 29–30
 reconstruction of, vein grafts for, 109–110
 renal
  accessory versus anomalous, 138–139
  preoperative determination modalities, 139
  retroperitoneal surgery cautions, 138–139
  traumatic hematoma of, 83, *83*
Ascites
 in cirrhotic patients, operative risks with, 345–346
 medication contraindications, 186–187
Aspartate aminotransferase (AST), for intra-abdominal trauma, in children, 325
Aspiration
 of loose teeth, 57, *58*
 through needle tip
  for biopsy of neck mass, 406
  during central venous access, 275–276
  before intravascular injection, 176
Aspirin
 allergic reaction to, 177
 for amputation reimplantation, 39
 for diabetic myocardial infarction, 386

for DVT prophylaxis, 106
perioperative bleeding risks, with anticoagulation history, 318
retroperitoneal bleeding related to, 321
Asplenia, overwhelming sepsis risks, 208–209
Assault, human bites associated with, 36
Asystole, verapamil-associated, 229
Atelectasis, post-abdominal surgery, 354
Atenolol, for perioperative cardiac ischemia, 217
Atrial fibrillation, perioperative thromboembolic risks, 319
Atrioventricular (AV) node
 depolarization physiology, 229
 digoxin effects on, 240
 verapamil effects on, 229–230
Atropine
 as antidote, 237, 238t
 antidote for, 238, 238t
 for beta-blocker toxicity, 241
 for digoxin toxicity, 240
 for verapamil-associated arrhythmias, 229
Attending staff, ruptured abdominal aortic aneurysm management, 3–4
Auscultation, for nasogastric tube placement, 254
Autoimmune disorders, factor VIII inhibitor associated with, 429
Autologous (vein) grafts, 109
 for penetrating vessel injuries, 81
 prep recommendations, 109–110
Avoparcin, 199
Avulsion
 of appendix, 152
 cystic artery, 126
 of hair, from adhesive tape, 403
 hernia sac, 336
 with open fractures, 17
Axillary artery, cannulation of, 371
Axillary lymph node dissection, avoid arm procedures following, 366–367
Axillary nerve injury
 in humeral fractures, 14–15, *15*
 with IM injections, 176
 in shoulder dislocations, 14–15

Azathioprine (Imuran), for transplant patients, IV versus PO dosages, 183

Azithromycin, for bite wounds, 37

Azole antifungals
for fungal infection prophylaxis, 210
sildenafil inhibition by, 213

Aztreonam
CNS side effects of, 191
P. aeruginosa resistance to, 205

B

Babesiosis, postsplenectomy risks, 208

Back pain
infectious etiologies workup for, 395–397
retroperitoneal bleeding and, 320
ruptured abdominal aortic aneurysm and, 2

Bacteremia
with IV site thrombophlebitis, 390
P. aeruginosa, two-drug regimen for, 205

Bacterial colonization, of pulmonary artery catheters, 295

Bacterial endocarditis, IV site thrombophlebitis causing, 390–391

Bacterial infections
anaerobic (*see* Anaerobic bacteria)
blood transfusion screening for, 435
mycotic aneurysm risks for, 29–30
in overwhelming postsplenectomy sepsis, 208
in perirectal abscess, 31, 33
in vertebral osteomyelitis, 396

Bacteroides fragilis, in perirectal abscess, 31

Bag mask ventilatory support, 375

Balloon occlusion
pulmonary artery catheter cautions, 293–295, *294*
for vascular injuries evaluation, 146

B antigens, in ABO blood groups, 436, 436t

Barbiturate coma, for head trauma, 416

Barbiturates, delirious withdrawal reaction to, 385

Bariatric surgery, postoperative complications of, 355
anastomotic, 398–399

Barium contrast studies
high-density, gastrointestinal contraindications, 338
upper gastrointestinal, for midgut volvulus in infants, 91–92

Basal cell carcinoma, shave biopsy of, 165

Basophils, ampicillin-sulbactam effect on, 245

Benign inflammatory disorders, of breast, 93–95

Benzodiazepines
delirious reactions to, 384–385
toxicity reversal, 238t, 239–240

Beta-agonists, leukocytosis associated with, 243

Beta-blockers
for aortic dissection, 6
for diabetic myocardial infarction, 386
post-abdominal surgery indications, 355
prophylactic perioperative, for cardiac ischemia, 216–217
toxicity reversal, 238t, 241–242
for transplant patients, IV versus PO dosages, 183
verapamil cautions, 230

β-Subunit, of human chorionic gonadotropin, 424

Betadine, for sterile field, 252

β-Lactam penicillins, for *P. aeruginosa* infections, 205

Betaxolol, for perioperative cardiac ischemia, 217

Bethesda assay, 422

Bevantolol, for perioperative cardiac ischemia, 217

Biceps brachii, weakness of, 16

Bile duct(s)
common, injury repair techniques, 117–118
extrahepatic, blood supply to, 117
injuries to, with laparoscopic cholecystectomy, 125

Biliary tree
blood supply to, intrahepatic versus extrahepatic, 117
injuries to, with laparoscopic cholecystectomy, 125
reconstruction techniques for, 117–118

Bilious vomiting, in infants, differential diagnosis of, 91–92
Bioavailability, of drugs, 434
Biopsy(ies)
  breast
    closure precautions, 159–160
    for malignant inflammatory disorders, 95–96
    prodrug analgesia coadministration, 214
  excisional
    breast, 159–160
    incisional versus, 161, 164
    of lymph node in neck, 405–406
    preoperative marking for, 161–162
    of proven melanomas, 166
  incisional
    breast, 159–160
    excisional versus, 161, 164
  needle aspiration, for anterior neck mass, 406
  punch, 164, 166
  shave, of skin lesions, 164–165
Bird's Nest filter, 271
Bisoprolol, for perioperative cardiac ischemia, 217
Bites
  mangement of (see Animal bites; Human bites)
  tetanus prophylaxis for, 37, 47–48
Bladder (see also Urinary entries)
  augmentation of, 148–149
  distention of, decompression cautions, 257
  distinguishing from colon, 149–150
  Foley catheter placement into, 255–256
  palpation of, 150
  perforation of, femoral vessel cannulation cautions, 269
Bladder outlet obstruction, 257
Bladder wall, anatomy variations, 149
Bleeding (see also Hemorrhage)
  with acquired factor VIII inhibitor, 428–429
  duodenal, 312
  gastrointestinal (see Gastrointestinal bleeding)
  jejunal, 312
  in liver trauma
    abdominal aortic aneurysm and, 136
    control strategies for, 122–124
    parenchymal venous, 119–122
  perioperative risk with anticoagulation history, 105, 318
    contributing factors, 318–319
  retroperitoneal
    diagnosis of, 320
    hematoma with, 82, 84, 321
    mortality rate, 321
    signs and symptoms of, 320
    treatment of, 321
Bleeding scan, radiolabeled, 313–314
"Blind colectomy," 313
Blisters, with frostbite, 50
Bloodborne infections
  glove protection against, 97
  occupational transmission of, 97–98, 98t
    response to, 98
  screening transfusions for, 435
Blood culture, for overwhelming postsplenectomy sepsis, 208
Blood dyscrasias, chloramphenicol side effect, 189, 190t
Blood flow
  collateral, arterial cannulation and, 371–373, 372
  coronary, verapamil effects on, 229
Blood gases (see Arterial blood gas)
Blood pregancy tests, 424
Blood pressure
  aortic dissection and, 6
  Dilantin effects on, 232
  intracranial injury outcomes and, 63–64
  intraoperative factors of, 114, 139
  postoperative arm measurement contraindications, 366
  ranges for, 64
  sudden cavity decompressions impact on, 257–258
  verapamil effects on, 229–230
  Viagra cautions, 212–213
Blood products (see also specific transfusion)
  for ruptured abdominal aortic aneurysm, 3
Blood samples, drawing from IV lines, 248

Blood transfusions
  for acquired factor VIII inhibitor, 428
  infection screening tests, 435
  for intra-abdominal trauma, in
      children, 325–326
  for retroperitoneal bleeding, 321
  typing for compatibility, 436, 436t
Blood urea nitrogen (BUN), bladder
      distention and, 257
Blunt trauma
  to abdomen, 71–72
    in children, 325–326
  to bowel wall, 130
  to chest
    imaging findings, 65–66
    sternal fracture complications,
        10–12
  complete examination of, 60
  to liver
    bleeding control strategies,
        120–124
    in children, 325–326
    grading of, 119
    Pringle maneuver for, 120, 123
    surgical perils, 119–120, 122
  to urethra, 73–74
Body fluids
  glove protection against, 97–98
  initial 500 ml drainage limitation,
      257–258
Body parts (see Amputation(s))
Body water, total versus current, in
      hypernatremia, 382
Body weight, sedative infusions based
      on, 415
Boerhaave's syndrome, esophageal
      rupture in, 330–331
Bogata bag, ventilator weaning
      contraindication, 412
Bone spike, with open fractures, 17
Bovine factor VIII, factor VIII inhibitor
      associated with, 429
Bovine spongiform encephalopathy
      (BSE), blood transfusion
      screening for, 435
Bowel loops
  bladder differentiation from,
      149–150
  devitalized, postoperative signs of,
      354–355
  enterotomy repair and, 130

Brachial artery
  aneurysm of, mycotic, 29
  cannulation of, 371
  traumatic injury evaluation, 145
Brachial plexus injuries, from lateral
      decubitus positioning, 111–113
Brachiocephalic artery, trachea fistula to,
      316–317
Bradycardia
  beta-blocker toxicity and, 241
  digoxin-associated, 240
  Dilantin-associated, 232
  intraoperative etiologies of, 114
  vasovagal reactions causing, 257–258
  verapamil-associated, 229–230
Brain injuries
  complete examination of, 59–60
  C-spine fractures associated with, 69
  hypotension etiologies with, 63–64
  intra-abdominal trauma assessment
      and, 76
Breast(s)
  abscess of
    lactation-related, 93–94
    recurring subareolar, 94
  biopsy of
    closure precautions, 159–160
    indications for, 95–96
    prodrug analgesia coadministration,
        214
  inflammation disorders of
    benign, 93–95
    malignant, 95–96
  mastitis of, 93–94
    plasma cell, 94
  thrombophlebitis of veins of, 94–95
Breast cancer, benign inflammatory
      disorders versus, 93–95
Breastfeeding
  abscesses from, 93–94
  inflammatory disorders and, 93–94
  probiotic therapy cautions, 194
Breathing circuit, anesthetic,
      disconnecting for patient
      repositioning, 116
Breslow stages, of melanoma invasion,
      163
Bridge prosthetic graft, vascular, for
      hemodialysis access, 267
Bridging therapy, for perioperative
      anticoagulation, 318–319

Bronchi
  endotracheal tube positioned in, 116
  teeth lodged in, 57, *58*
  traumatic injuries of, 9, 10, 65
Bronchodilators, leukocytosis associated
    with, 243
Bronchoscopy
  diagnostic, for inhalation injury,
      45–46
  therapeutic, for aspirated teeth
      removal, 57
Bulb suction, for Jackson-Pratt drains,
    260, *261*
Bullae, necrotizing fasciitis causing,
    378–379
Bumetanide (Bumex), urine electrolyte
    alterations associated with,
    424–425
Bundle-branch block (BBB)
  left, myocardial ischemia versus,
      376–377
  from pulmonary artery catheter,
      290–292
Burn centers, patient transfer
    indications, 45–46, 178
Burns
  of dorsal foot, 43, *44*
  inhalation injuries with, 45–46
  rhabdomyolysis with, 89
  tape, 403
  tetanus prophylaxis for, 47–48
Burst abdomen, 306
Bypass graft, of mycotic aneurysm, 29
Bypass surgery, gastric, postoperative
    complications of, 355
  anastomotic, 398–399

C
Calcium, serum, rhabdomyolysis impact
    on, 90
Calcium channel-blockers
  for transplant patients, IV versus PO
      dosages, 183
  verapamil mechanisms, 229–230
Calcium chloride
  intravenous, for life-threatening
      hyperkalemia, 180
  for verapamil-associated hypotension,
      229
Caloric intake, metformin cautions,
    223

Canadian C-spine Rule (CCR), for neck
    trauma clearance, 68–69
Cancer/carcinoma
  breast, 95–96
  colorectal, screening rectal exams for,
      333–334
  skin (*see* Melanomas)
  squamous cell cancer, 95, 165, 402
Candida albicans infections, prophylaxis
    for high-risk patients, 210
Cannulation needle, for jugular vein
    catheterization, 277–278, *278*
  checking for arterial placement,
      279–281
Capnocytophaga canimorsus, in
    overwhelming postsplenectomy
    sepsis, 208
Carbapenems
  CNS side effects of, 191
  for *P. aeruginosa* infections, 205
Carbon monoxide, effects on healing, 41
Carboxyhemoglobin, serum, inhalation
    injury and, 45
Carbuncles, 378
Cardiac conduction
  digoxin effects on, 240
  verapamil effects on, 229–230
Cardiac ischemia (*see* Coronary artery
    disease)
Cardiac output, 290, 293, 360
Cardiac pacing
  for beta-blocker toxicity, 242
  for digoxin toxicity, 240
  preoperative investigation of
      implantable devices, 364–365
  for pulmonary artery catheter-induced
      heart block, 291
Cardiac resynchronization therapy-
    defibrillators (CRT-Ds),
    364–365
Cardiac resynchronization therapy-
    pacemakers (CRT-Ps),
    364–365
Cardiac tamponade, 10
  from central venous catheterization,
      277, 288
Cardiology consult, for pulmonary artery
    catheter-induced arrhythmias,
    292
Cardiopulmonary reserve, endotracheal
    intubation consideration of, 374

Cardiopulmonary resuscitation (CPR)
for beta-blocker toxicity, 241
liver injury with
in adolescents and young adults,
326
in children, 325–326
Cardiovascular system
sudden cavity decompressions impact
on, 257–258
Viagra cautions, 212–213
Carotid artery
C-spine injury and, 70
inadvertent catheterization of, 274,
279, 281, 288
Catecholamines, for beta-blocker
toxicity, 241–242
Catheter-related sepsis
prevention of, 264–265
with TPN, 262
Catheters
central access (*see* Central venous
catheters (CVCs))
heparin-coated, thrombocytopenia
contraindication, 225–226
initial 500 ml drainage limitation,
257–258
pulmonary artery
balloon manipulation cautions,
293–295, *295*
complications of, 290, 293, 295
heart blocks induced by, 290–292
indications for, 290
red rubber, placement in Witzel
jejunostomy, 132–133
single- versus double-lumen
guidewire choices, 278
indications for, 264
for parenteral nutrition, 262
stopcocks for, 265
urinary (*see* Foley catheter)
Cattell-Braasch maneuver, 138
Cecum
distinguishing landmarks of, 128
in laparoscopic appendectomy,
151–152
mobilization in retroperitoneal
procedures, 138
Cefepime, *P. aeruginosa* resistance to, 205
Cefoperazone, *P. aeruginosa* resistance
to, 205

Cefoxitin
for bite wounds, 37
for vancomycin-resistant enterococci,
200
Ceftazidime, *P. aeruginosa* resistance to,
205
Ceftriaxone
for overwhelming postsplenectomy
sepsis, 208
for vancomycin-resistant enterococci,
200
Cefuroxime, prophylactic, for open
fractures, 17
Celiac axis, traumatic hematoma of, 82,
83
Cellulitis
abscess versus, 34
decubitus ulcer signs of, 305
mycotic aneurysm and, 29
in necrotizing fasciitis, 378–379
wound infections and, 300–301
Central nervous system (CNS)
atropine effects on, 237–238, 238t
depressants
delirious reactions to, 384–385
respiratory depression cautions,
368–369
hepatic encephalopathy of, 383–384
delirium versus, 384–385
stages of, 384t
medication toxicities in
antibiotics, 191
fluoroquinolones, 190, 190t
meperidine, 188
pain perception physiology, 370
stimulants, delirious reactions to, 385
Central serotonin syndrome, 215, 385
Central venous catheters (CVCs)
complications of, 277, 281, 290
Cordis, 278
dedicated, for parenteral nutrition,
262
infection prevention with, 264–265
insertion technique (*see also* Seldinger
technique)
aspirating needle while advancing,
275–276
check for venous versus arterial
blood, 279–281
dilator insertion, 282, *283*

internal jugular, 273–274
patient positioning for, 273, 275, 279
sterile procedure for, 265, 273
sutures for securing, 284, *285*
J-tip guidewire for placement, 270, 272
IVC filter ensnarement with, 271–272
prepackaged kits, 278
sites for insertion, 262, 264
vascular injuries from, 275–276
arterial puncture, 274, 279, 281, 288
back wall rupture, 282, *283*
Cephalosporins
for bite wounds, 36
CNS side effects of, 191
for *P. aeruginosa* infections, 205
prophylactic, for open fractures, 17
for vancomycin-resistant enterococci, 200
Cerebral perfusion, intracranial injury outcomes and, 63–64
Cervical collar, for neck trauma, 69
Cervical spine
fractures of, clinical clearance of, 68–70
osteomyelitis of, 395–396
Cesarean section, bladder identification for, 150
Chagas' disease, blood transfusion screening for, 435
Chance fracture, 72
Cheek laceration, nerve injuries with, 55–56
Chemical warfare, antidotes for, 237, 238t
Chemotherapy (*see also specific agent*)
skin fragility related to, 403
Chest compressions, liver injury with
in adolescents and young adults, 326
in children, 325–326
Chest pain (*see* Angina)
Chest radiograph (CXR)
of blunt sternal trauma, 11, 65–66
for chest tube position verification, 251
following central venous catheterization, 275
for vein wall rupture, 282
when switching sides, 288–289

post-abdominal surgery, 355, 399
for preoperative investigation of cardiac devices, 364
Chest trauma
blunt
imaging findings, 11, 65–66
sternal fracture complications, 10–12
great vessel injuries with, 8–9
Chest tube
manipulating cautions, 251–252
proper placement of
anatomical landmarks, 249–250, *250*
tips for, 251–252
radiograph verification of positioning, 251
Chest wall, ecchymosis of, 71
Child abuse
perineal trauma with, 60
suspicion of, reporting requirements for, 52
Childbearing age, pregnancy screening for, 424
Child-Pugh score, for liver disease, 345
Children
incarcerated hernia in, 337
laceration repair
scalp, 80
sutures for, 25
liver injuries with CPR, 325–326
overwhelming postsplenectomy sepsis risks, 207–208
perfusion indicators in, 63
probiotic therapy cautions, 195
Child-Turcotte score, for liver disease, 345
Chloramphenicol
blood dyscrasias related to, 189, 190t
increased use of, 189, 191
side effects of, 189, 190t
for vancomycin-resistant enterococci, 200
Chlorhexidine solution 4% (Hibiclens)
for central venous catheter insertion, 264
facial injuries related to, 107
for sterile field, 252
Chloride excretion, with diuretics, 431
Cholangiogram dye, 114

Cholecystectomy
  in cirrhotic patients, 345–346
  common duct injury risk, 118
  laparoscopic
    contraindications to, 125
    converting to open, 125–126
Choledochojejunostomy, 117
Cholestyramine, for *C. difficile* colitis,
  194
Cholinesterase inhibitors,
    organophosphate, antidote for,
    237–238, 238t
Chromic gut suture
  for laceration repair
    eyebrow, 24
    lip, 21–22
    in young child, 25
  for urologic procedures, 147
Chronotropic effects, negative
  of beta-blockers, 238t, 241
  of verapamil, 229
Cigarette smoking
  benign breast inflammation related to,
    94
  cessation programs, 41
  effects on healing, 41
Ciprofloxacin
  P. aeruginosa resistance to, 205
  prophylactic, for open fractures, 18
Cirrhosis
  abdominal surgery cautions, 345–346
  gastrointestinal bleeding with,
    322–324
  hemorrhoids associated with, 346
  hernias occurring with, 345–346
  medication contraindications
    aminoglycosides, 187
    NSAIDs, 186–187
  perioperative mortality based on class,
    345
Citalopram (Celexa), 214–215
"Clamp injury," 143
Clamps (*see* Vascular clamps)
Clarithromycin, sildenafil inhibition by,
  213
Clark levels, of melanoma invasion, 163,
  164
Clindamycin
  for bite wounds, 37
  C. difficile colitis from, 193

  prophylactic, for open fractures, 17
  for vancomycin-resistant enterococci,
    200
Clips (*see* Surgical clips)
Clopidogrel (Plavix)
  perioperative bleeding risks, with
    anticoagulation history, 318
  retroperitoneal bleeding related to,
    321
Clostridial myonecrosis, 379
  crepitus associated with, 379–380
Clostridium difficile
  antibiotic-related colitis
    clinical presentations, 193, 202
    diagnosis of, 193, 202
    probiotic therapy for, 192–193
    recurrent, 203
    treatment of, 202–203
  normal versus pathologic flora,
    192–193, 202
Clostridium perfringens, in necrotizing
    soft tissue infection, 304, 379
Clostridium spp.
  open fracture contamination with, 17
  in soft tissue infections, 304, 379–380
Clostridium tetani, wound contamination
    with, 47
Clotting cascade, intrinsic versus
    common pathways of, 427
Clotting factors
  PTT evaluation of, 427–428
  vitamin K dependent, 241
C-maneuver, for central vein rupture,
  282
Coagulation profile
  for intra-abdominal trauma, in
    children, 325
  preoperative, 427
  for protamine administration, 233
  PTT elevations, with normal PT,
    427–429
Coagulopathy
  acquired factor VIII inhibitor,
    428–429
  idiosyncratic, with Coumadin
    initiation, 241
  upper gastrointestinal bleeding
    accentuation, 324
Cocaine, delirious reactions to, 385
Codeine, for postoperative pain, 394

Colitis
  C. *difficile,* 192
    clinical presentations, 193, 202
    diagnosis of, 193, 202
    probiotic therapy for, 192–193
    recurrent, 203
    treatment of, 202–203
  ischemic
    full-thickness versus recoverable,
      343–344
    postoperative abdominal aorta
      repair, 343–344
  pseudomembranous, 193, 202
Collateral blood flow, arterial
      cannulation and, 371–373, *372*
Colon
  aortic fistula to, 315
  bleeding from
    blind resection of, 313
    nuclear imaging localization of, 314
    occult, 332–334
  distinguishing landmarks of, 128
  mobilization in retroperitoneal
      procedures, 138
  necrosis of, from Kayexalate-sorbitol
      enemas, 179
  perforation of, contrast studies for,
      338
Colonoscopy, serial, for ischemic colitis
      diagnosis, 343
Colorectal adenomas, 333
Colorectal cancer
  epidemiology of, 333
  familial link, 333
  rectal exams detection of, 333–334
Colostomy, diverting, for perirectal
      abscess, 33
Common bile duct, injury repair
      techniques, 117–118
Communication
  on disputed patient care issues, 363
  operating room etiquette, 171
Comorbidities
  cirrhotic ascites and renal function,
      186
  endotracheal intubation consideration
      of, 374
  of fascial dehiscence, 169, 307–308
  with mechanical ventilation, 412, 416
  of necrotizing fasciitis, 378

  with perirectal abscess, 31, 33
  in postoperative complications,
      392–393
  of vertebral osteomyelitis, 395
Compartment syndrome
  abdominal, 124
  complications of, 153
  diagnosis of, 153–154
  fasciotomy for
    with tibial fracture, 20
    wound closure, 154–155
  nontraumatic etiologies of, 153
  pathophysiology of, 153
  patient-controlled analgesia cautions,
      20
  pressure evaluation criteria for, 19–20,
      154
  signs and symptoms of, 19
  traumatic etiologies of, 153
  tibial fractures, 19–20
Competency (*see* Patient competency)
Complete blood count (CBC)
  in acute abdomen, 339
  for intra-abdominal trauma, in
      children, 325–326
Complete heart block, from pulmonary
      artery catheter, 291–292
Compression devices, intermittent, for
      DVT prophylaxis, 105–106
Compression fractures, of pelvic ring, 67
Compression packing, for traumatic
      hepatic hemorrhage, 120–123
Computed tomography (CT)
  appendicitis characteristics on, 341,
      342
  of blunt sternal trauma, 11, 66
  for brain injury assessment, 63
  contrast
    for abdominal arterial fistula
      detection, 316
    gastrointestinal contraindications,
      338
    gastrointestinal indications, 339
    for post-abdominal surgery
      infection diagnosis, 355
  of drain malfunction, 259
  for esophageal perforation detection,
      330
  helical chest, for great vessel trauma,
      8, 66

for hernia diagnosis, 350, *351*
of intra-abdominal trauma, 76
in children, 325–326
for Ludwig's angina evaluation, 88
for midgut volvulus detection, in
infants, 91
for neck trauma evaluation, 69
of pelvic injuries, *66, 67*
of peritonitis, in postoperative obese
patients, 398–399
for retroperitoneal bleeding
localization, 320–321
of ruptured abdominal aortic
aneurysm, 3, 6
of seat belt-related trauma, 71–72
for vertebral osteomyelitis evaluation,
396
Computed tomography angiography
for great vessel trauma, 8
mycotic aneurysm evaluation, 29
"Conditions of Participation for
Hospitals," on physical restraint
regulations, 383
Consultations (*see also specific discipline*)
importance of asking for, 408–409
Contrast dyes
intravascular
metformin administration
recommendations, 223–224
operating room protocol, 114
for retroperitoneal bleeding
localization, 320
Contrast-induced nephropathy
characteristics of, 219
metformin contributing to, 223
risk reduction regimens for, 219–220
Contrast studies
barium (*see* Barium contrast studies)
Gastrograffin, for gastric bypass
anastomosis complications,
398–399
imaging (*see specific modality*)
intravascular (*see* Contrast dyes)
iodine (*see* Iodine contrast)
water-soluble, gastrointestinal
indications, 338
Cooley vascular clamp, 142–143, *144*
Cooling, of amputated body parts, 40
Cooper's ligament, 350
Cordis catheters, 279

Corneal injury
chlorhexidine prep causing, 107
complete examination of, 59
with metallic debris, tetanus
prophylaxis for, 47–48
Coronary artery disease (CAD)
pain absence in diabetics, 386
perioperative risks with, 216
prophylactic beta-blockers for,
216–217
Viagra cautions, 212–213
Coronary blood flow, verapamil effects
on, 229
Corticosteroids
for acquired factor VIII inhibitor, 428
acute abdomen resulting from, 339
Addisonian insufficiency and,
401–402
intravenous, for adverse drug
reactions, 178
for IV vitamin K pretreatment,
227–228
skin fragility related to, 403
for transplant patients, IV versus PO
dosages, 182, 182t
Corticotropin stimulation test, low-dose,
for Addisonian insufficiency,
401–402
Cortisol, serum, in Addisonian
insufficiency, 401–402
Cortisone, for transplant patients, IV
versus PO dosages, 182, 182t
Cosmetic repair, of lacerations
eyebrow, *23,* 23–24
facial, 26
lip, *21,* 21–22
in young child, 25
Coudé catheter, 255
Cough reflex, loss of, endotracheal
intubation for, 374
Couinaud segments, in liver trauma, 119
CPK-MB isoenzymes, myocardial
contusion and, 12
Cranial nerves
C5, 14, 16
C6, 14–15
C8, 15–16
Creatine kinase (CK), in myoglobinuria
diagnosis, 89–90
Creatinine clearance

aminoglycoside dosing and, 197, 198t
fractional excretion formula, 428
post-bladder distention, 257
Crepitus, with soft tissue infections, 378–380
Cribiform fractures, nasotracheal/nasogastric intubation contraindications, 61
Cricothyroidotomy, for airway, with facial fractures, 61
Crohn's disease
enterocutaneous fistulae with, 130
gastrointestinal characteristics of, 128
Cruetzfeldt-Jakob disease, blood transfusion screening for, 435
Crushing clamps, 143
Crush injury
with open fractures, 17
of pelvic ring, 67
rhabdomyolysis with, 89–90
C-spine (*see* Cervical spine)
Cullen's sign, ruptured abdominal aortic aneurysm and, 2
Cultures
blood, for overwhelming postsplenectomy sepsis, 208
chest pain indications, 88
tissue, for *C. difficile* colitis, 193, 202
Cyanide, serum, inhalation injury and, 45
Cyclooxygenase-2 (COX-2) inhibitors, nephrotoxicity risk, 187
Cyclophosphamide, for acquired factor VIII inhibitor, 428
Cyclosporine
cytochrome metabolism of, 182–183
IV administration reactions, 227
microemulsion (Neoral, Gengraf), 181, 431
oral (Sandimmune), 181
peak and trough levels for, 433–434
phenytoin contraindication, 183
St. John's wort contraindication, 184
for transplant patients
IV versus PO dosages, 181
magnesium depletion and seizures, 232
CYP3A4, 182–183
Cystic artery, 118, 126
Cystoplasty, 148–149

Cytochrome P450 2D6 enzyme, prodrug metabolism role, 214
Cytochrome P450 3A4 enzyme, drug metabolism role
immunosuppressives, 182–183
sildenafil, 213
St. John's wort effect on, 184
streptogramin antibiotics, 200–201
Cytomegalovirus (CMV), blood transfusion screening for, 435

D

Dactinomycin (Cosmegen), inadvertent extravascular administration of, 174
Danaparoid, 225
PTT results with, 427
Daptomycin (Cubicin), for vancomycin-resistant enterococci, 201
Daunorubicin (Daunomycin), inadvertent extravascular administration of, 174
DeBakey vascular clamp, 143, *144*
Debridement
of amputated body parts, 40
of decubitus ulcer, 305
of frostbite, 49
of IV site thrombophlebitis, 390
of vertebral osteomyelitis, 397
of wound infection, 300
necrotizing, 304, 380
Deceleration injuries, imaging evaluations for, 66
Decompression procedures
for retroperitoneal bleeding, 321
sudden cavity, impact on cardiovascular system, 257–258
Decubitus ulcer, debridement cautions, 305
Deep vein thrombosis (DVT)
asymptomatic versus symptomatic incidence, 104
perioperative risks, 104–105, 319
postoperative, prophylaxis for, 104–106
of superficial femoral vein, 388
Defibrillators, implanted, preoperative investigation of, 364–365
Dehiscence (*see* Wound dehiscence)

Delirium, drug-related etiologies of, 384–385

Deltoid muscle
IM injections of, nerve injury with, 176
numbness in, 14–15

Dental infections, Ludwig's angina with, 87–88

Depolarization, cardiac, verapamil effects on, 229–230

Depression
agitation fluctuating with, 383–384
quinolone-induced, 190

Desmopressin acetate (DDAVP)
for acquired factor VIII inhibitor, 428
for retroperitoneal bleeding, 321

Dexamethasone, for transplant patients, IV versus PO dosages, 182, 182t

Dexmedetodomidine (Precedex), leukocytosis associated with, 243

Dexon suture, for laceration repair, in young child, 25

Dextromethorphan, 215

Diabetes mellitus
myocardial infarction and, 386
perirectal abscess associated with, 31, 33
skin fragility related to, 403–404
stomach dilatation associated with, 347

Dialysis patients (*see* Hemodialysis)

Diaphragm
abdominal, mechanical ventilation and, 412
urogenital, in males, 73

Diaphragmatic hernia, 66

Diarrhea, antibiotic-associated
clinical presentations, 193, 202
diagnosis of, 193, 202
probiotic therapy for, 192–193
recurrent, 203
treatment of, 202–203

Dicloflenac sodium (Voltaren), leukocytosis associated with, 243

Dietary supplements
organ transplant cautions, 184
sildenafil found in, 213

Dieulofoy's lesions, bleeding from, 312–313

Digital examination
for anterior neck mass, 406
of rectum
for colorectal cancer screening, 333–334
technique for, 332
of vascular injuries, 145

Digits (*see* Fingers)

Digoxin
beneficial effects of, 240
toxicity reversal, 238t, 240–241
for transplant patients, IV versus PO dosages, 183

Digoxin immune Fab (ovine) (Digifab), for digoxin toxicity, 238t, 240–241

Dilation, venous, for central line placement
checking for arterial versus, 279–281
jugular, 277–278

Dimethyl sulfoxide (DMSO), for extravasation necrosis prevention, 175

Diphtheria immunization, childhood protocol for, 47

Discharge, wound (*see* Exudate)

Discharges
"against medical advice" policies for, 362–363
responsibility for, 362

Disk injuries, intervertebral, in neck trauma, 69

Diskitis, pain complaints with, workup strategies, 395–397

Dislocation(s)
elbow, nerve injuries in, 14–16
glenohumeral, nerve injuries in, 14–16
hip, mechanisms of, 67
knee
classifications of, 27, *28*
popliteal artery injury with, 27–28
lumbar spine, 72

Dislodgment
of drains, 259
prevention of
for central lines, 284, *285*
for chest tubes, 251, 259

Disulfiram (Antabuse), intoxicated patient contraindication, 85

Diuretics, urine electrolyte alterations associated with, 430–432

Diverticulum, Meckel's, 128

Dobutamine, leukocytosis associated with, 243

Documentation, on disputed patient care issues, 363

Dolasetron (Anzemet), 235

Domestic violence
  perineal trauma with, 60
  reporting requirements for, 52

Dopamine
  inadvertent extravascular administration of, 174
  "renal dose"
    nonbeneficial in surgical patients, 221
    side effects of, 221–222

Doppler ultrasonography
  of femoral vein phlebitis, 388
  for hemodialysis access screening, 267
  mycotic aneurysm detection by, 29
  popliteal artery injury screening, 28

Dorsalis pedis artery, cannulation of, 371

"Double bubble" sign, 91

Double gloves, 98

Double-lumen catheters (*see* Multiple-lumen catheters)

Doxazosin (Cardura), 213

Doxorubicin (Adriamycin), inadvertent extravascular administration of, 174
  antidote for, 175

Doxycycline, for facial lacerations, 56

Drains
  abdominal cavity, for bleeding varices, 124
  initial 500 ml fluid limitation, 257–258
  Jackson-Pratt, 260, *261*
  malfunctioning workup for, 259

Dressings
  gauze, for dorsal foot burns, 43
  sterile, for central venous catheter site, 265
  tape cautions, 404
  for wounds (*see* Wound dressings)

Drug allergy (*see* Medication allergies)

Drug concentrations, pharmacokinetic
  equivalent to level (C), 433
  level at time zero (C_o), 433
  maximum (peak) (C_{max}), 433
  minimum (trough) (C_{min}), 433
  at x hours after drug ingestion (Cx), 433

Drug hypersensitivity, 177

Drug interactions, 434

Drug intolerance, 178

Drug overdose
  of acetaminophen, 220
  of MAO inhibitors, 385
  of narcotics, 368
  with patient-controlled analgesia, 368–369
  rhabdomyolysis with, 89

Drug side effects
  allergies versus, 178
  severe and irreversible, 189–191, 190t

Drug therapy (*see* Medications)

Drug use/abuse
  human bites associated with, 36
  intravenous (*see* IV drug users)
  tetanus prophylaxis for, 48

DTaP immunization, 47

Dt immunization, 47

DTP immunization, childhood protocol for, 47

DTwP immunization, 47

Duffy antigens, in ABO blood groups, 436

Duodenum
  aortic fistula to, 315–316
  bleeding from, 312, 314
  obstruction of distal, in infants, 91–92
  ulcers of, bleeding from, 323

E

Ear amputation, traumatic, 38

Ecchymosis
  with posterior urethral injury, 74
  retroperitoneal bleeding and, 320
  in seat belt–related trauma, 71–72

Echocardiography
  IV site thrombophlebitis indication for, 390
  of myocardial contusion, 12
  transesophageal, of aortic pathology, 6, 8

Ecstasy, delirious reactions to, 385

Efalizumba (Raptiva), leukocytosis associated with, 243

Eikenella corrodens, in human bite wounds, 36

Elbow dislocation
  radial nerve injuries in, 14–16
  ulnar nerve injuries in, 16

Elderly patient, perfusion indicators in, 63

Elective surgery, metformin administration recommendations, 223–224

Electrocardiogram (ECG)
myocardial contusion findings, 12
normal wave morphology, 376
post-abdominal surgery indications, 355
verapamil effects on, 230

Electrocautery
bile duct injuries from, 117
bowel wall injuries from, 130
cardiac pacemakers disturbed by, 364
for traumatic hepatic hemorrhage, 122

Electrolyte imbalances (*see also specific electrolyte or imbalance*)
serum
digoxin toxicity amplified with, 240–241
post-bladder distention, 257
rhabdomyolysis causing, 90
urine
conditions associated with, 428
diuretics impact on, 430–432

Electrolyte panel, for intra-abdominal trauma, in children, 325

Elevation
for dorsal foot burns, 43
for frostbite, 50
for hand injuries, 42

Embolism
air (*see* Air embolism)
catheter- and wire-tip, prevention of, 276–277
deep vein (*see* Deep vein thrombosis (DVT); Thromboembolism)
fat, post-abdominal surgery, 354–355
pulmonary (*see* Pulmonary embolism (PE))

Embolization, vascular
for intra-abdominal trauma, in children, 326
for pelvic hemorrhage, 67
for retroperitoneal bleeding, 321
for retroperitoneal hematoma, 84
for traumatic hepatic hemorrhage, 123
for vascular injuries evaluation, 146

Emergency room (ER)
gloves for examinations in, 97–98
sharps disposal, 100–101

Encephalopathy
endotracheal intubation for, 374
hepatic (*see* Hepatic encephalopathy)

Endocarditis, bacterial, IV site thrombophlebitis causing, 390–391

Endoscopy
for abdominal arterial fistula detection, 316
esophageal perforation related to, 330
stent placement for, 331
for gastrointestinal bleeding
diagnostic uses, 313, 322
therapeutic uses, 322–323

Endotracheal intubation
clinical criteria for, 374–375
comorbidities of, 412
for hemorrhaging tracheostomy, 316
for inhalation injury, 45–46
for Ludwig's angina, 87–88
moving/repositioning patient with, 116
for pulmonary artery rupture, 295

Endotracheal tube, positioned in bronchus, 116

Endovascular stents, for abdominal aortic aneurysm, 315–316, 344
renal artery use, 139

Enteric bacteria, in perirectal abscess, 31

Enteric infections, 312

Enterococcus faecalis, vancomycin-resistant, 200

Enterococcus faecium, vancomycin-resistant, 200

Enterococcus spp., vancomycin-resistant
control strategies, 200
epidemiology of, 199–200
genetic types of, 199
incidence of, 189, 195, 199
nosocomial trends, 199–200
treatment of, 200–201

Enterocutaneous fistula
causes of, 130
enterotomy repair and, 130–131

Enterotomy
for feeding tube placement, 132–133
inadvertent
postoperative signs of, 355
repair techniques for, 130–131

Enterotoxins A and B, in *C. difficile* colitis, 193, 202

Enzymatic creams, for decubitus ulcer, 305

Enzyme-linked immunosorbent assay (ELISA), for *C. difficile* colitis diagnosis, 193

Eosinophils, ampicillin-sulbactam effect on, 245

Epidermoid carcinoma (*see* Squamous cell cancer)

Epidural catheter, narcotic infusion cautions, 369

Epinephrine
for adverse drug reactions, 178
inadvertent extravascular administration of, 174
inadvertent intra-arterial administration of, 114, 175
leukocytosis associated with, 244
in local anesthetics, 114

ePTFE (Goretex), for fascial suturing, 170

Erectile dysfunction
mechanism categories, 212
vasodilator agents for, 212–213

Erosive lesions, gastric, bleeding from, 323

Erysipelas, 378

Erythema
adverse drug reactions causing, 177
necrotizing fasciitis causing, 378
wound infections and, 300

Erythromycin
ototoxicity of intravenous, 190
sildenafil inhibition by, 213

Eschar, noninfected decubitus, debridement guidelines, 305

Escitalopram (Lexapro), 214–215

Esmolol
for perioperative cardiac ischemia, 217
verapamil cautions, 230

Esophageal varices, 312, 322–323
operative risks with, 345

Esophagogastric junction, intraoperative differentiation of, 150

Esophagography, contrast, for esophageal perforation localization, 330

Esophagus
aortic fistula to, 315
rupture of, mediastinitis associated with, 330–331

Ethanol consumption (*see* Alcohol consumption)

Etiquette
communication, 171
instrument, 170

Euvolemic hypernatremia, 382

Evisceration, wound dehiscence versus, 306–307

Excision, surgical, of IV site thrombophlebitis, 390

Excisional biopsies
breast, 159–160
incisional versus, 161, 164
of lymph node, with anterior neck mass, 405–406
preoperative marking for, 161–162
of proven melanomas, 166

Exercise-induced rhabdomyolysis, 89

Exsanguination, from hemorrhaging tracheostomy, 316

External transcutaneous cardiac pacemaker, 291

Extravasation necrosis, from intravenous medications, 174–175
antidotes for, 175
Dilantin, 231

Extremity vascular procedure, surgical prep for, 109–110

Extubation, airway
abdominal restrictive devices and, 411
unintentional in operating room, 116

Exudate
necrotizing fasciitis causing, 379
pink gush of, wound dehiscence and, 306–308
purulent
VAC system for, 301, 302–303
wound infections and, 300–301
pus, wound infections and, 306

Eyebrow laceration, cosmetic repair of, *23,* 23–24

Eye injury
in children, 52
vision threatening
emergency room management of, 51–53, *52*
ophthalmologic surgery consult, 51, 53

Eyelid
  laceration of
    emergency room management of,
      52–53
    presentations of, 51, *52*
  layers of, 51

F
Facial fractures
  injuries associated with, 69
  nasotracheal/nasogastric intubation
    contraindications, 61
Facial nerve injuries, with facial
    lacerations, 55–56
Facial wounds
  human bites, 37
  lacerations
    cosmetic repair of, 26
    deep, surgical repair of, 54–56, *55*
    nerve injuries with, 55–56
    teeth assessment for, 57–58
    traumatic amputations, 38
Factor IX
  in clotting cascade, 427
  deficiency testing of, 427–428
Factor V, in clotting cascade, 427
Factor VII, in clotting cascade, 427
Factor VIII
  acquired inhibitors of, 428–429
  in clotting cascade, 427
  deficiency testing of, 427–428
Factor VIII assay, indications for, 428
Factor VIII infusions, for acquired factor
    VIII inhibitor, 428
Factor VIII inhibitor assay, indications
    for, 428
Factor XI
  in clotting cascade, 427
  deficiency testing of, 427–428
Factor XII
  in clotting cascade, 427
  deficiency testing of, 427–428
Failure to thrive, in infants, 92
Falls, blunt trauma from, 66–67
Familial adenomatous polyposis (FAP),
    333
Fascia, edges of, in enterotomy repair,
    130
Fascial dehiscence, 306–308
  diagnosis of, 306–308
  etiopathology of, 169, 307–308

incidence of, 306
management of, 307
mortality after, 308
presentations of, 306–307
suture failure prevention, 168–169
Fasciitis (*see* Necrotizing fasciitis)
Fasciotomy, for compartment syndrome
    with tibial fracture, 20
  wound closure, 154–155
FAST (Focused Abdominal Sonogram
    for Trauma) exam
  of intra-abdominal trauma, 76
  of seat belt-related trauma, 71
Fasting, metformin cautions, 224
Fat embolism, post-abdominal surgery,
    354–355
Fecal blood (*see* Occult fecal blood)
Fecal contamination
  of open fractures, 17
  of wounds, tetanus prophylaxis for,
    48
Fecal diversion, for perirectal abscess, 33
Feeding intolerance, in infants, 92
Feeding tubes
  nasogastric, 132
  surgically placed, 132–133
  in Witzel jejunostomy, 132–133
Femoral artery
  aneurysm of, mycotic, 29
  angiographic access injuries of,
    145–146
  cannulation technique for, 269–270,
    371
  pseudoaneurysm of, percutaneous
    thrombin for, 146
  retroperitoneal bleeding involvement,
    320
Femoral hernia
  incidence of, 349–350
  physical examination of, 350
Femoral vein
  catheterization of
    cutdown versus percutaneous
      puncture, 158
    for hemodialysis, 266–267
    for parenteral nutrition, 262
    technique for, 269–270
  superficial, thrombosis of, 388
Fenoldopam (Corlopam), leukocytosis
    associated with, 245
Fentanyl, for postoperative pain, 394

Fertility drugs, false positive pregnancy test with, 424
Fever
    with necrotizing fasciitis, 378–379
    phlebitis causing, 388
    postoperative, differential diagnosis of, 304
    with vertebral osteomyelitis, 395
    wound infections and, 300, 304
Fibrin glue, factor VIII inhibitor associated with, 429
Fingers
    paralysis of, 16
    traumatic amputation of, 38
First degree (superficial) burns, of dorsal foot, 43, *44*
Fish allergy, protamine administration risks and, 233
Fistula(e)
    aortoenteric, 309
        signs and symptoms of, 313–314
    arterial (*see* Arterial fistula)
    arteriovenous, as puncture complication, 281
    enterocutaneous
        causes of, 130
        enterotomy repair and, 130–131
    ileocolic, 315
    tracheobrachiocephalic, 316–317
    vascular, for hemodialysis access, 267
Flank pain
    aortic dissection and, 6
    retroperitoneal bleeding and, 320
    ruptured abdominal aortic aneurysm and, 2, 5
Fluconazole, fungal infection prophylaxis indications, 210
Fluid resuscitation
    inadequate intraoperative, with Foley catheter problems, 255
    isotonic, for brain injury, 63–64
    for overwhelming postsplenectomy sepsis, 209
    for retroperitoneal bleeding, 321
    for ruptured abdominal aortic aneurysm, 3
    for soft tissue infection-associated crepitus, 379–380
    for upper gastrointestinal variceal bleeding, 322–323

Flumazenil (Romazicon), for benzodiazepine reversal, 238t, 239–240
Fluoroquinolones
    CNS side effects of, 190, 190t
    for *P. aeruginosa* infections, 205
Fluoroscopy
    for central venous cannulation, 272, 280
    for drain malfunction, 259
Fluorouracil, leukocytosis associated with, 245
Fluoxetine (Prozac), 214–215
Fluvoxamine (Luvox), 214–215
Fold of Treves, 128
Foley catheter
    for intraoperative bladder differentiation, 150
    placement of, 255
        confirmation of, 255–256
Follow up care, responsibility for, 363
Foot, dorsal, second degree burns of, 43, *44*
Foreign bodies
    aspirated teeth as, 57–58
    esophageal perforation related to, 330
    in eye, 53
Fosphenytoin (Cerebyx), 232
Fournier's gangrene, perirectal abscess and, 32–33
    mortality rate, 31
Fractional excretion (FE), of urine electrolytes, 430–431, 431t
Fracture(s)
    acetabular, mechanisms of, 67
    compression, of pelvic ring, 67
    cribiform, nasotracheal/nasogastric intubation contraindications, 61
    facial, nasotracheal/nasogastric intubation contraindications, 61
    humeral, nerve injuries in, 14–16
    open
        injury grades, 17
        prophylactic antibiotics for, 17–18
    pelvic ring, *66,* 66–67
        urethral injuries with, 73–74
    rib, great vessel injuries with, 8–9, 66
    scapula, 9
    skull base, nasotracheal/nasogastric intubation contraindications, 61
    smoking impact on, 41

spinal (*see* Spinal fractures)
sternal
    cardiovascular injuries with, 10–12, *11*
    imaging findings, 65–66
tibial
    compartment syndrome after, 19–20
    vascular injuries with, 27
Free water, sterile IV, hypernatremia contraindication, 381–382
Freezing, of amputated body parts, 40
Fresh frozen plasma (FFP)
    compatibility rules, 436
    for retroperitoneal bleeding, 321
Frostbite
    early debridement cautions, 49
    tetanus prophylaxis for, 47–48
    treatment regimen, 49–50
Frozen section, of anterior neck mass, 406
Full-barrier protection, for central venous catheter insertion, 265
Furosemide (Lasix), urine electrolyte alterations associated with, 430–432
Furuncles, 378

G
Gag reflex, loss of, endotracheal intubation for, 374
Gallbladder infundibulum, in common bile duct surgery, 118
Gallstones
    in cirrhotic patients, 345
    staplers and clips associated with, 147
γ-Aminobutyric acid (GABA), in drug-induced seizures, 190–191
Gangrene
    gas, crepitus associated with, 379–380
    intestinal, with incarcerated inguinal hernia, 336
Gardner's syndrome, 333
Gas gangrene, 379
    crepitus associated with, 379–380
Gastric aspirate, blood testing for, 426
Gastric bypass surgery, postoperative complications of, 355
    anastomotic, 398–399
Gastric dilatation/distention
    abdominal radiograph for, 347, *348*

respiratory difficulty with, 347
    sudden decompression cautions, 258
Gastric erosions, superficial, bleeding from, 323
Gastric outlet obstruction, stomach dilatation with, 347
Gastric pouch anastomosis, leak detection, 399
Gastric ulcers, bleeding from, 323
Gastric varices, 312, 322–323
    drains for continual bleeding from, 124
Gastritis
    bleeding with, 323–324
    erosive, 323
    hemorrhagic, 323
    in ICU patients, 323
Gastroccult test kit, 426
Gastroenteritis, acute, in infants, 92
Gastrograffin contrast study, for gastric bypass anastomosis complications, 398–399
Gastrointestinal bleeding (*see also* Lower gastrointestinal (LGI) bleeding; Upper gastrointestinal (UGI) bleeding)
    endoscopy for
        diagnostic uses, 312, 322
        therapeutic uses, 322–323
    herald (sentinel), 315, 317
    nasogastric lavage for diagnosis, 312, 314
    nuclear imaging localization of, 313–314
    occult fecal blood testing, 332
        for colorectal cancer screening, 333–334
    occult gastric blood testing, 426
    upper tract sites of, 322–324
        lower tract versus, 312
    variceal, 312–313
        control strategies, 124
        differential diagnosis of, 322–324
        mortality rate, 322
        rebleeding incidence, 322
Gastrointestinal (GI) system/tract
    contrast studies
        high-density barium
            contraindications, 338
            indications for, 339

drug side effects in, 178
lavage of, for bleeding, 312, 314, 322
perforation of, corticosteroids and, 339
Gastrojejunostomy, anastomotic leak detection, 399
Gastropathy, portal hypertensive, 323
Gatifloxacin, for bite wounds, 37
Gauze
  for abscess packing, 35
  dressing, for dorsal foot burns, 43
Generic medications, patient education on, 187
Genetics
  of colorectal cancer, 333
  of vancomycin-resistant enterococci, 199
Gentamicin
  for bacterial endocarditis, 391
  for open fractures, prophylactic, 17
  peak and trough levels for, 195, 197t
    with impaired renal function, 197, 198t
  properties of, 196
  toxic side effects of, 196
GI tract (*see* Gastrointestinal (GI) system/tract)
Glasgow Coma Score
  in neck trauma evaluation, 68–70
  worsening, endotracheal intubation for, 374
Glenohumeral joint dislocation, axillary nerve injuries in, 14–15
Glomerular diseases, urine electrolyte alterations with, 430–431
Gloves
  double, 98
  for emergency room examinations, 97–98
Glucagon, for beta-blocker toxicity, 238t, 241–242
Glucocorticoids
  for extravasation necrosis prevention, 175
  leukocytosis associated with, 243
  for transplant patients, IV versus PO dosages, 182, 182t
Glucose, intravenous, for life-threatening hyperkalemia, 180
Glucose control, in ICU patients, 417

Gluteal IM injections, nerve injury with, 176
P-Glycoprotein transporter, St. John's wort effect on, 184
Gonadal vein, left renal vein relationship to, 135–136
Goretex (ePTFE), for fascial suturing, 170
Grafts and grafting
  bridge prosthetic graft, for hemodialysis access, 267
  bypass, of mycotic aneurysm, 29
  nonprosthetic, disadvantages of, 110
  prosthetic, infection risks with, 109
  skin (*see* Skin grafts)
  vascular, secondary abdominal fistulae of, 315–316
  vein (autologous), 109
    for penetrating vessel injuries, 81
    prep recommendations, 109–110
Gram-negative microbes
  aminoglycosides for, 196
  chlorhexidine effectiveness for, 107
  in human bite wounds, 36
  in IV site thrombophlebitis, 390
  in necrotizing fasciitis, 379–380
  in necrotizing soft tissue infection, 304
  in overwhelming postsplenectomy sepsis, 208
  in perirectal abscess, 31
  in vertebral osteomyelitis, 396
  in wound infections, 301
Gram-positive microbes
  chlorhexidine effectiveness for, 107
  in human bite wounds, 36
  in IV site thrombophlebitis, 390
  in necrotizing fasciitis, 379–380
  in necrotizing soft tissue infection, 304
  in overwhelming postsplenectomy sepsis, 208
  vancomycin for, 195
Granisetron (Kytril), 235
Granny knots, in fascial suturing, 168–169
Granulocyte colony-stimulating factor (g-CSF), 245
Granulocytopenia, chloramphenicol side effect, 189
Granulomas, high-density barium contrast studies causing, 338

Greater omentum, 128

Great vessels, thoracic, traumatic
injuries of, 8–9, 10
imaging findings, 65–66

Greenfield filter, 271–272

Groin abscess, emergency room
management of, 29

Groin hematoma, from angiographic
access, 145–146

Group A β-hemolytic streptococci
in necrotizing fasciitis, 379–380
in overwhelming postsplenectomy
sepsis, 208

Guaiac test, for occult fecal blood, 332
for colorectal cancer screening,
333–334

Guanine monophosphate (GMP), cyclic,
in sexual stimulation physiology,
212

Guidewires, for central line insertion
control in Seldinger technique,
277–278, *278*
J-tip (*see* J-tip guidewire)

Gunshot wounds, tetanus prophylaxis
for, 47

Gunther Tulip filter, 271

Gut suture
chromic (*see* Chromic gut suture)
plain, for laceration repair, 25

H

Haemophilus infection, in Ludwig's
angina, 87

Haemophilus influenzae type B, in
overwhelming postsplenectomy
sepsis, 208
antibiotics for, 208
preoperative vaccine for, 207, 209

Hair, avulsion of, from adhesive tape, 403

Hand(s)
human bite wounds on, 36–37
injuries of
elevation importance for, 42
smoking impact on, 41
traumatic amputations of, 38

Hand surgeon consult, 42

Headache, migraine management of, 235

Head and neck (*see also* Neck)
bacterial infection of, Ludwig's angina
with, 87–88

examination of, for anterior neck
mass, 405–406

Head trauma
barbiturate coma for, 416
complete examination of, 59–60
C-spine fractures associated with, 69
hypotension management with, 63–64
intra-abdominal trauma assessment
with, 76

Healing, tobacco use effects on, 41

Heart blocks (*see also* Bundle-branch
block (BBB))
diabetic myocardial infarction and,
386
digoxin-associated, 240
pulmonary artery catheter-induced,
291–292
verapamil-associated, 229–230

Heart rate (*see also* Bradycardia;
Tachycardia)
sudden cavity decompressions impact
on, 257–258
verapamil effects on, 229–230

Heart valves
IV site phlebitis precautions, 390–391
prosthetic
Lactobacillus infections of, 192
perioperative thromboembolic risks
with mechanical, 319

Helicobacter pylori, in peptic ulcer
disease, 323

Hematemesis, 312

Hematochezia, 312

Hematogenous osteomyelitis, of spine,
395–397

Hematoma(s)
breast, post-biopsy, 159–160
pelvic, with urethral injuries, 73–74
retroperitoneal
management of, 82, 84
zone classifications, 82–84, *83*
subcapsular, in liver trauma, 119
wound, 307
vascular control for examination of,
145

Hematuria
gross, with posterior urethral injury,
73–74
microscopic, in appendicitis, 341

Hemobilia, 312

Hemoccult test kit
  for fecal blood, 332
    in colorectal cancer screening,
      333–334
  gastric aspirate contraindication, 426
Hemodialysis
  access catheters for, percutaneous
    temporary versus permanent,
      266–267
  bloodborne infections related to, 97
  heparin-induced thrombocytopenia
    contraindication, 226
  incidence in U.S., 266
  for life-threatening hyperkalemia, 180
  vancomycin serum levels for, 196
Hemodynamics
  diabetic myocardial infarction and, 386
  direct versus indirect measurements
    of, 290, 293
    indications for, 290
  sudden cavity decompressions impact
    on, 257–258
Hemoglobin level
  blood loss indication limitations, 78
  retroperitoneal bleeding drop in,
    320–321
Hemorrhage
  abdominal trauma and
    blunt, 71–72
    control strategies, 82–84
  aortic dissection causing, 6
  central vein wall rupture causing, 282,
    283
  chest trauma and, blunt, 10, *11*, 65
  exsanguinating
    with liver injury, 122–124
    from tracheostomy, 316
  pelvic
    with fractures, 66–67
    versus intra-abdominal, 67
  with penetrating knife wounds, 81
  pulmonary interstitial, as balloon
    complication, 295
  VAC system contraindication, 303
  vitamin K for, IV administration, 227
Hemorrhagic shock
  intracranial injury outcomes and,
    63–64
  from scalp lacerations, 77–78
  treatment of, 63–64

Hemorrhoids, in cirrhotic patient, 346
Hemostasis
  clips and clamps for, 140–141
  postoperative, for liver injury, 123
  with retroperitoneal bleeding, 321
  scalp laceration device, 77
  topical agents, for traumatic hepatic
    hemorrhage, 122
Hemothorax
  from central venous catheterization,
    277, 288
  chest trauma and, 9, 10, 65–66
Heparin (*see also* Low-molecular-weight
    heparin (LMWH))
  bleeding related to, 105
    retroperitoneal, 320
  immune-mediated response to, 225
  low-dose, for DVT prophylaxis,
    105–106
  operating room protocol, 114
  for perioperative anticoagulation, 318
  protamine reversal of, 233, 238t, 239
Heparin-coated invasive lines,
    thrombocytopenia
    contraindication, 225–226
Heparin flushes, IV, thrombocytopenia
    contraindication, 227–228
Heparin-induced thrombocytopenia
    (HIT), 105, 227–228
Hepatic arteries, 117
  abdominal surgery impact on, 345
  common, ligation for continued
    bleeding, 123
  injuries to, laparoscopic treatment of,
    125
  in Pringle maneuver, 120, 123
  proper, ligation contraindications,
    123
Hepatic encephalopathy
  barbiturate coma for, 416
  classic stage-based signs of, 384, 384t
  delirium versus, 384–385
  physical restraints for combative
    patient, 383
Hepatic flexure, bleeding from, 314
Hepatic insufficiency, demerol toxicity
    cautions, 188
Hepaticojejunostomy, 117–118
Hepatic panel, for intra-abdominal
    trauma, in children, 325

Hepatic veins
  clips versus clamps for, 140
  traumatic bleeding from, 119–120
    compression control of, 120–121
    Pringle maneuver for, 120, 123
Hepatitis A virus, blood transfusion
    screening for, 435
Hepatitis B virus (HBV)
  blood transfusion screening for, 435
  occupational transmission of, 97–98,
    98t
Hepatitis C virus (HCV)
  blood transfusion screening for, 435
  occupational transmission of, 97–98,
    98t
Hepatobiliary system
  arteries of, 117
    ligation for continued bleeding,
      123
    in Pringle maneuver, 120, 123
  injuries to, with laparoscopic
    cholecystectomy, 125
  reconstructive surgery of, 117–118
Herald (sentinel) bleeding,
    gastrointestinal, 315, 317
Herbal remedies, St. John's wort
    cautions, 184
Hereditary nonpolyposis colorectal
    cancer (HNPCC), 333
Hereditary polyposis syndromes,
    colorectal, 333
Hernia(s)
  diaphragmatic, 66
  elective surgery for, cirrhosis
    contraindication, 345–346
  femoral
    incidence of, 349–350
    physical examination of, 350
  incisional, in cirrhotic patient,
    345–346
  inguinal
    in cirrhotic patient, 345–346
    incidence of, 349
    physical examination of, 349–350
  inguinal, incarcerated
    in children, 337
    imaging of, 351, 352
    manual reduction of, 335–337, 351
    physical examination of, 335, 350
    strangulated, 336–335, 349

lumbar, 349, 351
manual reduction of, 351–353
obturator, 349–350
recurrent (multiloculated), 336, 351
Richter's, 335
small bowel obstructions related to
  in children, 352
  incidence of, 349–350
  manual reduction contraindications,
    351
  manual reduction of, 352–353
  physical examination of, 349–350
  signs and symptoms of rarer,
    350–351, *352*
spigelian, 349–351
umbilical, 349
  in cirrhotic patient, 345–346
Hernia sac, problems with hernia
    reduction, 336
Herpes viruses, blood transfusion
    screening for, 435
Hesselbach's triangle, 349
High frequency ventilation, for acute
    lung disorders, 414
Hilar plate, in common bile duct repair,
    117–118
Hip dislocation, 67
Hirudin, 225
  PTT results with, 427
Histamine-2 (^{2}H) blockers, for "stress
    gastritis" prevention, 323
Histamine release, in adverse drug
    reactions, 177
History taking, for anterior neck mass,
    405–406
Homans' sign, 388
Howship-Romberg sign, 350
Human bites, emergency room
    management of
  on face, 37
  on hand, 36–37
Human chorionic gonadotropin (hCG)
  pregnancy tests for, 424
  as tumor marker, 424
Human immunodeficiency virus (HIV)
  Addisonian insufficiency related to,
    401
  blood transfusion screening for, 435
  occupational transmission of, 97–98,
    98t

Humerus fractures
  condylar, 16
  mid-shaft, 15
  nerve injuries with, 14–16, *15*
  proximal, 14, *15*
  supracondylar, 16
Hyaluronidase, for extravasation necrosis
      prevention, 175
Hydrocodone (Vicodin)
  drug contraindications, 214
  for postoperative pain, 394
Hydrocortisone (SoluCortef), for
      transplant patients, IV versus PO
      dosages, 182, 182t
Hydrogen cyanide, effects on healing, 41
Hydromorphone (Dilaudid)
  for amputation reimplantation, 39
  for frostbite, 49
  hydrocodone relationship to, 214
  for postoperative pain, 394
5-Hydroxytryptamine (5-HT)
  migraine management and, 235
  physiologic effects of, 235
5-Hydroxytryptamine (5-HT)
      antagonists, vasodilation caused
      by, 235
Hyperbaric oxygen therapy
  for necrotizing soft tissue infection,
      304, 380
  for perirectal abscess, 33
Hypercoagulable state
  deep vein thrombosis risks, 104–105
  perioperative bleeding risks, with
      anticoagulation history, 319
Hyperglycemia, in ICU patients, 417
Hyperkalemia
  compartment syndrome and, 153
  life-threatening, Kayexalate-sorbitol
      enemas for, 179–180
Hypernatremia
  pathophysiology of, 381
  sterile water contraindication,
      381–382
  treatment parameters for, 381–382
Hyperosmolar state, hypernatremia as,
      381–382
Hypertension
  aortic dissection and, 6
  intraoperative etiologies of, 114, 139
  pulmonary, protamine risk for, 233

Hypervolemia, urine electrolyte
      alterations with, 430–431
Hypervolemic hypernatremia, 382
Hypoglycemia, in ICU patients, 417
Hypokalemia, digoxin toxicity and,
      240–241
Hypoperfusion, metformin cautions, 223
Hypophyseal fossa, floor fractures of,
      61–62
Hypotension, 64
  diabetic myocardial infarction and, 386
  Dilantin-associated, 232
  intracranial injury outcomes and, 63–64
  protamine risk for, 233
  ruptured abdominal aortic aneurysm
      and, 2–3, 5
  vasovagal reactions causing, 257–258
  verapamil causing, 229
    calcium reversal of, 230
  Viagra cautions, 212–213
Hypothermia
  gastrointestinal lavage causing, 322
  traumatic injury examination and, 60
Hypovolemia, urine electrolyte
      alterations with, 430–431
Hypovolemic hypernatremia, 382
Hypoxia
  digoxin toxicity amplified with, 240
  metformin cautions, 223

I
Ibuprofen (Advil)
  for frostbite, 50
  leukocytosis associated with, 243
Ileocolic fistula, 315
Ileum
  distinguishing landmarks of, 128
  terminal, mobilization in
      retroperitoneal procedures, 138
Ileus, postoperative
  abdominal aorta repair, 344
  complications related to, 392
  gastric dilatation with, 347
  infections related to, 355
Iliac arteries
  femoral vessel cannulation cautions,
      269
  ruptured abdominal aortic aneurysm
      and, 6
  traumatic hematoma of, 83, *83*

Imaging (*see specific modality*)

Imipenem, *P. aeruginosa* resistance to, 205

Imipenem–cilastatin, for vancomycin-resistant enterococci, 200

Immunizations (*see* Vaccines)

Immunocompromised patients
C. *difficile* colitis risks, 202
fungal infection prophylaxis for, 210
IV site phlebitis in, 390–391
P. *aeruginosa* infection risk, 204–205

Immunoglobulins
in adverse drug reactions, 177
IgE-mediated, in adverse drug reactions, 177
intravenous, for acquired factor VIII inhibitor, 428

Immunosuppressant drugs
acute abdomen resulting from, 339
peak and trough levels for, 433–434
for transplant patients, 181–183, 182t
C. *difficile* colitis related to, 192–193
IV versus PO dosages, 181–183, 182t
St. John's wort contraindication, 184

Implantable cardiac defibrillators (AICDs), 364–365

Incarcerated inguinal hernia
in children, 337
imaging of, 351, *352*
manual reduction of, 335–337
contraindications to, 351
examination after, 336–337
problems with successful, 335–336
physical examination of, 350
signs and symptoms of, 335
strangulated, 336–337, 349

Incarcerated ovary, in children, 337

Incisional biopsies
breast, 159–160
excisional versus, 161, 164

Incisional hernia, in cirrhotic patient, 345–346

Incision and drainage (I and D)
of abscesses
breast, 93–95
emergency room cautions per anatomical type, 29

emergency room technique for, 34–35
perirectal, 31–32
of bite wounds, 37
of mycotic aneurysm, 29
of soft tissue infections, 378
for wound infection, 300–301

Infants, bilious vomiting in, differential diagnosis of, 91–92

Infection(s)
abscessed (*see* Abscess(es))
bite wounds risk for, 36–37
bloodborne
glove protection against, 97
occupational transmission of, 97–98, 98t
response to, 98
screening transfusions for, 435
catheter-related
IV sites, 390–391
prevention of, 264–265
with TPN, 262
of decubitus ulcer, 305
enteric, 312
with hand injuries, 42
high-density barium contrast studies causing, 338
intra-abdominal
early signs of, 354–355
enterocutaneous fistulae with, 130
late signs of, 354
mediastinitis associated with, 330
necrotic, of breast, 95
nosocomial bloodstream, 199
overwhelming postsplenectomy, 207–209
postoperative complications related to, 392
rhabdomyolysis with, 89

Inferior mesenteric artery (IMA), ligation in abdominal aorta repair, 343–344

Inferior polar arteries
infrarenal inferior vena cava relationship to, 138
retroperitoneal surgery cautions, 138–139

Inferior vena cava (IVC)
clips versus clamps for, 140

filter for
  designs available, 271
  J-tip guidewire ensnarement of,
    271–272
  infrarenal, inferior polar arteries
    relationship to, 138
  traumatic hematoma of, 82, *83*
Infiltrative diseases, Addisonian
  insufficiency related to, 401
Inflammation
  of breasts
    benign disorders, 93–95
    malignant disorders, 95–96
  mycotic aneurysm and, 29
Inflammatory bowel disease, 312
Influenza vaccine, preoperative, 207, 209
Informed consent, patient competency
  and, 360–361
Inframesocolic hematomas, 82, *83*
Infrarenal anomalies, vascular, imaging
  of, 139
Infrarenal inferior vena cava, inferior
  polar arteries relationship to, 138
Infrarenal reconstruction, of abdominal
  aorta, 343–344
Inguinal hernia
  in cirrhotic patient, 345–346
  incarcerated (*see* Incarcerated inguinal
    hernia)
  incidence of, 349
  physical examination of, 349–350
Inguinal ligament
  in femoral artery injury evaluation, 146
  femoral vessel cannulation cautions,
    269–270
Inhalation injury, early intubation for,
  45–46
Inlet radiographic view, for pelvic
  injuries, 67
Innominate veins, traumatic injuries of,
  10
Inotropic effects
  negative
    of beta-blockers, 238t, 241
    of verapamil, 229
  positive
    of digoxin, 240
    of glucagon, 238t, 241
Insecticides, antidotes for, 237, 238t
In situ repair, of mycotic aneurysm, 29

Instruments, operating room, etiquette
  for, 170
Insulin resistance, in ICU patients, 417
Insulin therapy
  intensive, for ICU patients, 417
  intravenous, for life-threatening
    hyperkalemia, 180
Intellectual functioning, in hepatic
  encephalopathy stages, 384t
Intensive care unit (ICU) patients
  Addisonian insufficiency risks,
    401–402
  central venous catheter infection
    prevention, 264–265
  fungal infection prophylaxis
    indications, 210
  glucose control guidelines, 417
  sedated, management of, 411–412
  "stress gastritis" and, 323
  ventilator managed
    lung protective paradigms, 414
    weaning contraindications, 412
Intercostal space, chest tube placement
  and, 249–250, *250*
Interferon, bloodborne pathogen
  transmission and, 98
Intermittent compression devices, for
  DVT prophylaxis, 105–106
International normalized ratio (INR),
  vitamin K effect on, 227, 241
Inter-sphincteric perirectal abscess, 32t
Interventional radiology
  dye study, for retroperitoneal bleeding
    localization, 320
  for vascular injuries evaluation, 146
Intervertebral disks
  infections of, pain complaints with,
    395–397
  in neck trauma, 69
Intestines
  malrotation of, in infants, 91–92
  perforation of, 71
    Chance fracture and, 72
    femoral vessel cannulation cautions,
      269
Intoxicated patient
  disulfiram contraindication, 85
  intra-abdominal trauma assessment,
    76
  metronidazole contraindication, 85–86

Intra-abdominal infection
early signs of, 354–355
fascial dehiscence related to, 307–308
late signs of, 354
Intra-abdominal trauma
with CPR in children, 325–326
intoxicated patient assessment, 76
seat belt-related, 71–72
Intra-arterial administration,
inadvertent, of epinephrine, 114,
175
Intra-articular medications, inadvertent
IV administration of, 175–176
Intracranial injuries (*see* Brain injuries)
Intrahepatic vein, traumatic hematoma
of, 82, *83*
Intramuscular (IM) medications
inadvertent IV administration of,
175–176
nerve injuries from, 176
Intrathoracic pleural pressure, 286
Intrathoracic venous pressure, 286
Intravascular blood volume
intracranial injury outcomes and,
63–64
urine electrolytes indication of, 428
diuretics impact on, 430–431
Intravenous drug users (*see* IV drug users)
Intravenous fluids
for amputation reimplantation, 38
for iodine contrast nephrotoxicity,
219–220
for myoglobinuria, 89–90
Intravenous immunoglobulin, for
acquired factor VIII inhibitor,
428
Intravenous (IV) lines
bloodborne pathogen transmission, 97
central (*see* Central venous catheters
(CVCs))
drawing blood samples from, 248
for hemodialysis access, percutaneous
temporary versus permanent,
266–267
for penetrating knife wounds, 81
for ruptured abdominal aortic
aneurysm, 3
thrombophlebitis of sites, aggressive
treatment indications, 390–391
venous cutdown for, 156–157

Intravenous medications
extravascular administration of
antidotes for, 175
aspiration before injecting, 176
caustic consequences of, 174–175
immunosuppressive, converting to
oral dosages, 181–183, 182t
Intubation
airway (*see* Endotracheal intubation)
nasotracheal, facial fracture
contraindication, 61–62
Invasive lines, heparin-coated,
thrombocytopenia
contraindication, 225–226
Invasive procedures
anticoagulation reversal for, 233
warfarin management, 318–319
gloves for, 97–98
Iodine contrast, nephrotoxicity of
characteristics of, 219
metformin contributing to, 223
risk reduction regimens for, 219–220
urine electrolyte alterations with, 425
Iodine gauze, for abscess packing, 35
Ipsilateral nipple, as jugular vein
catheterization landmark,
273–274
Ischemia
of amputated body parts, 40
aortic dissection causing, 5–6
with arterial injuries, 27
cardiac (*see* Coronary artery disease)
extremity, arterial cannulation and,
371–373
intestinal, in infants, 91–92
mesenteric, 312
musculoskeletal, rhabdomyolysis with,
89–90
myocardial, electrocardiogram signs
of, 376
left bundle branch block and,
376–377
ureteral, with kidney transplant, 139
Ischemic colitis
full-thickness versus recoverable,
343–344
postoperative, abdominal aorta repair,
343–344
Ischemic heart disease (*see* Coronary
artery disease)

Ischiorectal abscess, 32, 32t
Isoniazid
   CNS side effects of, 191
   rhabdomyolysis related to, 89
Isoproterenol, leukocytosis associated
     with, 243
Isosorbide, Viagra contraindication, 212
Isosulfan blue, 114
IV drug users
   bloodborne infections in, 97–98
   mycotic aneurysms in, 29
   vertebral osteomyelitis in, 396

J

Jackson-Pratt (JP) drains
   removal of, 260
   suction for, 260, *261*
Jejunostomy, Witzel, feeding tube
     placement, 132–133
Jejunum
   bleeding from, 312, 314
   proximal versus distal marker, 132
Joint Commission on Accreditation of
     Healthcare Organizations
     (JCAHO), on physical restraint
     regulations, 383
J-tip guidewire
   for femoral vessel cannulation, 270
   for right internal jugular vein
     catheterization, 274
   vena cava filter contraindication,
     271–272
Jugular veins, catheterization of
   check for venous versus arterial blood,
     279–281
   for hemodialysis, 266–267
   for parenteral nutrition, 262
   technique for, 273–274

K

Kanamycin
   peak and trough levels for, 195, 197t
   properties of, 196
   toxic side effects of, 196
Kayexalate-sorbitol enema
   alternatives to, 180
   colonic necrosis from, 179
   proper administration of, 179–180
Kell antigens, in ABO blood groups, 436
Keratitis, chlorhexidine treatment of, 107

Ketoconazole, sildenafil inhibition by,
   213
Ketorolac (Toradol)
   leukocytosis associated with, 243
   for postoperative pain, 394
Kidd antigens, in ABO blood groups,
   436
Kidney(s)
   arterial supply to (*see* Renal arteries)
   right, vascular anomalies involving,
     138
   urine electrolyte alterations with
     diseases of, 430–431
     diuretics impact on, 430–432
     prerenal state versus intrinsic renal
       dysfunction, 431t
Kidney function (*see* Renal *entries*)
Kidney stones, staplers and clips
     associated with, 147–148
Kidney transplant
   Foley catheter placement cautions,
     256
   Kayexalate-sorbitol enema
     contraindication, 176
   vascular anomalies and, 139
Knee dislocation
   classifications of, 27, *28*
   popliteal artery injury with, 27–28
Knife wounds (*see* Stab wounds)
Knot-tying technique, for fascial
     suturing, 168–169

L

Laboratory tests (*see also specific test or
     specimen*)
   for acute abdomen workup, 339
   for blood transfusions
     infection screening, 435
     typing, 436, 436t
   for *C. difficile* colitis, 193, 202
   coagulation profiles
     for anticoagulation monitoring,
       241
     preoperative, 427–429
     vitamin K effect on, 227, 241
   for drug dosing
     antibiotics, 195, 198, 197t
     immunosuppressants, 433–434
   for intra-abdominal trauma, in
     children, 325–326

for occult gastrointestinal bleeding
fecal, 332–334
gastric aspirate, 426
for occupational exposures, 98
for overwhelming postsplenectomy
sepsis, 208
for pregnancy status, 424
unexplainable abnormal results, 248,
427
Laceration(s)
cheek, nerve injuries with, 55–56
eyebrow, cosmetic repair of, *23,* 23–24
eyelid, emergency room management
of, 51–53, *52*
facial
cosmetic repair of, 26
deep, surgical repair of, 54–56, *55*
nerve injuries with, 55–56
lip, cosmetic repair of, *21,* 21–22
liver
from CPR, in children, 325–326
signs and symptoms of, 325
scalp
bleeding control, 77–78
deep, 77, *78*
full-thickness, 79
galea closure for, 79–80
skin, with open fractures, 17
in young child, suture for, 25
Lactation (*see* Breastfeeding)
Lactation abscess, 93–94
Lactic acid level, in acute abdomen, 339
Lactic acidosis
metformin-associated, 223
physiology of, 223
Lactiferous ducts, benign inflammatory
disorders of, 93–94
Lactinex
contraindications to, 193–194
for patients on antibiotics, 192
Lactobacillus therapy
contraindications to, 193–194
for patients on antibiotics, 192
Lactose-intolerance, probiotic therapy
cautions, 193–194
Lamivudine, bloodborne pathogen
transmission and, 98
Laparoscopic appendectomy, 151–152
Laparoscopic cholecystectomy
contraindications to, 125

converting to open, 125–126
stone formation risks, 147
Laparoscopic nephrectomy, stone
formation risks, 147–148
Laparoscopy, diagnostic, for intra-
abdominal trauma, 76
Laparotomy
emergency
for anastomosis leak detection,
398–399
for retroperitoneal hematoma, 82
for ruptured abdominal aortic
aneurysm, 2–3
for intra-abdominal trauma, in
children, 326
Large bowel (*see* Colon)
Laryngeal mask airway (LMA), for facial
fractures, 61
Larynx, teeth lodged in, 57
Lateral decubitus position/positioning
of anesthetized patient
general rules for, 111
specific recommendations for,
111–113
for rectal examination, 332
Latex allergy, 293
Left bundle-branch block (LBBB)
etiologies of, 377
myocardial ischemia versus, 376
from pulmonary artery catheter,
291
Left ventricular function, verapamil
effects on, 229
Leg(s)
surgical prep of, for vascular
procedures, 109–110
venous drainage systems of, 388
Legal consultation, for disputed patient
care issues, 363
Legal reporting (*see* Reporting
requirements)
Leishmaniasis, blood transfusion
screening for, 435
Leukocytosis
in acute abdomen, 339
in appendicitis, 341
drug-induced, 243–244
Level of consciousness (*see also* Glasgow
Coma Score)
in neck trauma evaluation, 68

Lidocaine injection, for chest tube insertion, 249–250

Ligament injuries, in neck trauma, 69

Ligament of Trietz, 312
feeding tube placement marker, 132–133

Ligation, arterial
hepatic, for continued bleeding, 123
inferior mesenteric, in abdominal aorta repair, 343–344
for mycotic aneurysm, 29

Linear staplers, clip interference with, 140–141

Lines
central (*see* Central venous catheters (CVCs))
pulmonary (*see* Pulmonary artery (PA) catheter)
venous (*see* Intravenous (IV) lines)

Linezolid (Zyvox), 215
for vancomycin-resistant enterococci, 201

Lip(s)
laceration of, cosmetic repair of, *21, 21*–22
traumatic amputation of, 38

Lipase
in acute abdomen, 339
intra-abdominal trauma impact on, in children, 325

Lithium
leukocytosis associated with, 243
rhabdomyolysis related to, 89

Litigation, malpractice, patient competency evaluation and, 360–361

Liver (*see also* Hepatic *entries*)
blunt trauma to
bleeding control strategies, 120–124
in children, 325–326
grading of, 119
Pringle maneuver for, 120, 123
surgical perils, 119–120, 122
drug clearance role (*see* Cytochrome P450 *entries*)
hilum of
in common bile duct repair, 117–118
left renal vein relationship to, 136
in Pringle maneuver, 120

lacerations of, signs and symptoms of, 325
lobectomy of, hemostasis challenges with, 140
penetrating trauma to, 122–124
traumatic injuries to
abdominal aortic aneurysm and, 136
chest trauma and, 11
with CPR, 325–326
excessive bleeding control, 120–121, 123–124
management improvements for, 119
minor bleeding control, 122–123

Liver function/panel
abdominal surgery impact on, 345–346
in acute abdomen, 339

Liver transplantation, biliary reconstruction with, 118

Lobectomy, hepatic, hemostasis challenges with, 140

Local anesthetic
for breast biopsy, 159
for chest tube insertion, 249–250
for deep abscess incision and drainage, 34
inadvertent intravascular injection of, 175
operating room protocol, 114

Loop diuretics, urine electrolyte alterations associated with, 430–432

Loupe magnification, for laceration repair
facial, 26
lip, 21

Low-dose corticotropin stimulation test, for Addisonian insufficiency, 401–402

Low-dose heparin, for DVT prophylaxis, 105–106

Lower gastrointestinal (LGI) bleeding
nuclear imaging localization of, 313–314
rule out upper tract source, 312, 314
sites of, 312

Low-molecular-weight heparin (LMWH)
for DVT prophylaxis, 105–106

heparin-induced thrombocytopenia and, 105, 225
for perioperative anticoagulation, 318
PTT results with, 427
retroperitoneal bleeding related to, 320
Ludwig's angina
complications of, 87
early airway control for, 87–88
pathology of, 87
signs and symptoms of, 87
treatment of, 88
Lumbar hernia, 349, 351
Lumbar spine
fractures of, 72
osteomyelitis of, 395–396
Lumbar veins, left renal vein relationship to, 135–136
Lumpectomy, avoid arm procedures following, 366–367
Lung(s)
abdominal restrictive devices impact on, 412
injuries to
blunt chest trauma and, 10, 65–66
ventilation protocols for, 414
Lung protective paradigms, 414
Lyme disease, blood transfusion screening for, 435
Lymphedema, postoperative arm procedures and, 366–367
Lymph nodes
dissection of axillary, avoid arm procedures following, 366–367
enlarged, with anterior neck mass, 405–406
Lymphocytes
ampicillin-sulbactam effect on, 244
mapping dye for, 114
Lymphoma, anterior neck mass as, 406
Lynch syndrome, 333

M

Mad cow disease, blood transfusion screening for, 435
Magnesium depletion, in transplant patients, seizures with, 232
Magnetic resonance imaging (MRI)
of aortic pathology, 6–7
for hemodialysis access screening, 267

for neck trauma evaluation, 69
non-iodine contrast agents for, 220
of seat belt-related trauma, 72
for vertebral osteomyelitis evaluation, 396
Malaria
blood transfusion screening for, 435
postsplenectomy risks, 208
Malgaigne fractures, 73
Malignancy(ies)
anterior neck, 405–406
excisions biopsies of, 161–162
factor VIII inhibitor associated with, 429
inflammatory breast, 95–96
renal, retroperitoneal bleeding related to, 320
VAC system contraindication, 303
Mallory-Weiss tears, gastrointestinal bleeding with, 322–324
Malpractice litigation, patient competency evaluation and, 360–361
Mammary duct ectasia, 94
Mammary vessels, internal, traumatic injuries of, 10
Mannitol, for myoglobinuria, 90
Manual reduction, of hernias, 335, 352–353
in children, 352
contraindications to, 351
examination after, 336–337
problems with successful, 335–336
Manubrium sterni, fractures of, 10
Margins, in excisional biopsies, 161–162
of melanomas, 166
Mass(es)
anterior neck, workup guidelines, 405–406
pulsatile abdominal, ruptured abdominal aortic aneurysm and, 2, 5
Masseter muscle, parotid duct injuries and, 54, *55*
Mastectomy, radical, avoid arm procedures following, 366–367
Mastitis, 93–94
plasma cell, 94
Maxillofacial trauma, teeth assessment for, 57–58

Mayo stand, scrub nurse responsibility
for, 170
Mechanical ventilation (*see* Ventilatory
support)
Mechlorethamine (Mustargen),
inadvertent extravascular
administration of, 174
antidote for, 175
Meckel's diverticulum, 128
Median nerve injury, in humeral
fractures, 16
Mediastinitis
esophageal perforation causing,
330–331
signs and symptoms of, 330
Mediastinum, widened, great vessel
trauma and, 9, 10, *11*, 66
Medicaid, physical restraint regulations,
383
Medic Alert bracelets, for asplenic
patients, 209
Medicare, physical restraint regulations,
383
Medication allergies
manifestations of, 177
physiologic responses, 177
side effects versus, 178
treatment of, 178
verbal orders and, 177
Medications (*see also specific agent or class*)
antidotes for (*see* Antidotes)
extravascular, inadvertent
intravascular administration of,
114, 175–176
factor VIII inhibitor associated with,
429
intravenous, inadvertent extravascular
administration of, 174–175
patient education on
contraindications, 184, 187
peak and trough levels for
antibiotics, 195–198, 197t
immunosuppressants, 433–434
pharmacokinetics of
factors influencing, 434
terminology for, 433
side effects of (*see also specific toxicity*)
allergies versus, 178
severe and irreversible, 189–191,
190t

for transplant patients (*see*
Immunosuppressant drugs)
verbal orders for, allergy inquiries
with, 177–178
Melanomas
ABCDE mnemonic for, 166, *166*
of anterior neck, 406
biopsies of
shave, 164–165
types of, 164
incidence of, 163
prognosis for, 163
staging of, 163, *164*
warning signs of, 165–166
Melena, 312
Mental status
depressed fluctuating with agitated,
383–384
endotracheal intubation consideration
of, 374
Meperidine hydrochloride (Demerol)
CNS toxicity with renal insufficiency,
188
MAOIs cautions, 215
for postoperative pain, 394
Meropenem, *P. aeruginosa* resistance to,
205
Mesenteric arteries
inferior, ligation in abdominal aorta
repair, 343–344
superior
occlusion of, in infants, 91–92
traumatic hematoma of, 82, *83*
Mesenteric vein (*see* Superior mesenteric
vein)
Mesentery
inspection of, with enterotomy repair,
131
ischemia of, 312
vascular injury to, 171
Mesoappendix, in laparoscopic
appendectomy, 151–152
Metabolic acidosis, urine electrolyte
alterations with, 431
Metabolic panel, complete, in acute
abdomen, 339
Metacarpophalangeal (MCP) joints
positioning in hand splinting, 42
puncture wounds of, 36
Metastatic mass, in anterior neck, 406

Metformin (Glucophage)
  in combination drugs (Glucovance,
    Metaglip), 223
  contraindications to, 223
  discontinuation prior to procedures,
    223–224
  extended release (Glucophage XR), 223
  liquid (Riomet), 223
  mechanism of actions, 223
Methicillin, for bite wounds, 36
Methicillin-resistant *Staphylococcus*
    aureus, 195, 199
Methylene dimethamphetamine
    (MDMA, Ecstasy), delirious
    reactions to, 385
Methylphenidate (Ritalin), delirious
    reactions to, 385
Methylprednisolone (Solu-Medrol), for
    transplant patients, IV versus PO
    dosages, 182, 182t
Metoprolol
  intravenous, for diabetic myocardial
    infarction, 386
  for perioperative cardiac ischemia, 217
Metronidazole (Flagyl)
  for *C. difficile* colitis, 193, 203
  CNS side effects of, 191
  intoxicated patient contraindication,
    85–86
  neuropathy related to, 189, 190t
  for vancomycin-resistant enterococci,
    200
Mezlocillin, *P. aeruginosa* resistance to,
    204
Middle ear injury, chlorhexidine prep
    causing, 107
Midgut, volvulus of, in infants, 91–92
Migraine, pharmacologic management
    of, 235
Milk allergy, Lactinex cautions, 193–194
Minocyline, ototoxicity of, 190
Minute ventilation, for acute lung
    disorders, 414
"Mississippi Mud," 195
Mithramycin (Mithracin), inadvertent
    extravascular administration of,
    174
Mitomycin C (Mutamycin), inadvertent
    extravascular administration of,
    174
  antidote for, 175

Mixed venous oxygen saturation, 290
Mondor's disease, 94–95
Monoamine oxidase (MAO) activity,
    oxazalidinones cautions, 201
Monoamine oxidase (MAOI) inhibitors
  overdose reactions, 385
  SSRI contraindication, 217
Monocryl suture, for laceration repair
  scalp, 79
  in young child, 25
Monocytes, ampicillin-sulbactam effect
    on, 245
Morphine
  for amputation reimplantation, 39
  intravenous, for diabetic myocardial
    infarction, 386
  meperidine potency versus, 188
  for postoperative pain, 394
Mortality (*see* Perioperative mortality)
Motor vehicle accident (MVA)
  blunt trauma with
    abdominal injuries, 71–72
    imaging evaluations of, 65–67
  spinal injury evaluation for
    cervical, 68–70
    lumbar, 71–72
Moxifloxacin, for bite wounds, 37
Mucosa
  oral
    in lip laceration repair, 21
    panendoscopy for anterior neck
      mass, 406
  rectal, digital examination of, 332
Multiple-lumen catheters
  capping for removal of, 286–287
  guidewire choice for, 278
  indications for, 264
  for parenteral nutrition, 262
  stopcocks for, 265
Muscles (*see also specific muscle*)
  oral, in lip laceration repair, 21
Musculocutaneous nerve injury, in
    humeral fractures, 16
Mycophenolate mofetil (CellCept), for
    transplant patients, IV versus PO
    dosages, 183
Mycotic aneurysm
  antibiotic therapy for, 29–30
  diagnosis of, 29
  differential diagnosis of, 29
  surgical treatment of, 29

Myocardial contractility
 digoxin effects on, 240
 verapamil effects on, 229–230
Myocardial contusion
 diagnostic criteria for, 12
 sternal fractures and, 10, 12
Myocardial infarction (MI)
 electrocardiogram signs of, 376
  left bundle branch block and,
   376–377
 pain absence in diabetics, 386
 perioperative, prophylactic beta-
  blockers for, 216–217
 silent, 386
 standard workup for, 386
 Viagra cautions, 212
Myocardial ischemia, electrocardiogram
 signs of, 376
 left bundle branch block and, 376–377
Myoglobinuria
 compartment syndrome and, 153
 etiopathologies of, 89
 signs and symptoms of, 89–90

N

Nabumetone (Relafen), leukocytosis
 associated with, 243
N-Acetylcysteine (NAC)
 for acetaminophen overdose, 220
 for iodine contrast nephrotoxicity,
  219–220
Naloxone (Narcan)
 for narcotic toxicity, 238t, 239
 patient-controlled analgesia
  indications, 368–369
Naproxen (Naprosyn), leukocytosis
 associated with, 243
Narcotics
 for amputation reimplantation, 39
 for frostbite, 49
 hydrocodone relationship to, 214
 meperidine potency versus, 188
 overdose signs and symptoms, 368
 post-abdominal surgery, 355
 toxicity reversal, 238t, 239
Nasal cavity, anatomy of, 61
Nasogastric lavage, for gastrointestinal
 bleeding, 312, 314, 322
Nasogastric (NG) tube
 confirmation of placement, 347
 for feedings, 132
 for gastric dilatation, 347
 for gastrointestinal bleeding, 312, 314
 for intraoperative anatomy
  differentiation, 150
 irrigation of, 254
 trauma contraindications, 61–62
 vomiting around, 253
  problem solving, 253–254
Nasotracheal intubation, facial fracture
 contraindication, 61–62
Nausea, 5-HT$_3$ antagonists for, 237
Neck
 abscess of, emergency room
  management of, 29
 anterior mass of, workup guidelines,
  405–406
 bacterial infection of, Ludwig's angina
  with, 87–88
 pain, infectious etiologies workup for,
  395–397
 trauma to
  clinical clearance of, 68–70
  mechanisms of, 68
Necrosis
 in breast inflammatory disorders, 95
 extravasation, 174–175
 intestinal
  with incarcerated inguinal hernia,
   335–336
  in infants, 91–92
 of wound infections, 304
  VAC system contraindication,
   303
Necrotizing fasciitis
 crepitus associated with, 379–380
 pathology of, 304, 378
 signs and symptoms of, 378–379
 types of, 379
Necrotizing pancreatitis, fungal infection
 prophylaxis for, 210
Necrotizing soft tissue infection (NIST),
 304
 "second look" operation for, 304, 380
Needle aspiration biopsy, for anterior
 neck mass, 406
Needlestick pain, acupressure for, 370
Needlesticks, occupational
 bloodborne infection transmission, 98,
  98t
 expert consultation for, 98, 100
 post exposure prophylaxis for, 100

prevention of
in emergency room, 100–101
in operating room, 170
Nefazodone (Serzone), 215
Neisseria meningitidis, in overwhelming
postsplenectomy sepsis, 208
antibiotics for, 208
preoperative vaccine for, 207, 209
Neomycin, ototoxicity of, 190
Neoplasms
anterior neck, 405–406
enterocutaneous fistulae with, 130
gastrointestinal, bleeding from,
312–313
trophoblastic, hCG marker of, 424
Nephrectomy
laparoscopic, stone formation risks,
147–148
open, hemostasis challenges with, 140
Nephropathy, contrast-induced
characteristics of, 219
metformin contributing to, 223
risk reduction regimens for, 219–220
Nephrotoxicity
of aminoglycosides, 187, 190, 196–197
iodine contrast-associated
characteristics of, 219
metformin contributing to, 223
risk reduction regimens for, 219–220
urine electrolyte alterations with,
431
of NSAIDS, 186–187
of vancomycin, 196
Nerve blocks
for amputation reimplantation, 39
inadvertent intravascular injection of,
175
Nerve gases, antidotes for, 237, 238t
Nerve injuries
with humeral fractures, 14–16
from IM injections, 176
from lateral decubitus positioning, 111
prevention of, 111–113
Netilmicin
peak and trough levels for, 195, 197t
properties of, 196
toxic side effects of, 196
Neuromuscular blockade, from
aminoglycosides, 196
Neuromuscular functioning, in hepatic
encephalopathy stages, 384t

Neurons, pain perception physiology,
370
Neuropathy
diabetic, stomach dilatation associated
with, 347
metronidazole side effect, 189, 190t
nitrofurantoin-induced, 190
peripheral, from aminoglycosides, 196
Neurovascular injuries, intercostal, with
chest tube insertion, 249–250
Nicotine, effects on healing, 41
Nipple discharge, 93–94
Nissen's fundoplication, stomach
dilatation associated with, 347
Nitrates, Viagra contraindication,
212–213
Nitric oxide, in sexual stimulation
physiology, 212
Nitrofurantoin, side effects of, 191
Nitroglycerin
sublingual, for diabetic myocardial
infarction, 386
Viagra contraindication, 212
Nociception, 370
Nonautologous graft conduits,
nonprosthetic, disadvantages of,
110
Noncrushing clamps, 143–144, *144*
Non-group A streptococci, in
necrotizing fasciitis, 379
Nonprosthetic nonautologous graft
conduits, disadvantages of, 110
Nonsteroidal anti-inflammatory drugs
(NSAIDs)
for breast inflammatory disorders, 95
cirrhosis contraindication, 186–187
leukocytosis associated with, 243
peptic ulcer bleeding risks, 323
for postoperative pain, 394
Nontrophoblastic tumors, hCG marker
of, 424
Nonvascular clamps, 144
NORASEPT II study, 221
Norepinephrine
inadvertent extravascular
administration of, 174
leukocytosis associated with, 243
Normeperidine hydrochloride, toxicity
symptoms, 188
Normoglycemia
blood glucose range for, 417

improved ICU patient outcomes with, 417

Normovolemia, urine electrolyte values with, 430–431

Nosocomial infections
antibiotic resistance and, 199
enterococci, 199–200
Pseudomonas spp., 204–205
Staphylococcus spp., 199

Novarel, false positive pregnancy test with, 424

NPH insulin, protamine administration risks and, 233

Nuclear imaging (*see also specific modality*)
for gastrointestinal bleeding localization, 313–314
radiotracer criteria, 314
pulmonary, for inhalation injury, 45

Nucleic acid amplification (NAT) test, for blood transfusion screening, 435

Nurse anesthetist, addressing properly, 171

Nylon suture, for laceration repair
facial, 26, 55
lip, 21
in young child, 25

O

O antigens, in ABO blood groups, 436, 436t

Obese patients, morbidly
abdominal sepsis in, 398–399
femoral vessel cannulation technique for, 269–270
surgical treatment complications, 355, 398–399

Observation
for intra-abdominal trauma, in children, 325–326
for knee dislocation, rule out vascular injury, 27–28

Obstruction(s)
of drains, 259
gastric outlet, stomach dilatation with, 347
of nasogastric tubes, 253–254
small bowel
common etiologies, 349
gastric dilatation with, 347

hernias causing, 349–353
incarcerated hernia causing, 335–336
in infants, 91–92
of surgical feeding jejunostomy, 133

Obturator hernia, 349–350

Obturator nerve, 350

Occult fecal blood, guaiac test for, 332
in colorectal cancer screening, 333–334

Occult gastric blood, test kit for, 426

Occupational exposures
bloodborne infection transmission, 98, 98t
expert consultation for, 98, 100
post exposure prophylaxis for, 100
prevention of
in emergency room, 100–101
in operating room, 170
to viral infections, 98, 100

Occupational transmission, of bloodborne pathogens, 97–98, 98t
response to, 98

Ocular injuries (*see* Ophthalmologic trauma)

Oncologic procedures, leg preps for, 110

Ondansetron (Zofran), 235

Operating room (OR)
etiquette for
communication, 171
instrument, 170
injections protocol, 114
intubated patient repositioning, 116
patient positioning rules, 111–113
patient preps for (*see* Surgical preps)

Ophthalmologic surgery consult, for ophthalmologic trauma, 51, 53

Ophthalmologic trauma
in children, 52
emergency room management of, 51–53
vision threatening
emergency room management of, 51–53, *52*
ophthalmologic surgery consult, 51, 53

Opiates/opioids
delirious withdrawal reaction to, 385
for postoperative pain, 394

Oral cavity, bacterial infection of, Ludwig's angina with, 87–88

Oral immunosuppressive medications, converting to intravenous dosages, 181–183, 182t
Oral surgeon consult, for facial lacerations, 56
Orbicularis oris muscle, in lip laceration repair, 21
Organophosphate cholinesterase inhibitors, antidote for, 237–238, 238t
Organ transplantation (*see also specific organ*)
    drug-induced nephrotoxicity cautions, 186–187
    immunosuppressive drugs for
        IV versus PO dosages, 181–183, 182t
        St. John's wort contraindication, 184
    recipients of, bloodborne infections in, 97
Oropharyngeal edema, endotracheal intubation for, 374
Orotracheal tube, for airway, with facial fractures, 61
Osmolality
    in hypernatremia management, 381–382
    urine, in prerenal state versus intrinsic renal dysfunction, 431t
Osmolarity, serum, post-bladder distention, 257
Osteomyelitis, vertebral, 395–397
Otolaryngology consult, for facial lacerations, 56
Ototoxicity
    of aminoglycosides, 190, 190t, 196–197
    miscellaneous drug-related, 190
    of vancomycin, 196
Ovary(ies)
    incarcerated, in children, 337
    torsion of, 337
Overcoagulation
    antidotes for, 233, 321
        warfarin management, 318–319
    retroperitoneal bleeding related to, 318
    vitamin K for, 227–228, 238t, 241
Overdose (*see* Alcohol overdose; Drug overdose)

Oversedation
    of ICU patients, 415
    reversal agents for, 238t, 239–240
Over-the-counter medications, organ transplant cautions, 184
Overwhelming postsplenectomy sepsis (OPSS)
    antibiotic prophylaxis for, 209
    causative organisms, 208
    characteristics of, 207
    diagnosis of, 208
    incidence of, 207–208
    patient education on, 209
    preoperative vaccines for, 207, 208–209
Oxacillin, for bite wounds, 36
Oxazalidinones, for vancomycin-resistant enterococci, 201
Oxycodone, for postoperative pain, 394
Oxygen
    100% supplementary, for air embolism, 287
    hyperbaric (*see* Hyperbaric oxygen therapy)
    partial pressure of, 280
        arterial, 279–281
Oxygen consumption, peripheral, 290
Oxygen saturation
    endotracheal intubation indications, 375
    pulmonary artery (mixed venous), 290

P
Pacemakers, cardiac
    for beta-blocker toxicity, 242
    for digoxin toxicity, 240
    implantable, preoperative investigation of, 364–365
    temporary
        for pulmonary artery catheter-induced heart block, 291
        types of, 291
Packing
    compression, for traumatic hepatic hemorrhage, venous, 120–123
    wound
        for drained abscesses, 34–35
        for infected wounds, 300–301
Paclitaxel (Taxol)
    inadvertent extravascular administration of, 174
    IV administration reactions, 227

Padding, for positioning anesthetized patient, 111–112

Pain
aortic dissection and, 6
appendicitis characteristics, 341–342
with arterial injuries, 27
back
infectious etiologies workup for, 395–397
retroperitoneal bleeding and, 320
ruptured abdominal aortic aneurysm and, 2
blunt sternal trauma and, 11–12
chest (*see* Angina)
compartment syndrome evaluation, 19
with incarcerated inguinal hernia reduction, 336
neck
infectious etiologies workup for, 395–397
in trauma evaluation, 68
with necrotizing fasciitis, 378–379
needlestick, acupressure for, 370
postoperative
complications related to, 392–394
inadequate control of, 394
retroperitoneal bleeding and, 320
ruptured abdominal aortic aneurysm and, 2, 5
wound infections and, 300–301, 304

Pain control (*see also specific agent*)
for amputation reimplantation, 39
for frostbite, 49
for ICU patients, oversedation cautions, 415–416
inadequate postoperative, 394
post-abdominal surgery, 354–355

Pain perception, neurophysiology of, 370

Pallor, with arterial injuries, 27

Pancreas, injuries to, blunt chest trauma and, 11

Pancreaticoduodenal arteries, 117

Pancreaticoduodenectomy, biliary reconstruction with, 118

Pancreatitis, necrotizing, fungal infection prophylaxis for, 210

Panendoscopy, of aerodigestive tract, for anterior neck mass, 406

Papaverine, 114

Parenchyma
disease of, urine electrolyte alterations with, 430–431, 431t
disruption in liver trauma, 119
venous bleeding with, 119–122
left renal vein relationship to, 136

Parenteral nutrition, dedicated central venous catheter for, 262

Parotid duct
anatomic sections of, 54, *55*
laceration of, surgical repair of, 54–56

Parotid gland, anatomical location of, 54

Paroxetine (Paxil), 214–215

Partial pressure of arterial oxygen (PaO_2), 279–281

Partial pressure of oxygen (PO_2), 280

Partial thromboplastin time (PTT)
acquired factor VIII inhibitor results, 428–429
coagulation measures, 427
mixing study outcomes, 427–428
normal prothrombin time and, 427

Pasteurella spp., in animal bite wounds, 37

Patient competency
in disputed patient care issues, 363
psychiatric evaluation for, 360–361

Patient-controlled analgesia (PCA), 415
commonly used medications, 368
compartment syndrome masked by, 20
meperidine toxicity cautions, 188
naloxone at bedside for, 368–369

Patient education
on medication contraindications, 184, 187
for overwhelming postsplenectomy sepsis, 208–209

Patient positioning (*see* Positioning)

PCP (phencyclidine), delirious reactions to, 385

Peak and trough levels
for antibiotics, 195–198, 197t
for immunosuppressants, 433–434

Peau d'orange, 95

Pelvic ring, fractures of, *66*, 66–67
urethral injuries with, 73–74

Pelvis
procedures on, bladder differentiation for, 149–150
retroperitoneal hematomas and, 82–84, *83*

Penetrating trauma
  complete examination of, 59–60
  foreign object removal, 81
  to liver, bleeding control strategies,
    122–124
Penicillin(s)
  for bite wounds, 36–37
  CNS side effects of, 191
  factor VIII inhibitor associated with,
    429
  for overwhelming postsplenectomy
    sepsis, 208–209
  P. aeruginosa resistance to, 204–205
Penicillin G, prophylactic, for open
    fractures, 17
Peptic ulcers, gastrointestinal bleeding
    from, 312–313, 322–323
Percutaneous decompression, for
    retroperitoneal bleeding, 321
Perforation
  colonic, contrast studies for, 338–339
  esophageal, 330–331
  gastrointestinal, corticosteroids and,
    339
  intestinal, 71
    Chance fracture and, 72
    femoral vessel cannulation cautions,
      269
Perianal abscess, 32t
Pericardial effusion, post-abdominal
    surgery, 354–355
Pericardial tamponade, with central vein
    wall rupture, 282
Pericolic gutter hematomas, 82–83, *83*
Perineal examination
  for posterior urethral injury, 74
  for traumatic injuries, 59–60
Perioperative management
  of beta-blockers, 217
  of long-term anticoagulation therapy,
    318–319
  thromboembolism risks during,
    104–105, 319
Perioperative mortality, of cirrhotic
    patients based on class, 345
Perirectal abscesses
  comorbidities with, 31, 33
  Fournier's gangrene with, 32–33
  infection severity spectrum, 31
  mortality rate, 31

surgical drainage of, 31–32, *32*
types of, 31, 32t
Peritoneum
  abdominal aortic aneurysm rupture
    into, 3, 5
  free air in, 125, 339
  lavage of, in laparoscopic
    appendectomy, 152
Peritonitis
  fungal infection prophylaxis for, 210
  high-density barium contrast studies
    causing, 338
  with incarcerated inguinal hernia,
    335–336
  in morbidly obese patient, 398–399
  post-abdominal surgery, 355
  traumatic causes of, 71
Personality changes, quinolones and, 192
Personal names, etiquette regarding, 171
Personal protective equipment, for
    emergency room examinations,
    97–98
Pertussis immunization, childhood
    protocol for, 47
Pharmacokinetics
  factors influencing, 434
  terminology for, 433
Phencyclidine (PCP), delirious reactions
    to, 385
Phenelzine (Nardil), 215
Phenobarbital, for transplant patients,
    IV versus PO dosages, 183
Phentolamine mesylate (Regitene), for
    extravasation necrosis
    prevention, 174
Phenytoin sodium (Dilantin)
  cyclosporine contraindication, 183
  factor VIII inhibitor associated with,
    429
  IV administration cautions, 231–232
  pharmacokinetics of, 231
  for transplant patients, IV versus PO
    dosages, 183
Phlebitis (*see* Deep vein thrombosis
    (DVT); Thrombophlebitis)
Phlebotomy, postoperative
    contraindications, 366
Phosphodiesterase type 5 (PDE-5), in
    sexual stimulation physiology,
    212

Phosphorus, serum, rhabdomyolysis
impact on, 90
Phrenic vein, inferior, left renal vein
relationship to, 135
Physical examination
for anterior neck mass, 406
complete, for traumatic injuries,
59–60
Physical restraints
for combative patient, with hepatic
encephalopathy, 383
essential order requirements, 383
Physiologic stress
Addisonian insufficiency related to,
401–402
patient risks for (*see* Intensive care
unit (ICU) patients)
Physostigmine, for atropine reversal,
238, 238t
Piperacillin, *P. aeruginosa* resistance to,
204
Piperacillin-tazobactam, for
vancomycin-resistant
enterococci, 200
Plain gut suture, for laceration repair, in
young child, 25
Plasma cell mastitis, 94
Plasmapheresis, for acquired factor VIII
inhibitor, 426
Plastic surgery consult
for amputated body part, 38–39
for lip laceration repair, 22
for ophthalmologic trauma, 51, 53
Platelet count
ampicillin-sulbactam effect on, 244
in heparin-induced
thrombocytopenia, 225–226
Platelet factor four (PF4), 225
Platelet transfusions, for retroperitoneal
bleeding, 321
Pleural effusions, drainage cautions,
257
Pleural fluid analysis, for esophageal
perforation diagnosis, 330
Pleural space
chest tube placement into, 249–252
complications of, post-abdominal
surgery, 354–355
Pleurevac-tubing connection, avoid
breaking, 251

Plicamycin (Mithracin), inadvertent
extravascular administration of,
174
Pneumococcal vaccine, preoperative,
207, 209
Pneumococci, antibiotic resistance of,
199, 209
Pneumonia
aspirated teeth causing, 58
community-acquired, 199, 209
post-abdominal surgery, 354
Pneumoperitoneum, 125, 339
Pneumothorax
from central venous catheterization,
275, 277
chest radiograph indications,
288–289, *289*
chest trauma and, 10, 66
tension, *289*
PO immunosuppressive medications,
converting to intravenous
dosages, 181–183, 182t
Poison(s), antidotes for, 237
Polar arteries, inferior
infrarenal inferior vena cava
relationship to, 138
retroperitoneal surgery cautions,
138–139
Polydioxanone (PDS) suture, for fascial
suturing, 169
Polyethoxylated castor oil (Cremophor
EL), 227
Popliteal artery injuries, with knee
dislocations, 27–28
Porta hepatis, in Pringle maneuver, 123
Portal hypertension
abdominal surgery risks with, 345–346
gastrointestinal bleeding with, 322–323
Portal hypertensive gastropathy, 323
Portal triad, in Pringle maneuver, 123
Portal vein
injuries to, laparoscopic treatment of,
125
in Pringle maneuver, 120, 123
traumatic hematoma of, 82, *83*
Positioning
of anesthetized patient
general rules for, 111
specific recommendations for,
111–113

for central venous catheterization, 273, 275, 279
 removal or replacement, 286–287
for chest tube placement, 249
for rectal examination, 332
Positive end–expiration pressure (PEEP), for pulmonary artery rupture tamponade, 295
Positive-pressure ventilation, endotracheal intubation for, 374
Postanal abscess, 32t
Posterior urethral injury, in males, 73–74
Post exposure prophylaxis, for needlesticks, 100
Postoperative fever, differential diagnosis of, 304
Postoperative pain
 complications related to, 392–394
 inadequate control of, 394
Postoperative recovery, undiagnosed complication presentations, 392–393
Postphlebitic syndrome, 104
Potassium, serum
 decreased, digoxin toxicity and, 240–241
 elevated
  compartment syndrome and, 153
  Kayexalate-sorbitol enemas for, 179–180
 rhabdomyolysis impact on, 90
Prednisolone, for transplant patients, IV versus PO dosages, 182, 182t
Prednisone, for transplant patients, IV versus PO dosages, 182, 182t
Pregnancy/pregnant patient
 factor VIII inhibitor associated with, 429
 laparoscopic procedure contraindication, 125
 perfusion indicators in, 63
 testing guidelines, 424
Pregnancy testing
 false positives with, 424
 guidelines for, 424
Pregnyl, false positive pregnancy test with, 424
Prekallikrein
 in clotting cascade, 427
 deficiency testing of, 427

Preload, 293
Preoperative evaluation
 of coagulation status, 427–428
 of pregnancy status, 424
Preoperative marking, for excisional biopsies, 161–162
Prerenal state, urine electrolyte alterations with, 430–431, 431t
Pressure points, on anesthetized patient, 112
Primary closure, for esophageal perforations, 331
Primary sclerosing cholangitis (PSC), 186
Pringle maneuver, 120, 123
P-R interval, verapamil effects on, 230
Probiotic therapy, for patient on antibiotics, 192–194
Profasi, false positive pregnancy test with, 424
Professional titles, etiquette regarding, 171
Prolene (polypropylene) suture
 for fascial suturing, 169
 for laceration repair
  facial, 26
  lip, 21
  scalp, 79
  in young child, 25
Prone positioning, for acute lung disorders, 414
Propofol, rhabdomyolysis related to, 89
Prostate, enlargement of, catheter placement cautions, 255
Prostate exam, rectal examination in, 332–333
Prosthetic graft material, infection risks with, 109
Prosthetic heart valves
 Lactobacillus infections of, 192
 mechanical, perioperative thromboembolic risks, 319
Protamine sulfate
 for heparin reversal, 233, 238t, 239
 monitored administration of, 233
Protein C resistance, deep vein thrombosis risks, 104–105
Prothrombin complex, for acquired factor VIII inhibitor, 428

Prothrombin time (PT)
  partial thromboplastin time versus, 427–429
  vitamin K effect on, 241
Proton pump inhibitors, for "stress gastritis" prevention, 323
"P's," of arterial injuries, 27
Pseudoaneurysm
  femoral artery, percutaneous thrombin for, 146
  pulmonary artery, as balloon complication, 295
Pseudomembranous colitis, 193, 202
Pseudomonas aeruginosa
  antibiotic resistance of, 204–205
  infectious properties of, 204
  nosocomial infections of, 204
  sepsis, two-drug regimen for, 205
Psychiatric evaluation, for patient competency, 360–361
Pubic rami, fractures of, 67
  urethral injuries with, 73
Pulmonary artery
  aortic trauma and, 9
  pressure measurements in, 290, 293
  rupture of, with balloon inflation, 295
Pulmonary artery (PA) catheter
  balloon manipulation cautions, 293–295, *294*
  bundle-branch block cautions, 290–292
  complications of, 290, 293, 295
  indications for, 290
Pulmonary capillary wedge pressure, 290, 293
  balloon manipulation cautions, 293–295, *294*
Pulmonary contusion, chest trauma and, 66
Pulmonary edema, reeexpansion, 257
Pulmonary embolism (PE)
  perioperative risks, 104–105, 319
  postoperative
    abdominal surgery, 354, 399
    prophylaxis for, 104–106
  signs and symptoms of, 388
Pulmonary hypertension, protamine risk for, 233
Pulmonary scans, radioisotope, for inhalation injury, 45

Pulselessness, with arterial injuries, 27
Pulse oximetry, post-abdominal surgery indications, 357
Punch biopsies, 164, 166
"Purple glove" syndrome, 231
P waves, normal, 376

Q
QRS complex, normal versus ischemic, 376
Quinolones
  for bite wounds, 36–37
  CNS side effects of, 190, 190t
Quinupristin-dalfopristin (Synercid), for vancomycin-resistant enterococci, 200–201

R
Rabies prophylaxis, for animal bites, 52
Radial artery
  Allen's test for patency, 371–372
    reliability limitations, 372
  cannulation of, 371–372, *372*
Radial nerve injury
  in elbow dislocations, 15–16
  in humeral fractures, 15–16
Radical mastectomy, avoid arm procedures following, 366–367
Radiography
  of aspirated teeth, 57, *58*
  of blunt sternal trauma, 11, 65–66
  chest (*see* Chest radiograph (CXR))
  C-spine, for neck trauma evaluation, 68–70
  for esophageal perforation evaluation, 330
  of gastric dilatation, 347, *348*
  of great vessel trauma, 8, 10, *11*, 66
  intravascular contrast, metformin administration recommendations, 223–224
  of lumbar spine fracture, 72
  for midgut volvulus, in infants, 91
  for nasogastric tube placement, 254
  pelvic, for fall injuries, 67
  for peritonitis, in postoperative obese patients, 398–399
  of seat belt-related trauma, 71–72
Radio-iodinated contrast nephropathy, 431

Radioisotopes
commercial kits of, 313
diagnostic applications of (*see* Nuclear imaging)
Radiologist consult, for gastrointestinal bleeding localization, 314
Rainey clips, for scalp lacerations, 77
Range of motion
exercises, for frostbite, 50
in neck trauma evaluation, 68–69
Rash, maculopapular, adverse drug reactions causing, 177
Recombinant factor VIIa, for acquired factor VIII inhibitor, 428
Rectal examination
for posterior urethral injury, 74
routine screening, for colorectal cancer, 333–334
technique for, 332
Rectal sphincters
anatomy of, 332
inter-sphincteric abscess of, 32t
Recurrent (multiloculated) hernia, 336, 351
Red blood cells
radiolabeled, for gastrointestinal bleeding localization, 313–314
transfusions of
compatibility rules, 434, 434t
for intra-abdominal trauma in children, 326
"Red man" syndrome, 177, 195
Red rubber catheter, placement in Witzel jejunostomy, 132–133
Reentrant arrhythmias, verapamil-associated, 230
Reexploration surgery, for traumatic hepatic hemorrhage, 123
Reflux surgery, stomach dilatation associated with, 347
Renal arteries
accessory
infrarenal inferior vena cava relationship to, 138
retroperitoneal surgery cautions, 138–139
preoperative determination modalities, 139
traumatic hematoma of, 83, *83*
Renal colic, ruptured abdominal aortic aneurysm versus, 5

"Renal dose" dopamine
nonbeneficial in surgical patients, 221
side effects of, 221–222
Renal failure (*see also* Kidney transplant)
in nephrotoxic insult with cirrhosis, 186–187
rhabdomyolysis causing, 90
in surgical patients, "renal dose" dopamine for, 221
Renal function
aminoglycoside dosing and, 197, 197t
cirrhotic ascites comordidity, 186
urine electrolytes indication of, 428
diuretics impact on, 430–432
prerenal state versus intrinsic renal dysfunction, 431t
Renal insufficiency
demerol toxicity cautions, 188
iodine contrast nephrotoxicity risks, 219–220
Renal malignancies, retroperitoneal bleeding related to, 320
Renal veins, left
abdominal aortic surgery cautions, 136
complex anatomy of, 135–136
Renin-angiotensin axis, ascites role, 345–346
Reperfusion therapy, AHA recommendations, 377
Reporting requirements
for animal bites, 52
for child abuse suspicion, 52
for domestic violence, 52
Resection, for esophageal perforations, 331
Resident staff, ruptured abdominal aortic aneurysm management, 4
Respiratory depression, with narcotic infusions, 368–369
Respiratory distress
endotracheal intubation for, 374–375
with gastric dilatation, 347
post-abdominal surgery, 354–355
Restraint (*see* Physical restraints)
Restrictive devices, abdominal circumferential, ventilator weaning contraindication, 412
Resuscitation
ACLS protocols, 407
cardiopulmonary (*see* Cardiopulmonary resuscitation (CPR))

drug choices for, with implanted cardiac devices, 365
fluid (*see* Fluid resuscitation)
Retinitis pigmentosa, Viagra cautions, 213
Retroduodenal arteries, 117
Retrograde urethrogram, for male urethral injury evaluation, 74
Retroperitoneal hematomas
    serial imaging for bleeding localization, 320
    signs and symptoms of, 320
    traumatic, management of, 82, 84
    Zone 1, 82, *83*
    Zone 2, 82–83, *83*
    Zone 3, *83*, 83–84
Retroperitoneum
    abdominal aortic aneurysm rupture into, 3, 5
    bleeding into
        diagnosis of, 320
        hematoma with, 82, 84, 321
        mortality rate, 321
        signs and symptoms of, 320
        treatment of, 321
    vascular anomalies found in, 138–139
Retropubic space, bladder wall landmark, 149–150
Retroviruses (*see also* Human immunodeficiency virus (HIV))
    blood transfusion screening for, 435
Revascularization procedures, for mycotic aneurysm, 29
Reversal agents (*see* Antidotes; *specific agent*)
Reverse Trendelenberg position, for anesthetized patient, 113
Rewarming, of frostbite tissue, 49
Rhabdomyolysis
    diagnosis of, 89–90
    etiologies of, 89
    management of, 90
Rh antigens, in ABO blood groups, 434
Ribs
    chest tube placement and, 249–250, *250*
    fractures of, great vessel injuries with, 8–9, 66
Richter's hernia, 335
Rifampin
    for *C. difficile* colitis, 193, 203

for vancomycin-resistant enterococci, 200–201
Right bundle-branch block (RBBB)
    nonpathologic, 377
    from pulmonary artery catheter, 290–291

S
Sacroiliac joint, traumatic disruption of, 67
Sacrum
    fractures of, 67
    retroperitoneal hematomas and, 82–84, *83*
Saddle fractures, urethra injury with, 73
Saddle-type injuries, to urethra, 73
Safety precautions
    for anesthetized patient positioning
        general rules for, 111
        moving/repositioning, 116
        specific recommendations for, 111–113
    for med injections by surgical team, 114
St. John's wort, coadministration contraindications, 184
Sales representatives, consultation on implanted cardiac devices, 364–365
Saline gauze
    for abscess packing, 34–35
    for amputated body parts, 38, 40
        reimplantation wound dressing, 39
    for eyelid laceration, 52–53
Saline intravenous fluids
    for iodine contrast nephrotoxicity, 219–220
    for myoglobinuria, 89–90
Saline preservation procedure, for amputated body parts, 38, 40
Saline solution, for amputated body parts, 38
    freezing cautions, 40
Salt-wasting, urine electrolytes
    indication of, 430–431
    diuretics impact on, 430–431
Saphenous vein
    as graft conduit, 109
    venous cutdown of, 156–157
Sarcoidosis, of breasts, 95
Satinsky vascular clamp, 142

Scalp
  lacerations of
    bleeding control, 77–78
    deep, 77, *78*
    full-thickness, 79
    galea closure for, 79–80
  tissue layers of, 79
  traumatic amputation of, 38
Scapula, fractures of, 9
Sciatic nerve injuries, with IM
        injections, 176
Scrub nurse, Mayo stand responsibility,
        170
Seat belts
  three-point, 12
  two-point, 71
Seat belt sign, 71
Seborrheic keratoses, shave biopsy of, 165
Secondary intention, in wound healing,
        300, 307
Second degree (partial-thickness) burns,
        of dorsal foot, 43, *44*
Second-degree heart block, verapamil-
        associated, 229–230
"Second look" operation, for necrotizing
        soft tissue infection, 304, 380
Sedatives/sedation
  of ICU patients
    continuous infusion protocols, 415
    emergence time strategies, 415
    for mechanical ventilation
        management, 415–416
  reversal agents for, 238t, 239, 240
Seizures
  Cerebyx for, 232
  Dilantin for, 231
  drug-related, 188, 190–191
Seldinger technique
  check for venous versus arterial blood,
        279–281
  complications of, 277, 281
  dilator insertion, 282–283
  for femoral vessel cannulation, 269
  guidewire control during, 277–278, *278*
  for right internal jugular vein catheter
        placement, 273–274
  vena cava filter cautions, 271–272
Selective serotonin reuptake inhibitors
        (SSRIs)
  monoamine oxidase inhibitor
        contraindication, 215

oxazalidinones cautions, 201
  prodrug analgesia compatibility, 214
Selegiline (Deprenyl), 215
Senior staff
  asking for help from, 408–409
  notification of, for ruptured AAA, 3–4
Sensorium, altered, intra-abdominal
        trauma assessment with, 76
Sentinel (herald) bleeding,
        gastrointestinal, 315, 317
Sepsis
  abdominal (*see* Peritonitis)
  Addisonian insufficiency versus, in
        ICU patient, 401–402
  arterial fistulae causing, 315
  catheter-related
    IV sites, 390–391
    prevention of, 264–265
    with TPN, 262
  intra-abdominal, enterocutaneous
        fistulae with, 130
  overwhelming postsplenectomy,
        207–209
  P. aeruginosa, two-drug regimen for,
        205
Serotonin, physiologic effects of, 235
Serotonin agonists, vasodilation caused
        by, 235
Serotonin antagonists, vasoconstriction
        caused by, 235
Serotonin receptors, in migraine
        management, 235
Serotonin reuptake inhibitors, 385
Serotonin syndrome, central, 215, 385
Sertraline (Zoloft), 214–215
Sexual enhancement products, nitrates
        caution, 213
Sexual trauma
  complete examination of, 59–60
  human bites as, 36–37
Sharps disposal
  emergency room, 100–101
  operating room, 170
Shave biopsies, 164
  melanoma contraindication,
        165–166
  of skin lesions, 165
Shaving, for laceration repair
  eyebrow, 23
  scalp, 79
Shear stress, in fascial suturing, 168

Shock
  hemorrhagic
    intracranial injury outcomes and, 63–64
    from scalp wounds, 77–78
    treatment of, 63–64
  life-threatening causes of, 77
  nonhemorrhagic causes of, 63
  signs of impending, 63
Shoulder dislocation
  axillary nerve injuries in, 14–15
  musculocutaneous nerve injuries in, 16
Sick sinus syndrome, 229
Sigmoidoscopy, for ischemic colitis, postoperative, 344
Sildenafil (Viagra)
  half-life of, 213
  nitrates contraindication, 212–213
  vasodilatation actions of, 212
Silent myocardial infarction, 386
Silver sulfadiazine (Silvadene)
  for burns, of dorsal foot, 43
  for frostbite, 50
Single-lumen catheters
  guidewire choice for, 278
  indications for, 264
  for parenteral nutrition, 262
  stopcocks for, 265
Sinoatrial (SA) node, depolarization physiology, 229
Sirolimus (Rapamune)
  cyclosporine interactions with, 182
  St. John's wort contraindication, 184
  for transplant patients, IV versus PO dosages, 182
SiteRite, for central vessel cannulation, 279
Skeletal muscle trauma, myoglobinuria with, 89–90
Skin allergic reactions, to medications, 177
Skin fragility
  adhesive tape contraindication, 403–404
  causes of, 403–404
Skin grafts
  for dorsal foot burns, 43
  for fasciotomy closure, 155
  full thickness, for amputation reimplantation, 38
  split-thickness, VAC system and, 302

Skin laceration, with open fractures, 17
Skin lesions, biopsies of, 164–166
Skin tags, shave biopsy of, 165
Skin tears, from adhesive tape, 403–404
Skull base fractures, nasotracheal/nasogastric intubation contraindications, 61
Sliding knots, in fascial suturing, 168
Slip knots, in fascial suturing, 169
Small bowel
  aortic fistula to, 315–316
  bleeding from, nuclear imaging localization of, 313–314
  distinguishing landmarks of, 128
  hernias affecting
    incidence of, 349–350
    manual reduction of, 352–353
      contraindications to, 351
    physical examination of, 349–350
    signs and symptoms of rarer, 350–351, *352*
  obstruction of
    common etiologies, 349
    gastric dilatation with, 347
    hernias causing, 349–353
    incarcerated hernia causing, 335–336
    in infants, 91–92
  perforation injuries of, 71
Smoke
  inhaled, physiologic toxicity of, 45
  tobacco (*see* Cigarette smoking)
Snake bites, rhabdomyolysis with, 89
Sodium, serum, in hypernatremia management, 381–382
Sodium bicarbonate
  intravenous, for life-threatening hyperkalemia, 180
  for iodine contrast nephrotoxicity, 220
  for myoglobinuria, 90
Sodium excretion, renal, with diuretics, 431, 431t
Sodium polystyrene sulfonate (Kayexalate)
  enemas
    alternatives to, 180
    colonic necrosis from, 179
    proper administration of, 179–180
  kidney transplant contraindication, 179

Sodium thiosulfate, for extravasation necrosis prevention, 175
Soft tissue infection (*see also specific infection*)
crepitus associated with, 378–380
necrotizing, 304
"second look" operation for, 304, 380
wound infections and, 300–301
Soft tissue trauma
blunt chest trauma and, 10, *11*, 65–66
frostbite evaluation, 49–51
with open fractures, 17
smoking impact on, 41
Soil contamination, of wounds, tetanus prophylaxis for, 48
Solubilizing agent, in intravenous vitamin K anaphylaxis, 227
SonoSite, for central vessel cannulation, 279
Sorbitol
for hyperkalemia management (*see* Kayexalate-sorbitol enema)
laxative uses, 179
Space of Retzius, bladder wall landmark, 149
Specialty practitioners (*see also specific discipline*)
importance of consulting with, 408–409
Sphenoid fractures, 61–62
Sphincters, rectal
anatomy of, 332
inter-sphincteric abscess of, 32t
Spigelian hernia, 349–351
Spinal cord compression, with vertebral infections, 396–397
Spinal cord injury without radiologic abnormality (SCIWORA), 69
Spinal fractures
cervical, clinical clearance of, 68–69
lumbar, 72
noncervical, C-spine fractures associated with, 69
Spinal osteomyelitis, 395–397
Spinal reconstruction, for vertebral osteomyelitis, 397
Splenectomy, overwhelming sepsis following
antibiotic prophylaxis for, 209
causative organisms, 208

characteristics of, 207
diagnosis of, 208
incidence of, 207–208
patient education on, 209
preoperative vaccines for, 207, 208–209
Splinting, of hand injuries, 42
Squamous cell cancer
of anterior neck, 406
of breast, 95
shave biopsy of, 165
Square knots, in fascial suturing, 168–169
Stab wounds
knife removal guidelines, 81
tetanus prophylaxis for, 47
Staphylococcus aureus
methicillin-resistant, 199
in vertebral osteomyelitis, 396
Staphylococcus infection
in Ludwig's angina, 87
in mastitis, 93
in mycotic aneurysm, 30
wound infection and, 301
Staples (*see* Surgical staples)
Statins, rhabdomyolysis related to, 89
Stenosis, of cannulated veins, in hemodialysis patients, 266–267
Stensen's duct stent, for parotid duct injuries, 54, *55*
Stents
for central venous occlusion, 267
endovascular, for abdominal aortic aneurysm, 139, 315–316, 344
esophageal, for perforations, 331
Stensen's, for parotid duct injuries, 54, *55*
for vascular injuries evaluation, 146
Sterile dressing, for central venous catheter site, 265
Sterile procedure
for central venous catheter insertion, 265, 273
for chest tube insertion, 251–252
Sterile water, intravenous, hypernatremia contraindication, 381–382
Steristrips, in facial laceration repair, 26
Sternal fractures
body area involved, 10
cardiovascular injuries with, 10–11, *11*, 66

diagnosis of, 11–12
manubrium sterni, 10
myocardial contusion with, 10, 12
operative management of, 12
thoracic visceral injuries with, 11–12
xiphoid process, 10–11
Steroids (*see* Corticosteroids)
Stevens-Johnson syndrome, 177–178
Stomach
aspirate of, blood testing for, 426
decompression of
for facial and skull trauma, 61
vasovagal reactions with, 258
dilatation of, 347, *348*
disorders of (*see* Gastric *entries*)
intraoperative differentiation of, 150
Stool testing, for *C. difficile* colitis, 193,
202
Stopcocks, for central line lumen ports,
265
Streptococcus infection
in Ludwig's angina, 87
in mycotic aneurysm, 30
in necrotizing soft tissue infection, 304
wound infection and, 301, 379
Streptococcus pneumoniae, in
overwhelming postsplenectomy
sepsis, 208
antibiotics for, 208–209
preoperative vaccine for, 207, 209
Streptogramins, for vancomycin-
resistant enterococci, 200–201
"Stress gastritis," in ICU patients, 323
Strictures
common bile duct repair and, 117–118
with enterotomy repair, 130
Stridor, with Ludwig's angina, 87
Stroke
perioperative, prophylactic beta-
blockers for, 216
Viagra cautions, 212
Stroke volume, 293
Subareolar abscess, recurring, 94
Subcapsular hematoma, in liver trauma,
119
Subclavian artery
aortic trauma and, 8, 65
inadvertent catheterization of, 279, 281
Subclavian veins, catheterization of
dialysis contraindication, 266–267
for parenteral nutrition, 262

Subcutaneous (SQ) medications,
inadvertent IV administration of,
175–176
Subspecialty practitioners (*see also
specific discipline*)
importance of consulting with,
408–409
Succession splash, 347, *348*
Sucralfate, for "stress gastritis"
prevention, 323
Suction
for Jackson-Pratt drains, 260, *261*
for nasogastric tubes, proper
functioning of, 253–254
Sulbactam (Unasyn), for bite wounds, 37
Sulfa drugs, factor VIII inhibitor
associated with, 431
Sumatriptan succinate (Imitrex), 235
Sump port function, for nasogastric
tubes, 253–254
Superior mesenteric artery (SMA)
occlusion of, in infants, 91–92
traumatic hematoma of, 82, *83*
Superior mesenteric vein (SMV)
occlusion of, in infants, 91–92
traumatic hematoma of, 82, *83*
Superior vena cava (SVC), traumatic
injuries of, 10
Supralevator abscess, 32t
Supramesocolic hematomas, 82, *83*
Surgery (*see also specific anatomy or
procedure*)
Addisonian insufficiency related to, 401
DVT prophylaxis for, 104–106
medical management concerns (*see*
Perioperative *entries*)
prolonged, rhabdomyolysis with, 89
Surgical clips, for hemostasis, 140–141
stapling devices and, 140–141
vascular clamp cautions, 140
Surgical drainage (*see* Incision and
drainage (I and D))
Surgical preps
chlorhexidine solution cautions, 107
for extremity vascular procedure,
109–110
Surgical staples
facial laceration repair and, 26
for fasciotomy closure, 155
gastric anastomosis leaks with,
398–399

for laparoscopic appendectomy, 152
surgical clip cautions, 140–141
for traumatic hepatic hemorrhage, 122
for urologic procedures, 147–148
Surgical team
anesthesia members of, 171
med injections protocol, 114
permission to move intubated patient,
116
Suture and suturing
absorbable
for bladder or ureter, 147
types of, 25
use in children, 25, 26
anchoring
of central lines, 284, *285*
of chest tubes, 251
of excisional biopsies, 161–162
for fascial dehiscence prevention,
168–169
for laceration repair
eyebrow, 23–24
facial, 26, 54–56
lip, 21–22
scalp, 79–80
young child, 25
nonabsorbable
types of, 21
urologic contraindications, 21
for traumatic hepatic hemorrhage, 122
Swan-Ganz catheter
balloon manipulation cautions,
293–295, *294*
bundle-branch block cautions, 290–292
cardiac pacing capabilities of, 291
complications of, 290, 293, 295
indications for, 290
Symphis pubis
bladder wall relationship, 149–150
disruption injuries of, 67
urethral injuries with, 73
Syndrome of inappropriate antidiuretic
hormone secretion (SIADH),
urine electrolyte alterations with,
430–431
Syphilis, of breasts, 95
Systemic reactions, to IV
anticonvulsants, 231–232
Systemic vascular resistance, 290, 293
verapamil effects on, 229

T
Tachycardia
implanted cardiac devices and,
364–365
intraoperative etiologies of, 114
persistent post-abdominal surgery,
354–355
anastomotic complications and,
398–399
Tachypnea, persistent post-abdominal
surgery, 354–355
Tacrolimus (Prograf)
cytochrome metabolism of, 182
peak and trough levels for, 433–434
sildenafil inhibition by, 213
St. John's wort contraindication,
184
for transplant patients
IV versus PO dosages, 181–182
magnesium depletion and seizures,
232
Tadalafil (Cialis), nitrates
contraindication, 213
Tamponade
cardiac, 10
from central venous catheterization,
277, 288
for hemorrhaging tracheostomy, 316
pericardial, with central vein wall
rupture, 282
for pulmonary artery rupture, 295
with retroperitoneal bleeding, 321
Tamsulosin (Flomax), 213
Tape burns, 403
T-cell lymphotropic virus type 1
(HTLV-1), blood transfusion
screening for, 435
Td immunization, 47
Technetium-99m (^{99m}Tc) scan, for
gastrointestinal bleeding
localization, 313
delayed, 314
Teeth
abscessed, Ludwig's angina with,
87–88
accounting for, in maxillofacial
trauma, 57–58
aspirated, 57, *58*
discoloration, tetracyline-related,
190–191, 190t

Tenderness, wound infections and, 300–301

Teniposide, IV administration reactions, 227

Tensile force, in fascial suturing, 168

Tension pneumothorax, *289*

Terazosin (Hytrin), 213

Terbutaline, leukocytosis associated with, 243

Tetanus
mortality rate, 47
signs and symptoms of, 47

Tetanus immune globulin (TIG)
for bite wounds, 37, 47
indications for, 47–48

Tetanus immunization
for bite wounds, 37
childhood protocol for, 47

Tetanus toxoid (TT), 47
booster, wound indications for, 47–48, 49

Tetracyclines
for bite wounds, 37
side effects of, 190, 190t
tooth staining related to, 190–191, 190t
for vancomycin-resistant enterococci, 200

Third degree (full-thickness) burns, of dorsal foot, 43

Third-degree heart block, verapamil-associated, 229–230

Thoracic aorta
aneurysm of, 6
dissection of, 5–7
traumatic injuries of, 8–9, 10
imaging findings, 65–66

Thoracic nerves, T1, 16

Thoracic spine, osteomyelitis of, 395–396

Thoracotomy, for aspirated teeth removal, 57–58

Thrombin, percutaneous, for femoral artery pseudoaneurysm, 146

Thrombin inhibitors, retroperitoneal bleeding related to, 320

Thrombocytopenia, chloramphenicol side effect, 198

Thromboembolism
perioperative risk with anticoagulation history, 318
contributing factors, 104–105, 319

pulmonary versus systemic circulation of, 287
air embolism versus, 287

Thrombolytic therapy, for diabetic myocardial infarction, 386

Thrombophlebitis
of breast veins, 94–95
of IV sites, aggressive treatment indications, 390–391
of superficial femoral vein, 388

Thromboplastin, tissue, rhabdomyolysis impact on, 90

Thrombosis
of cannulated veins, in hemodialysis patients, 266–267
deep vein (*see* Deep vein thrombosis (DVT))
in heparin-induced thrombocytopenia, 105, 225

Tibia fractures, compartment syndrome after, 19–20

Tibial plateau fractures
compartment syndrome after, 19–20
vascular injury with, 27

Ticarcillin, *P. aeruginosa* resistance to, 204

Ticarcillin with clavulanate (Timentin), for bite wounds, 37

Tickborne diseases, blood transfusion screening for, 435

Tidal volumes, ventilatory, for acute lung disorders, 414

Tinea coli, 128

Tissue culture assay, for *C. difficile* colitis, 193, 202

Tissue perfusion
intracranial injury outcomes and, 63–64
metformin cautions, 223
reperfusion therapy recommendations, 377
VAC system and, 303
vital signs indicator limitations, 63

Tissue thromboplastin, rhabdomyolysis impact on, 90

Tobacco use (*see* Cigarette smoking)

Tobramycin
peak and trough levels for, 195, 197t
properties of, 196
toxic side effects of, 196

Toldt, white line of, 138

Topical agents, hemostatic, for traumatic hepatic hemorrhage, 122

Total parenteral nutrition (TPN), catheter-related sepsis with, 262

Toxic epidermal necrolysis, 177–178

Trachea
deviation of, great vessel trauma and, 9, 65
edema of, endotracheal intubation for, 370
teeth lodged in, 57

Tracheobrachiocephalic fistulae, 316–317

Tracheobronchial tree, traumatic injuries of, 9, 10
imaging findings, 65–66

Tracheostomy
comorbidities of, 412
fistulae formation with, 316–317
for Ludwig's angina, 87–88

Tramadol (Ultram), drug contraindications, 214

Transcutaneous cardiac pacemaker, external, 291

Transesophageal echocardiography (TEE), of aortic pathology, 6, 8, 66

Transplant patients (*see* Organ transplantation; *specific organ*)

Transposons, in vancomycin-resistant enterococci, 199

Transvenous cardiac pacemaker, 291

Tranylcypromine (Parnate), 215

Trauma
abdominal
liver injury in children, 325–326
retroperitoneal vascular injury with, 82–84, *83*
blunt (*see* Blunt trauma)
chest
blunt, 10–12, 65–66
vascular injuries with, 8–9
corneal, with metallic debris, 47–48
examination of, complete and undressed, 59–60
facial (*see* Facial wounds)
hepatic (*see* Liver)
intra-abdominal, 71–72, 76
intracranial, hypotension etiologies with, 63–64

maxillofacial, teeth assessment for, 57–58

musculoskeletal (*see* Dislocation(s); Fracture(s))

nerve (*see specific nerve*)

ophthalmologic, emergency room management of, 51–53

penetrating (*see* Penetrating trauma)

seat belt-related, 12, 71–72

soft tissue (*see* Soft tissue trauma)

thermal (*see* Burns)

urethral
in females, 74
in males, 73–74

vascular (*see* Vascular injuries)

Trauma surgeon consult, for hepatobiliary injuries, 118, 124

Trendelenberg position
for anesthetized patient, 113
for central venous catheter insertion, 273, 275, 279
air embolism and, 286–287
for hernia reduction, 353

Triangle of Calot, 125

Triazolam (Halcion), delirious reactions to, 385

Tricyclic antidepressants, 215

Trimethoprim-sulfamethoxazole
for overwhelming postsplenectomy sepsis, 209
for vancomycin-resistant enterococci, 200

Trophoblastic tumors, hCG marker of, 424

Trough levels
for antibiotics, 195–198, 197t
for immunosuppressants, 433–434

Tuberculosis, of breasts, 95

Tubes (*see specific anatomy, type, or indication*)

Tumors (*see* Neoplasms; *specific tumor*)

Turner's sign, ruptured abdominal aortic aneurysm and, 2

T waves, normal versus ischemic, 376

Tympanic membrane, nonintact, chlorhexidine prep cautions, 107

Type and cross-match, for intra-abdominal trauma, in children, 325

U

Ulcer(s)
  decubitus, 305
  duodenal, bleeding from, 323
  gastric, bleeding from, 323
  peptic, bleeding from, 312–313,
      322–323
Ulnar artery, cannulation of, 371–372, *372*
Ulnar nerve injury
  in humeral fractures, 16
  from lateral decubitus positioning,
      111–113
Ultrasonography
  abdominal, of ruptured abdominal
      aortic aneurysm, 3, 6
  of benign inflammatory disorders, 93
  for central vessel cannulation, 270,
      273, 279
  deep abscess detection by, 34
  Doppler
    of femoral vein phlebitis, 388
    for hemodialysis access screening,
        267
    mycotic aneurysm detection by, 29
    popliteal artery injury screening, 28
  of IV site thrombophlebitis, 390
  for midgut volvulus detection, in
      infants, 91
  of peritonitis, in postoperative obese
      patients, 398–399
Umbilical hernia, 349
  in cirrhotic patient, 345–346
Undressing of patient, for traumatic
      injury examination, 59–60
Universal donor, blood type for, 434–435
Universal recipient, blood type for,
      434–435
Upper gastrointestinal (UGI) bleeding
  endoscopy detection of, 313, 322
  incidence of, 322
  mortality rate, 322
  occult blood testing, 426
  sites of, 312
  variceal versus nonvariceal etiologies,
      322–324
Upper gastrointestinal contrast study, for
      midgut volvulus, in infants, 91–92
Ureters
  complications of
    with kidney transplant, 139
    with laparoscopic procedures, 147

strictures of, catheter placement
      cautions, 255
Urethral injury
  in females, 74
  with Foley catheter placement,
      255–256
  in males
    incidence of, 73
    posterior types of, 73
    retrograde urethrogram diagnosis
        of, 74
    signs and symptoms of, 73–74
Urethrogram, retrograde, for male
      urethral injury evaluation, 74
Urethroscopy, for female urethral injury
      evaluation, 74
Urinary catheterization
  difficult placement cautions,
      255–256
  in male trauma, urethral injury
      evaluation prior to, 73–74
  during surgery, 150–151
Urine dipstick, for gastric aspirate blood
      detection, 426
Urine electrolytes, conditions indicated
      by, 428
  diuretics impact on, 430–432, 431t
Urine output monitoring
  for intra-abdominal trauma, in
      children, 326
  polyuric, post-bladder distention, 257
Urine pregnancy tests, 424
Urogenital diaphragm, in males, 73
Urologic procedures
  surgical staples for, 147–148
  vascular clamps for, 142
Urology consult
  for Foley catheter placement,
      255–256
  for urethral injury, 74
Urticaria, adverse drug reactions
      causing, 177
Uterine surgery, bladder identification
      for, 150

V

Vaccines
  DPT protocol, 47
  for overwhelming postsplenectomy
      sepsis prophylaxis, 207, 208–209

VAC (Vacuum Assisted Closure) system
  application guidelines, 302
  contraindications for, 302
  indications for, 155, 301, 302–303
  ventilator weaning contraindication,
    412
Vacuum Assisted Closure (*see* VAC
    (Vacuum Assisted Closure)
    system)
Vaginal wall, rectal examination of, 332
Vancomycin
  for bacterial endocarditis, 391
  for *C. difficile* colitis, 193, 203
  indications for, 195
  for open fractures, prophylactic, 17
  peak and trough levels for, 195–196
  properties of, 195
  side effects of, 195–196
Vancomycin-resistant enterococci (VRE)
  control strategies, 200
  epidemiology of, 199–200
  genetic types of, 199
  incidence of, 189, 195, 199
  nosocomial trends, 199–200
  treatment of, 200–201
Vardenafil (Levitra), nitrates
    contraindication, 213
Varices
  esophageal, 312, 322–323
    operative risks with, 345
  gastric, 312, 322–323
    continual bleeding from, abdominal
      drains for, 124
    gastrointestinal bleeding from, 312–313
    control strategies, 124
    differential diagnosis of, 322–324
    mortality rate, 322
    rebleeding incidence, 322
Vascular anomalies
  accessory renal arteries versus, 138–139
  imaging of infrarenal, 139
Vascular clamps
  for abdominal aorta, 84
  check for appropriate jaws, 142–144
  surgical clip cautions, 140
Vascular consult, for central vein wall
    rupture, 282
Vascular grafts (*see also* Vein(s))
  secondary abdominal fistulae of,
    315–316

Vascular injuries
  with abdominal trauma, 82–84, *83*
  from angiography access, 145–146
  arterial cannulation and, 371–373
  brachial artery, 145
  central venous catheterization and,
    275–276
    arterial puncture, 274, 279, 281,
      288
    back wall rupture, 282, *283*
  control for examination of, 145
  enterocutaneous fistulae with,
    130
  intercostal, with chest tube insertion,
    249
  interventional radiologic management
    of, 146
  with open fractures, 17
  with penetrating knife wounds, 81
  pulmonary artery rupture, 293–295
Vascular lesions, retroperitoneal
    bleeding related to, 320
Vascular procedure, extremity, surgical
    prep for, 109–110
Vasculitis, gastrointestinal, 312
Vasectomy, protamine administration
    risks and, 233
Vasoconstrictors
  inadvertent extravascular
    administration of, 174
  in local anesthetics, inadvertent
    intravascular administration of,
    175
Vasodilation, migraine management and,
    235
Vasopressors (*see also* Dopamine;
    Epinephrine)
  leukocytosis associated with, 243
Vasovagal reaction
  with sudden bladder decompression,
    257
  with sudden gastric decompression,
    258
Vein(s)
  grafts of, 109
    for penetrating vessel injuries, 81
    prep recommendations, 109–110
  hemodialysis access techniques, 267
  infarction of, with inguinal hernia,
    335–336

injuries of
with abdominal trauma, 82–84, *83*
in liver trauma, 119–124
nonvariceal bleeding from, 323–324
Vena cava filter
designs available, 271
J-tip guidewire ensnarement of,
271–272
Vena Tech TrapEase filter, 271
Venipuncture, postoperative
contraindications, 366
Venlafaxine (Effexor), 215
Venography
for hemodialysis access screening, 267
iodine contrast nephrotoxicity with,
219–220
Venous blood, discriminating from
arterial blood, 279–281
Venous cutdown, for emergency access,
156–157
Venous drainage systems, deep versus
superficial, of leg, 388
Ventilatory support
bag mask, 375
endotracheal intubation for, 374
for inhalation injury, 45–46
invasive, comorbidities of, 412, 416
laryngeal mask, 61
lung protective paradigms for, 414
noninvasive as trend, 412
sedation and analgesia management,
415–416
weaning with abdominal binder in
place, 412
Verapamil, monitored administration of,
229–230
Verbal orders, for medication, allergy
inquiries, 177–178
Vermilion border, in lip laceration
repair, *21,* 21–22
Vertebral osteomyelitis, 395–397
Very-low-molecular-weight heparin
(very-LMWH), for DVT
prophylaxis, 106
Vibrio spp., in necrotizing fasciitis,
379–380
Vicryl suture, for laceration repair
lip, 22
scalp, 79
in young child, 25

Vinblastine (Velban), inadvertent
extravascular administration of,
174–175
Vincristine (Oncovin), inadvertent
extravascular administration of,
175
Vinorelbine (Navelbine), inadvertent
extravascular administration of,
175
Viral infections
blood transfusion screening for, 435
occupational transmission of, 97–98,
98t
response to, 98, 100
Vital signs
in neck trauma evaluation, 68
as perfusion indicators, special
population limitations, 63
Vitamin K
IV administration of
indications for, 227–228
pretreatment of, 227–228
reactions with, 227
for overcoagulation, 227–228, 238t,
241
PO administration of, 227
SQ administration of, 227
Vitamin K antagonists, retroperitoneal
bleeding related to, 320–321
Volvulus, midgut, in infants, 91–92
Vomiting
around nasogastric tube, 253
problem solving, 253–254
bilious, in infants, 91–92
5-HT$_3$ antagonists for, 235
spontaneous esophageal rupture with,
330

W

Ward care, 360–409 (*see also specific
aspect*)
Warfarin (Coumadin)
for DVT prophylaxis, 106
long-term therapy with, perioperative
management of, 318–319
vitamin K for overcoagulation with,
227, 238t, 241
Water deficit, total, 382
Water-soluble contrast studies,
gastrointestinal indications, 338

Wedge pressure, pulmonary capillary, 290, 293
  balloon manipulation cautions, 293–295, *294*
West Nile virus, blood transfusion screening for, 435
"Wet-to-dry" gauze, for abscess packing, 35, 300
White blood cell count
  drugs which elevate, 243–244
  in postoperative complications, 392
White line of Toldt, 138
Whole blood transfusions, compatibility rules, 434, 434t
Withdrawal reaction, delirium related to, 385
Witzel jejunostomy, feeding tube placement, 132–133
Witzel tunnel, 132–133
Wound(s)
  bite (*see* Bites)
  tetanus prophylaxis for, 37, 47, 49
Wound care, for IV site thrombophlebitis, 390
Wound closure
  for amputation reimplantation, 38
  for dehiscence, 307
  human bite cautions, 36–37
  wound infection and, 300–301
Wound dehiscence
  abdominal wound factors, 168–169
  diagnosis of, 306–308
  evisceration with, 306–307
  fascial, 306–308
  incidence of, 306

infections with, 308
  management of, 307
  mortality after, 308
  presentations of, 306–307
  timing of, 306
Wound dressings
  for amputation reimplantation, 39
  for decubitus ulcer, 305
  for frostbite, 50
  tape cautions, 404
Wound healing
  secondary intention, 300, 307
  smoking impact on, 41
Wound hematoma, 307
Wound infection
  etiopathologies of, 300
  incidence of, 300
  signs and symptoms of, 300
  treatment of, 300–301
Wound packing
  for drained abscesses, 34–35
  for infected wounds, 300–301
WoundVac system, 155
"Wrist-drop," 16

X
Xiphoid process fractures, 10–11

Y
Yogurt, for patients on antibiotics, 192
Young adults, slender, liver injuries with CPR, 326

Z
Zoll pacemaker, 291